Childhood Leukemia and Cancer

Editor

YADDANAPUDI RAVINDRANATH

PEDIATRIC CLINICS
OF NORTH AMERICA

www.pediatric.theclinics.com

Consulting Editor
BONITA F. STANTON

February 2015 • Volume 62 • Number 1

ELSEVIER

1600 John F. Kennedy Boulevard • Suite 1800 • Philadelphia, Pennsylvania, 19103-2899

http://www.theclinics.com

THE PEDIATRIC CLINICS OF NORTH AMERICA Volume 62, Number 1
February 2015 ISSN 0031-3955, ISBN-13: 978-0-323-35448-6

Editor: Kerry Holland
Developmental Editor: Casey Jackson

The Pediatric Clinics of North America (ISSN 0031-3955) is published bimonthly by Elsevier Inc., 360 Park Avenue South, New York, NY 10010-1710. Months of issue are February, April, June, August, October, and December. Periodicals postage paid at New York, NY and additional mailing offices. Subscription prices are $200.00 per year (US individuals), $493.00 per year (US institutions), $270.00 per year (Canadian individuals), $657.00 per year (Canadian institutions), $325.00 per year (international individuals), $657.00 per year (international institutions), $100.00 per year (US students and residents), and $165.00 per year (international and Canadian residents and students). To receive students/resident rare, orders must be accompanied by name of affiliated institution, date of term, and the signature of program/residency coordinator on institution letterhead. Orders will be billed at individual rate until proof of status is received. Foreign air speed delivery is included in all Clinics subscription prices. All prices are subject to change without notice. POSTMASTER: Send address changes to The Pediatric Clinics of North America, Elsevier Health Sciences Division, Subscription Customer Service, 3251 Riverport Lane, Maryland Heights, MO 63043. Customer Service: 1-800-654-2452 (US and Canada). From outside of the US and Canada: 1-314-447-8871. Fax: 1-314-447-8029. For print support, E-mail: JournalsCustomerService-usa@elsevier.com. For online support, E-mail: JournalsOnlineSupport-usa@elsevier.com.

Reprints. For copies of 100 or more, of articles in this publication, please contact the Commercial Reprints Department, Elsevier Inc., 360 Park Avenue South, New York, NY 10010-1710. Tel.: 212-633-3874; Fax: 212-633-3820; E-mail: reprints@elsevier.com.

The Pediatric Clinics of North America is also published in Spanish by McGraw-Hill Inter-americana Editores S.A., Mexico City, Mexico; in Portuguese by Riechmann and Affonso Editores, Rua Comandante Coelho 1085, CEP 21250, Rio de Janeiro, Brazil; and in Greek by Althayia SA, Athens, Greece.

The Pediatric Clinics of North America is covered in MEDLINE/PubMed (Index Medicus), Excerpta Medica, Current Contents, Current Contents/Clinical Medicine, Science Citation Index, ASCA, ISI/BIOMED, and BIOSIS.

Printed in the United States of America.

PROGRAM OBJECTIVE

The goal of the *Pediatric Clinics of North America* is to keep practicing physicians and residents up to date with current clinical practice in pediatrics by providing timely articles reviewing the state-of-the-art in patient care.

TARGET AUDIENCE

All practicing pediatricians, physicians and healthcare professionals who provide patient care to pediatric patients.

LEARNING OBJECTIVES

Upon completion of this activity, participants will be able to:

1. Discuss childhood oncological conditions including leukemias, sarcomas, retinoblastoms and neuroblastomas.
2. Discuss risk factors of childhood cancers and the impact of genome wide studies.
3. Review remaining challenges in childhood cancer and newer targeted therapeutics for pediatric cancers.

ACCREDITATION

The Elsevier Office of Continuing Medical Education (EOCME) is accredited by the Accreditation Council for Continuing Medical Education (ACCME) to provide continuing medical education for physicians.

The EOCME designates this enduring material for a maximum of 15 *AMA PRA Category 1 Credit*(s)™. Physicians should claim only the credit commensurate with the extent of their participation in the activity.

All other health care professionals requesting continuing education credit for this enduring material will be issued a certificate of participation.

DISCLOSURE OF CONFLICTS OF INTEREST

The EOCME assesses conflict of interest with its instructors, faculty, planners, and other individuals who are in a position to control the content of CME activities. All relevant conflicts of interest that are identified are thoroughly vetted by EOCME for fair balance, scientific objectivity, and patient care recommendations. EOCME is committed to providing its learners with CME activities that promote improvements or quality in healthcare and not a specific proprietary business or a commercial interest.

The planning committee, staff, authors and editors listed below have identified no financial relationships or relationships to products or devices they or their spouse/life partner have with commercial interest related to the content of this CME activity:

Carl E. Allen, MD, PhD; Saro Armenian, DO, MPH; Smita Bhatia, MD, MPH; Deepa Bhojwani, MBBS; Catherine Bollard, MD; Patrick Brown, MD; Murali Chintagumpala, MD; Stacy Cooper, MD; Christopher C. Dvorak, MD; Josephine H. HaDoung, MD; Kristen Helm; Meret Henry, MD, MS; Kerry Holland; Brynne Hunter; Meredith S, Irwin, MD; Justine Kahn, MD; Kara M. Kelly, MD; Indu Kumari; Wendy Landier, PhD, RN; Sandy Lavery; Lawrence G. Lum, MD, DSc; Kanwaldeep Mallhi, MD; Kelly Maloney, MD; Erin L. Marcotte, PhD; Andrew A. Martin, MD; Leo Mascarenhas, MBBS, MS; Soheil Meshinchi, MD, PhD; Frederic Millot, MD; Darren B. Orbach, MD, PhD; Nathan Pankratz, PhD; Julie R. Park, MD; Lindsay Parnell, Ching-Hon Pui, MD; Yaddanapudi Ravindranath, MBBS; Gregory H. Reaman, MD; Irene Roberts, MD; Carlos Rodriguez-Galindo, MD; Prakash Satwani, MD; Kirk R. Schultz, MD; Stephen X. Skapek, MD; Malcolm A. Smith, MD, PhD; Logan Spector, PhD; Megan Suerman; Lillian Sung, MD, PhD; Meinolf Suttorp, MD; Katherine G. Tarlock, MD; Jeffrey W. Taub, MD; Deborah VanderVeen, MD; Paresh Vyas, MRCP, FRCP, FRCPath; Jun J. Yang, PhD; Maxim Yankelevich, MD.

The planning committee, staff, authors and editors listed below have identified financial relationships or relationships to products or devices they or their spouse/life partner have with commercial interest related to the content of this CME activity:

Amar Gajjar, MD, is a consultant/advisor for AstraZeneca and Celgene Corporation.
Maxim Yankelevich, MD, is a consultant/advisor for Jazz Pharmaceuticals plc, sanofi-aventis, US LLC, Pfizer, Inc., and Sigma-Tau Pharmaceuticals, Inc.

UNAPPROVED/OFF-LABEL USE DISCLOSURE

The EOCME requires CME faculty to disclose to the participants:

1. When products or procedures being discussed are off-label, unlabelled, experimental, and/or investigational (not US Food and Drug Administration [FDA] approved); and

2. Any limitations on the information presented, such as data that are preliminary or that represent ongoing research, interim analyses, and/or unsupported opinions. Faculty may discuss information about pharmaceutical agents that is outside of FDA-approved labelling. This information is intended solely for CME and is not intended to promote off-label use of these medications. If you have any questions, contact the medical affairs department of the manufacturer for the most recent prescribing information.

TO ENROLL

To enroll in the *Pediatric Clinics of North America* Continuing Medical Education program, call customer service at 1-800-654-2452 or sign up online at http://www.theclinics.com/home/cme. The CME program is available to subscribers for an additional annual fee of USD 290.

METHOD OF PARTICIPATION

In order to claim credit, participants must complete the following:
1. Complete enrolment as indicated above.
2. Read the activity.
3. Complete the CME Test and Evaluation. Participants must achieve a score of 70% on the test. All CME Tests and Evaluations must be completed online.

CME INQUIRIES/SPECIAL NEEDS

For all CME inquiries or special needs, please contact elsevierCME@elsevier.com.

Contributors

CONSULTING EDITOR

BONITA F. STANTON, MD
Professor of Pediatrics and Vice Dean for Research, School of Medicine, Wayne State University, Detroit, Michigan

EDITOR

YADDANAPUDI RAVINDRANATH, MBBS
Professor of Pediatrics, Georgie Ginopolis Chair of Pediatric Cancer and Hematology, Division of Pediatric Hematology/Oncology, Children's Hospital of Michigan, Wayne State University School of Medicine, Detroit, Michigan

AUTHORS

CARL E. ALLEN, MD, PhD
Assistant Professor, Department of Pediatrics, Texas Children's Cancer Center, Baylor College of Medicine, Houston, Texas

SARO ARMENIAN, DO, MPH
Assistant Professor, Department of Population Sciences, City of Hope, Duarte, California

SMITA BHATIA, MD, MPH
Professor and Chair, Department of Population Sciences, City of Hope, Duarte, California

DEEPA BHOJWANI, MD
Department of Oncology, St. Jude Children's Research Hospital; Department of Pediatrics, University of Tennessee Health Sciences Center, Memphis, Tennessee

CATHERINE M. BOLLARD, MD
Professor of Pediatrics, Program for Cell Enhancement and Technologies for Immunotherapy, BMT Division, Department of Pediatrics, Children's National Health System, The George Washington University, Washington, District of Columbia

PATRICK A. BROWN, MD
Director, Pediatric Leukemia Program, Associate Professor of Oncology and Pediatrics, Sidney Kimmel Comprehensive Cancer Center, Johns Hopkins University School of Medicine, Baltimore, Maryland

MURALI CHINTAGUMPALA, MD
Texas Children's Cancer Center, Baylor College of Medicine, Houston, Texas

STACY L. COOPER, MD
Clinical Fellow, Pediatric Hematology/Oncology, Johns Hopkins/National Institutes of Health, Baltimore, Maryland

CHRISTOPHER C. DVORAK, MD
Associate Professor of Pediatrics, Department of Pediatrics, University of California, San Francisco, California

AMAR GAJJAR, MD
Department of Oncology, St Jude Children's Research Hospital, Memphis, Tennessee

JOSEPHINE H. HₐDUONG, MD
Assistant Professor, Division of Hematology, Oncology, and Blood & Marrow Transplantation, Department of Pediatrics, Children's Center for Cancer and Blood Diseases, Children's Hospital Los Angeles, University of Southern California Keck School of Medicine, Los Angeles, California

MERET HENRY, MD, MS
Division of Hematology/Oncology, Children's Hospital of Michigan/Wayne State University, Detroit, Michigan

NOBUKO HIJIYA, MD
Professor of Pediatrics, Division of Hematology, Oncology, and Stem Cell Transplantation, Ann & Robert H. Lurie Children's Hospital of Chicago; Professor, Department of Pediatrics, Northwestern University Feinberg School of Medicine, Chicago, Illinois

MEREDITH S. IRWIN, MD
Professor of Pediatrics, Division of Hematology-Oncology, Hospital for Sick Children, University of Toronto, Toronto, Ontario, Canada

JUSTINE KAHN, MD
Pediatric Hematology/Oncology Fellow, Department of Pediatrics, Columbia University, New York, New York

KARA M. KELLY, MD
Professor of Pediatrics, Herbert Irving Child and Adolescent Oncology Center, Morgan Stanley Children's Hospital, New York-Presbyterian, Columbia University Medical Center, New York, New York

WENDY LANDIER, PhD, RN
Assistant Professor, Department of Population Sciences, City of Hope, Duarte, California

LAWRENCE G. LUM, MD, DSc
Department of Oncology, Barbara Ann Karmanos Cancer Institute, Wayne State University, Detroit, Michigan

KANWALDEEP MALLHI, MD
BC Children's Hospital, Vancouver, British Columbia, Canada

KELLY W. MALONEY, MD
Center for Cancer & Blood Disorders, Children's Hospital Colorado, Aurora, Colorado

ERIN L. MARCOTTE, PhD
Postdoctoral Fellow, Division of Epidemiology/Clinical Research, Department of Pediatrics, University of Minnesota, Minneapolis, Minnesota

ANDREW A. MARTIN, MD
Assistant Professor, Division of Hematology/Oncology, Department of Pediatrics, Pauline Allen Gill Center for Cancer and Blood Disorders, Children's Medical Center, University of Texas Southwestern Medical Center, Dallas, Texas

LEO MASCARENHAS, MD, MS
Associate Professor, Division of Hematology, Oncology, and Blood & Marrow Transplantation, Department of Pediatrics, Children's Center for Cancer and Blood Diseases, Children's Hospital Los Angeles, University of Southern California Keck School of Medicine, Los Angeles, California

SOHEIL MESHINCHI, MD, PhD
Member, Clinical Research Division; Professor, Department of Pediatrics, Fred Hutchinson Cancer Research Center, University of Washington School of Medicine, Seattle, Washington

FREDERIC MILLOT, MD
Centre d'Investigation Clinique 802, Institut National de la Santé et de la Recherche Médicale (INSERM), University Hospital Poitiers, Poitiers, France

DARREN B. ORBACH, MD, PhD
Department of Radiology, Boston Children's Hospital, Harvard Medical School, Boston, Massachusetts

NATHAN PANKRATZ, PhD
Assistant Professor, Department of Lab Medicine and Pathology, University of Minnesota, Minneapolis, Minnesota

JULIE R. PARK, MD
Professor of Pediatrics, Division of Hematology-Oncology, Seattle Children's Hospital, University of Washington School of Medicine, Fred Hutchinson Cancer Research Center, Seattle, Washington

CHING-HON PUI, MD
Department of Oncology, St. Jude Children's Research Hospital; Department of Pediatrics, University of Tennessee Health Sciences Center, Memphis, Tennessee

YADDANAPUDI RAVINDRANATH, MBBS
Professor of Pediatrics, Georgie Ginopolis Chair of Pediatric Cancer and Hematology, Division of Pediatric Hematology/Oncology, Children's Hospital of Michigan, Wayne State University School of Medicine, Detroit, Michigan

GREGORY H. REAMAN, MD
Associate Director, Office of Hematology and Oncology Products, OND, Center for Drug Evaluation and Research, U.S. Food and Drug Administration, Silver Spring, Maryland

IRENE ROBERTS, MD
Department of Paediatrics and Molecular Haematology Unit, University of Oxford and Oxford University Hospitals NHS Trust, Oxford, United Kingdom

CARLOS RODRIGUEZ-GALINDO, MD
Department of Pediatric Oncology, Dana-Farber/Boston Children's Cancer and Blood Disorders Center, Harvard Medical School, Boston, Massachusetts

PRAKASH SATWANI, MD
Associate Professor of Pediatrics, Division of Pediatric Blood and Bone Marrow Transplantation, Department of Pediatrics, New York-Presbyterian Morgan Stanley Children's Hospital, Columbia University, New York, New York

KIRK R. SCHULTZ, MD
BC Children's Hospital, Vancouver, British Columbia, Canada

STEPHEN X. SKAPEK, MD
Professor, Division of Hematology/Oncology, Department of Pediatrics, Pauline Allen Gill Center for Cancer and Blood Disorders, Children's Medical Center, University of Texas Southwestern Medical Center, Dallas, Texas

MALCOLM A. SMITH, MD, PhD
Associate Branch Chief, Pediatrics, Cancer Therapy Evaluation Program, National Cancer Institute, Bethesda, Maryland

LOGAN G. SPECTOR, PhD
Associate Professor, Division of Epidemiology/Clinical Research, Department of Pediatrics, University of Minnesota, Minneapolis, Minnesota

LILLIAN SUNG, MD, PhD
Division of Haematology/Oncology, The Hospital for Sick Children, Toronto, Ontario, Canada

MEINOLF SUTTORP, MD
Professor, Division of Pediatric Hematology and Oncology, University Children's Hospital, Dresden, Germany

KATHERINE TARLOCK, MD
Research Associate, Clinical Research Division; Acting Instructor, Department of Pediatrics, Fred Hutchinson Cancer Research Center, University of Washington School of Medicine, Seattle, Washington

JEFFREY W. TAUB, MD
Division of Pediatric Hematology/Oncology, Children's Hospital of Michigan, Wayne State University School of Medicine, Detroit, Michigan

DEBORAH VANDERVEEN, MD
Department of Ophthalmology, Boston Children's Hospital, Harvard Medical School, Boston, Massachusetts

PARESH VYAS, MD
MRC Molecular Haematology Unit, Department of Haematology, Weatherall Institute of Molecular Medicine, Oxford University Hospitals NHS Trust, University of Oxford, Oxford, United Kingdom

JUN J. YANG, PhD
Department of Pediatrics, University of Tennessee Health Sciences Center; Department of Pharmaceutical Sciences, St. Jude Children's Research Hospital, Memphis, Tennessee

MAXIM YANKELEVICH, MD
Division of Hematology/Oncology, Children's Hospital of Michigan, Wayne State University, Detroit, Michigan

Contents

This article summarizes the adventures and explorations in the 1970s and 1980s in the treatment of children with leukemia and cancer that paved the way for the current success in childhood cancers. Indeed, these were adventures and bold steps into unchartered waters. Because childhood leukemia the most common of the childhood cancers, success in childhood leukemia was pivotal in the push toward cure of all childhood cancers. The success in childhood leukemia illustrates how treatment programs were designed using clinical- and biology-based risk factors seen in the patients.

The causes of childhood cancer have been systematically studied for decades, but apart from high-dose radiation and prior chemotherapy there are few strong external risk factors. However, inherent risk factors including birth weight, parental age, and congenital anomalies are consistently associated with most types of pediatric cancer. Recently the contribution of common genetic variation to etiology has come into focus through genome-wide association studies. These have highlighted genes not previously implicated in childhood cancers and have suggested that common variation explains a larger proportion of childhood cancers than adult. Rare variation and nonmendelian inheritance may also contribute to childhood cancer risk but have not been widely examined.

Advancements in the care of children with cancer have, in part, been achieved through improvements in supportive care. Situations that require prompt care can occur at the time of presentation as well as during treatment. This article discusses the approach to children with fever and neutropenia, a complication encountered daily by care providers, as well as oncologic emergencies that can be seen at the time of a child's initial diagnosis: hyperleukocytosis, tumor lysis syndrome, superior vena cava syndrome, and spinal cord compression.

made in understanding aspects of the molecular basis of JMML. How these molecular mechanisms may lead to targeted therapeutics and improved outcomes remains to be elucidated. Allogeneic hematopoietic stem cell transplant is the only curative option for children with JMML, and it is fraught with frequent relapse and significant toxicity.

Chronic myelogenous leukemia (CML) is a rare disease in children. Although there is little evidence of biological differences between CML in children and adults, host factors are very different. Children develop distinct morbidities related to the off-target effects of tyrosine kinase inhibitors. The goal of treatment in children should be cure rather than suppression of disease, which can be the treatment goal for many older adults. This article reviews data from the literature on the treatment of CML, discusses the issues that are unique to CML in children, and recommends management that takes these issues into consideration.

Children with Down syndrome (DS) and acute leukemias acute have unique biological, cytogenetic, and intrinsic factors that affect their treatment and outcome. Myeloid leukemia of Down syndrome (ML-DS) is associated with high event-free survival (EFS) rates and frequently preceded by a preleukemia condition, the transient abnormal hematopoiesis (TAM) present at birth. For acute lymphoblastic leukemia (ALL), their EFS and overall survival are poorer than non-DS ALL, and it is important to enroll them on therapeutic trials, including relapse trials; investigate new agents that could potentially improve their leukemia-free survival; and strive to maximize the supportive care these patients need.

Although there have been dramatic improvements in the treatment of children with non-hodgkin lymphoma, hodgkin lymphoma and histiocytic disorders over the past 3 decades, many still relapse or are refractory to primary therapy. In addition, late effects such as 2nd malignancies, cardiomyopathy and infertility remain a major concern. Thus, this review focuses on the current state of the science and, in particular, novel treatment strategies that are aimed at improving outcomes for all pediatric patients with lymphoma and histiocytic disorders while reducing treatment related morbidity.

The past 2 decades have witnessed a revolution in the management of childhood brain tumors, with the establishment of multidisciplinary teams and national and international consortiums that led to significant

improvements in the outcomes of children with brain tumors. Unprecedented cooperation within the pediatric neuro-oncology community and
sophisticated rapidly evolving technology have led to advances that are
likely to revolutionize treatment strategies and improve outcomes.

Malignant bone tumors (osteosarcoma, Ewing sarcoma) and soft-tissue
sarcomas (rhabdomyosarcoma, nonrhabdomyosarcoma) account for
approximately 14% of childhood malignancies. Successful treatment of
patients with sarcoma depends on a multidisciplinary approach to therapy,
including oncology, surgery, radiation oncology, radiology, pathology, and
physiatry. By combining systemic treatment with chemotherapy and
primary tumor control using surgery and/or radiation, survival rates for
localized disease range from 70% to 75%. However, children with metastatic or recurrent disease continue to have dismal outcomes. A better understanding of the biology underlying both bone and soft-tissue sarcomas
is required to further improve outcomes for children with these tumors.

Retinoblastoma is the most common neoplasm of the eye in childhood,
and represents 3% of all childhood malignancies. Retinoblastoma is a cancer of the very young; two-thirds are diagnosed before 2 years of age and
95% before 5 years. Retinoblastoma presents in 2 distinct clinical forms:
(1) a bilateral or multifocal, heritable form (25% of all cases), characterized
by the presence of germline mutations of the *RB1* gene; and (2) a unilateral
or unifocal form (75% of all cases), 90% of which are nonhereditary. The
treatment of retinoblastoma is multidisciplinary and is designed primarily
to save life and preserve vision.

Neuroblastoma (NB) is the third most common pediatric cancer. Although
NB accounts for 7% of pediatric malignancies, it is responsible for more
than 10% of childhood cancer-related mortality. Prognosis and treatment
are determined by clinical and biological risk factors. Estimated 5-year survival rates for patients with non–high-risk and high-risk NB are more than
90% and less than 50%, respectively. Recent clinical trials have continued
to reduce therapy for patients with non–high-risk NB, including the most
favorable subsets who are often followed with observation approaches.
In contrast, high-risk patients are treated aggressively with chemotherapy,
radiation, surgery, and myeloablative and immunotherapies.

Hematopoietic cell transplantation (HCT) represents the most common and
effective form of immunotherapy for childhood malignancies. The role of

the graft-versus-leukemia effect in allogeneic HCT has been well established in childhood malignancies, but is also associated with short-term and long-term morbidity. HCT may be ineffective in some settings at obtaining control of the malignancy, and as such, cannot be used as a universal cancer immunotherapy. Novel therapies using dendritic cell vaccinations, tumor-infiltrating lymphocytes, and chimeric antigen receptor T cells are being evaluated as potential adjuvants to HCT.

Wendy Landier, Saro Armenian, and Smita Bhatia

Treatment for childhood cancer with chemotherapy, radiation and/or hematopoietic cell transplant can result in adverse sequelae that may not become evident for many years. A clear understanding of the association between therapeutic exposures and specific long-term complications, and an understanding of the magnitude of the burden of morbidity borne by childhood cancer survivors, has led to the development of guidelines to support lifelong risk-based follow up for this population. It is important to develop interventions to reduce the impact of treatment-related late effects on morbidity and mortality and to continue research regarding the etiopathogenesis of therapy-related cancers and other late effects.

Malcolm A. Smith and Gregory H. Reaman

Despite the enormously important and gratifying advances in cancer treatment outcomes for children with cancer, cancer remains the biggest cause of death from disease in children. Because the etiology and biology of cancers that occur in children differ dramatically from those that occur in adults, the immediate extrapolation of efficacy and safety of new cancer drugs to childhood cancer indications is not possible. We discuss factors that will play key roles in guiding pediatric oncologists as they select lines of research to pursue in their quest for more effective treatments for children with cancer.

PEDIATRIC CLINICS OF NORTH AMERICA

Foreword

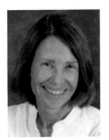

Bonita F. Stanton, MD
Consulting Editor

I have had the joy of practicing pediatrics for well over three decades. During this time, I have witnessed the remarkable achievements made possible through the collaboration of superb researchers and pediatric oncologists/hematologists across the country and, increasingly, the globe. Capitalizing on the strength of carefully structured clinical trials, building block by block on past successes, these scientists and clinicians have created bright futures for countless children and their families. For many of the former life-threatening conditions, the current challenges are seeking to minimize the long-term consequences of the successful treatments.

This issue is remarkable for the breadth and depth of the conditions described. Beginning with the childhood lymphohematopoietic tumors and then addressing several of the nervous system tumors, embryonal tumors, and sarcomas, the issue concludes with discussions addressing new and future therapeutic approaches. The final article discusses some of the major challenges confronting the field.

The authors contributing to this issue represent a broad and far-reaching array of the real heroes and heroines in the field of pediatric cancer research and treatment. The issue is highly readable and serves as a wonderful update for the practicing pediatrician.

An issue such as this that so clearly chronicles the major progress that has been made in far less than half a century provides great hope to pediatricians, parents, and children alike; today's great challenges will be tomorrow's great cures. As pediatricians, it is our privilege and duty to remain up-to-date with regard to these achievements. We must be able to recognize the disorders in a timely manner and refer patients to the specialized care that they need and that is available, while offering comfort and supportive care to our patients and their families as they receive what so often is now the life-saving treatment available. When I entered the field of

Pediatr Clin N Am 62 (2015) xv–xvi
http://dx.doi.org/10.1016/j.pcl.2014.10.004
0031-3955/15/$ – see front matter © 2015 Published by Elsevier Inc.

pediatric.theclinics.com

pediatrics, I never imagined how much could be accomplished for so many in such a relatively short time.

Bonita F. Stanton, MD
School of Medicine
Wayne State University
1261 Scott Hall
540 East Canfield, Suite 1261
Detroit, MI 48201, USA

E-mail address:
bstanton@med.wayne.edu

Preface

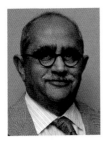

Yaddanapudi Ravindranath, MBBS
Editor

The progress made in curing children with cancer over the last 5 decades represents one of the great stories in modern medicine. Once predominantly fatal, cancer can now be cured in more than 85% children. This success is the culmination of efforts of a unique partnership of the child, the parents, the community, and the physicians. The child with cancer provided the inspiration for developing new treatment strategies for finding cures for incurable diseases; the parent helped develop community and governmental resources, and the physician and hospital systems responded to the challenges. Although many low-stage tumors were cured with surgery and/or radiation, it was not until the introduction of effective chemotherapy that cure as an achievable goal was not recognized. Many hurdles had to be overcome in the 1960s through the early 1980s, not the least of which was the widely held notion in both the hospital and the lay communities that cancer cannot be cured, and chemotherapy results only in prolongation of the suffering of innocent children. The success in curing a large number of children with acute lymphoblastic leukemia changed this notion, and subsequent progress could not be held back.

The story of the evolution of modern therapy in the 1970s and 1980s starts the issue, and an article on the remaining challenges in treating children with cancer closes the issue. In the pages in between there are articles on the genetic and nongenetic risk factors for child cancer, the need for early diagnosis and critical supportive care to minimize fatal complications from disease-related or infection-related causes, and long-term issues faced by childhood cancer survivors from the late sequelae of surgery/radiation and chemotherapy. Other articles discuss the biology and treatment of various common childhood cancers. I regret very much that time and space constraints led to the omission of a discussion on renal tumors (notably Wilm tumor) and certain rare tumors, such as germ cell tumors, adrenocortical cancer, and nasopharyngeal carcinoma. The advances made in these tumors are extraordinary, and Wilm tumor is one of the most curable of childhood cancers. Space limitations also did not permit us to have an article on the strategies being used to export systems for curing of children within low-income countries, where cure rates remain low for

Pediatr Clin N Am 62 (2015) xvii–xviii
http://dx.doi.org/10.1016/j.pcl.2014.10.003
0031-3955/15/$ – see front matter © 2015 Published by Elsevier Inc.

pediatric.theclinics.com

lack of resources. I apologize to the readers and, as well, my colleagues for this omission. Nevertheless, trainees and general pediatricians can appreciate the breadth and scope of the knowledge gained and the successes achieved in the last 5 decades in reading these articles. The story of cancer as a disease caused by gene aberrations emerges—a story of predisposing genes (cancer suppressor genes, DNA repair genes) that facilitate cancer-initiating mutations and enabling mutations (epigenetic mutations) that confer proliferative advantage to mutant clone and alter response to chemotherapy positively or negatively. The advances in the treatment of childhood cancer, a cellular and molecular disease, demonstrate that science (research) and clinical care are not opposing values. Thus, the credo followed by pediatric oncologists is (in paraphrase from the vision statements of the Children's Oncology Group) "improving patient care through scientific discovery." The ultimate goal is to "Cure Childhood Cancer Worldwide."

Yaddanapudi Ravindranath, MBBS
Georgie Ginopolis Chair of Pediatric Cancer and Hematology
Wayne State University School of Medicine
3901 Beaubien Boulevard
Detroit, MI 48201, USA

E-mail address:
ravi@med.wayne.edu

Acknowledgments

When Dr Bonita Stanton, former chair of the department of Pediatrics and current vice dean for Research at Wayne State University asked me to be the guest editor for this issue on childhood cancer for *Pediatric Oncology Clinics of North America*, I accepted this with some trepidation and with much appreciation. Rarely one gets an opportunity to present a story in which a person was so intimately involved over 5 decades. I am very much indebted to all the authors for their contributions to this monograph and painting the picture of the progress in curing childhood cancer so eloquently. I also acknowledge the help from Elsevier editorial staff in putting this issue together.

Evolution of Modern Treatment of Childhood Acute Leukemia and Cancer

Adventures and Battles in the 1970s and 1980s

Yaddanapudi Ravindranath, MBBS

KEYWORDS

- Treatment of Acute lymphoblastic leukemia • Central nervous system leukemia
- History of Childhood acute leukemia and cancer • Aminopterin • Subbarow

KEY POINTS

- The success in childhood leukemia illustrates how treatment programs were designed using clinical- and biology-based risk factors seen in the patients.
- In the mid-1960s a principal focus in curing childhood leukemia entailed control of the central nervous system part of the disease.
- New frontiers were explored and new supportive disciplines were established that paved the way for the current molecular era, which promises to discover new targets for therapy so that we can achieve high cure rates with low morbidity in children with cancer.

The search for understanding is an adventure or more commonly is a series of adventures...now that geographical boundaries in our own and in other civilized lands have been determined, the pioneering spirits found in scientific research find enticing vistas for adventure.
—Walter B. Cannon

The Way of an Investigator
—Quotation from the foreword to Pediatric Clinics of North America, v.9, no. 3, 1962, issue on Hematology by Editor Carl H. Smith.

When I received the invitation from *Pediatric Clinics of North America* to guest edit an issue on pediatric oncology, I gladly accepted this challenge, as it gave me an opportunity to present the advances from a perspective of one who started a career in pediatric hematology oncology when the cure rates were abysmally low in contrast to the

Supported by Georgie Ginopolis endowment, Melissa Ann Krinsky Memorial fund, David Carr memorial fund, Leukemia Research Life, Kids Without Cancer.
Department of Pediatrics, Wayne State University School of Medicine, 3901 Beaubien Boulevard, Detroit, MI 48201, USA
E-mail address: ravi@med.wayne.edu

Pediatr Clin N Am 62 (2015) 1–10
http://dx.doi.org/10.1016/j.pcl.2014.09.005
0031-3955/15/$ – see front matter © 2015 Published by Elsevier Inc.
pediatric.theclinics.com

optimism for curing all children with cancer now—current estimates project nearly 80% long-term survival rate for all children with leukemia and cancer. A quote from Dr Sanford Leiken's section in the 1962 issue of *Pediatric Clinics of North America* on Leukemia: Current Concepts In Therapy illustrates status of childhood cancer therapy in the early to mid-1960s, "At present acute leukemia of childhood is not curable, but it is treatable; although fatal, it can be controlled in varying periods of time so that the patient's life can be prolonged in a relatively comfortable and functional state."[1] It was in this milieu that I started my own career. The task of caring for children was grim indeed. Our standard opening dialogue with parents of a child with leukemia (most cancers) newly diagnosed started with the sentence "Your child has leukemia/cancer and there is no cure for it."

One of my first experiences was coming across several children with leukemia who were long survivors, many of whom were included in the original publication of long survivors written by Joseph Burchenal and M. Lois Murphy from Sloan-Kettering Institute of Cancer Research and Cornell University Medical College in New York.[2] In this publication, Drs Burchenal and Murphy attempted to list all of the known survivors of acute leukemia from direct correspondence with hematologists in the United States. There were 71 patients with acute leukemia living 5 years or more from diagnosis at that time. Of those, only 36 were living with no evidence of leukemia. A large cohort of these patients had come from Children's Hospital of Michigan and was treated under the direction of Wolf W. Zuelzer, my mentor, and mentor to noted pediatric oncologists - Sanford Lieken, William Newton, and Theresa Vietti.[3,4] One of the patients (GB) in the Burchenal cohort was a child with acute lymphoblastic leukemia (ALL) treated in 1952 who I tried to contact in preparation for a report on long survivors in childhood leukemia. To my disappointment, the parents did not permit me to contact the young man, as at that time the practice was to not tell the children of their diagnosis. He received aminopterin for a total of 10 months, the first generation of antifolates synthesized by Yellapragada Subbarow of Lederle Laboratories.[5] This is one of the antifolates first used by Sidney Farber; although, in his famous article, Dr Farber failed to include Dr Subbarow as coauthor, an astonishing omission considering that Subbarow synthesized the antifolates specifically for treatment of childhood leukemia at Dr Farber's request.[6] As things turned out, I discovered patient GB at a fundraising golf outing in 1998 and fortuitously earlier this year, through a colleague at another golf event, he reestablished contact with me.[7] Now 67, one of the longest survivors of childhood leukemia, he is doing well and has a thriving engineering business.

In the next few paragraphs I summarize the adventures and explorations in the 1970s and 1980s in the treatment of children with leukemia and cancer that paved the way for the current success in childhood cancers. Indeed, these were adventures and bold steps into unchartered waters. Because childhood leukemia is the most commonly known childhood cancer, success in childhood leukemia was pivotal in the push toward cure of all childhood cancers. The success in childhood leukemia illustrates how treatment programs were designed using clinical- and biology-based risk factors seen in the patients. Thus, in the mid-1960s, although the remission/induction rate was quite respectable by even current standards, relapse occurred frequently, and the overall cure rate still remained less than 10%. A major problem in child ALL was relapse at extramedullary sites, most often in the central nervous system (CNS). A collage of the types of extramedullary disease we were seeing is shown in **Fig. 1**. Hence, a principal focus in curing childhood leukemia entailed control of the CNS part of the disease. Concurrently with these attempts, new developments were occurring rapidly in the immunophenotyping and karyotyping of the childhood leukemias and thus a better definition of the molecular biology and risk factors for the type

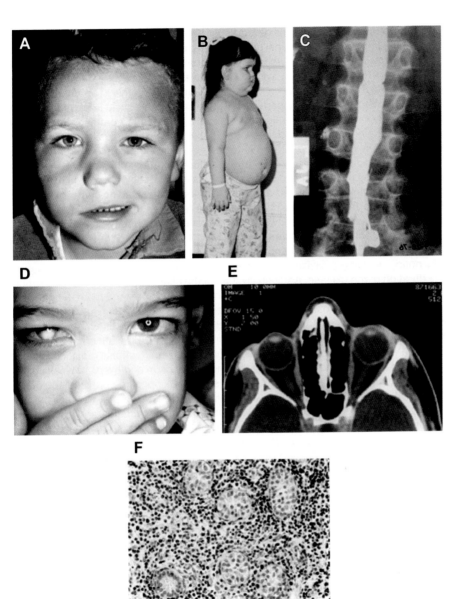

Fig. 1. Central nervous system and other extramedullary disease in childhood ALL. (A) Facial palsy. (B) Cushing's syndrome from hypothalamic involvement. (C) Epidural lesion causing cord compression. (D) Leukemic involvement of iris with cellular exudate in the anterior chamber. (E) Optic nerve (left) involvement causing blindness. (F) Testicular infiltration with leukemia.

of relapses seen. Investigators pursued varied strategies, and these initial forays remind me of an explorer of yesteryear who discovered new sea routes to India, discovered the New World, and changed the face of the earth.

The single most important event that changed the disease pattern undoubtedly is work by Donald Pinkel and his colleagues at St. Jude Children's Research Hospital.

I recall distinctly what was considered sensational at that time. The world came to know of the impact of craniospinal radiation as a means for preventing CNS leukemia one night on June 26, 1972 when Danny Thomas, founder of St. Jude Hospital, appeared on *The Tonight Show* with Johnny Carson and famously declared that the physicians at St. Jude's found a cure for childhood leukemia. The impact of this one television appearance is unparalleled by any other single event in the modern therapy of childhood cancer. Overnight there was a nationwide communication of this news and then no doubt around the world. Pinkel and his group used 2400 cGy radiation to the whole brain and 1200 cGy to the spinal axis immediately after remission induction and noted that nearly 50% of the children treated in that manner had initial remission lasting more than 3 to 5 years.[8–10] This news, of course, met with some expected skepticism at many levels and investigators at other leading centers attempted to duplicate the results or developed alternative methods for prevention of CNS disease. A debate ensued as to how the craniospinal radiation may be preventing CNS leukemia and achieving the cures noted. Those who accepted the sanctuary theory of cause of CNS disease attempted to duplicate the St Jude results. Skeptics of this notion, including Zuelzer felt that seeding of the CNS could occur throughout the duration of the disease. Additionally, half of the children still experienced relapses both in the CNS and extramedullary locations such as testes and marrow relapse.

Thus, 2 groups embarked on alternative approaches. Protocols were designed rapidly within a few days, and new methods of CNS prophylaxis were explored. In Detroit, we used the so-called intermittent intrathecal methotrexate and fractional radiation (IMFRA) regimen of intermittent methotrexate and fractional radiation in which intrathecal methotrexate was given at the end of induction and every 10 weeks thereafter, along with radiation of 200 cGy to the skull by 2 opposing ports and 100 cGy to the spinal axis.[11] Ten such courses were given, and the estimate was that the total dose of radiation approximated the 2400 cGy of cranial radiation and 1200 cGy to the spinal axis used by Pinkel and colleagues.[8] Simplistic as this notion may be, this approach also resulted in nearly 50% cure with long-term remissions at 3 years. At the same time, using the high-dose methotrexate therapy for treating children with leukemia devised by Isaac Djerassi, investigators at Roswell Park devised a CNS prophylaxis regimen that combined intrathecal methotrexate with 3 courses of intermediate-dose methotrexate at 500 mg/m^2 times a total of 3 courses with leucovorin rescue.[12–14] In a seminal publication in 1983, Freeman and colleagues[15] from CALGB (Cancer and Acute Leukemia Group B) showed that this approach yielded results comparable to that achieved with the cranial radiotherapy for childhood ALL. These 2 studies found that a strategy of intermittent CNS prophylaxis would be equally effective as the initial cranial radiation approach. An advantage of the regimen devised by Freeman and colleagues was that the methotrexate dose could be pushed to higher levels (up to 33 g/M^2 in one study),[16,17] whereas the initial 2400 cranial radiation approach was limiting subsequent therapy especially because use of high-dose methotrexate after prior cranial radiation resulted in high incidence of leukoencephalopathy. A potential benefit was the avoidance of long-term effects of cranial radiation during brain growth in small children and late complications of secondary malignancy. Thus, today, the preferred approach to prevention of CNS disease in childhood ALL is based on intrathecal methotrexate and high-dose intravenous methotrexate.

To summarize the experience with the first-generation CNS prophylactic regimens, it was evident that 50% long-term remissions can be achieved. Clinical risk factors for prediction of outcome were devised combining the initial white count, the original prognostic marker, with age at diagnosis and the newer markers were applied for classification of ALL.[18–20] The so-called lymphosarcoma variant of ALL with a thymic mass and poor-outcome thymic enlargement was identified as T-cell derived using E-rosettes, mature B phenotype was recognized by surface Ig staining, and the so-called null cell (neither T or B) leukemias could be identified as either B lineage (B precursor) or T lineage by the first-generation polyclonal antibodies.[21–25] These developments ushered in the era of immunophenotyping of ALL, completed by the development of monoclonal antibodies for the common ALL antigen marker CD10 (CALLA), T cell markers (OKT3, 5, 7), B lineage markers (Ia, Dr) and the CD34 stem cell marker.[26–30] The first wide-scale application of cytogenetics in childhood ALL led to the recognition that high hyperdiploidy was associated with good outcome.[31] We now know that the clinical markers of yesteryear are surrogate markers for biology of the disease—mediastinal mass indicates T-ALL, FAB L3 is associated with mature B phenotype, infant ALL is invariably CD10 negative, E2A- PBX all is CD34 negative, and MLL gene rearranged leukemia frequently expresses CD15.[24,25,32–35] The Children's Cancer Study Group (CCSG) defined ALL good prognostic group of age 3 to 7 years and white count less than 10,000 is within the 2 to 7 year age peak observed in childhood ALL and identifies most cases of high hyperdiploidy and ETV6/RUNX1 cases, the two subgroups of ALL associated with best outcome.[19,20,31,34,36] For a description of the current understanding of the biology of childhood ALL see the chapter by Bojwani and Pui in this issue.

The euphoria initially accompanying first-generation CNS prophylactic regimens in ALL was tempered with the recognition that half of precursor cases fail, results were lower in T-ALL, and the results in mature B-ALL were worse (**Fig. 2**). Based on these facts, several investigators, including the investigators from Pediatric Oncology Group (POG) and Nordic Pediatric Hematology/Oncology Society, explored increasing the dose intensity of high-dose methotrexate by increasing the dose per course and the number of doses, ultimately resulting in the current strategy of including 4 to 6 courses of high-dose methotrexate as a part of the consolidation strategy in childhood ALL.[36–39] This strategy improved the outcome over the 50% level achieved with the prior regimens, with a particular benefit to the group with E2A-PBX1–associated ALL and T-ALL. Over time, the intracellular mechanisms for methotrexate resistance

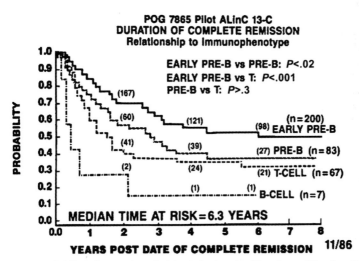

Fig. 2. Survival in childhood acute lymphoblastic leukemia. (*Courtesy of* Drs Jeantte Pullen, University of Mississipi Medical Center, Jackson, MS and James Boyett, St Jude Research Hospital, Memphi, TN.)

were defined (high content of dihydrofolate reductase, the target enzyme for methotrexate, and low folylpolyglutamate synthase in T-ALL blasts) thus explaining the improved outcome in T-ALL with dose intensification of methotrexate.[40–42] The concepts of age-based dosing of intrathecal methotrexate and triple intrathecal therapy added to improved CNS control.[43–45] Addition of L-asparaginase to the standard 2-drug regimen by Children's Cancer Study Group was another important development.[46] Although the initial remission induction rates were not different, there was improvement in long-term outcome by reducing CNS relapse. Other groups like the Berlin, Frankfurt, Munster (BFM) group who continued to use cranial radiotherapy for CNS prophylaxis, introduced the concepts of reintensification courses, and the Dana Farber consortium explored high-dose asparaginase, both resulting in significant improvements in outcome.[47–51] Mature B-ALL, once invariably fatal, suddenly became curable with the use of high-dose methotrexate and fractionated cyclophosphamide, concepts developed by investigators from France, St. Jude Research Hospital, and the Pediatric Oncology Group.[52,53]

Simultaneously, there were improvements in the treatment of other cancers as well. Many of these achievements are chronicled in the other sections of this issue. A notable achievement was a success in osteosarcoma with neoadjuvant/adjuvant multiagent chemotherapy including high-dose methotrexate,[14,54] cisplatin, and Adriamycin. Long-term control in osteosarcoma jumped from a historically low 20% to a near 65% in a single study such that the randomized study had to be closed because it was no longer ethical to randomly assign patients to the inferior standard arm.[55] Chemoreduction strategies in the treatment of retinoblastoma in the early 1990s triggered by the need to preserve vision in infants with bilateral cases (reviewed elsewhere in this issue by Rodriguez-Galindo) revolutionized the care in this disorder by

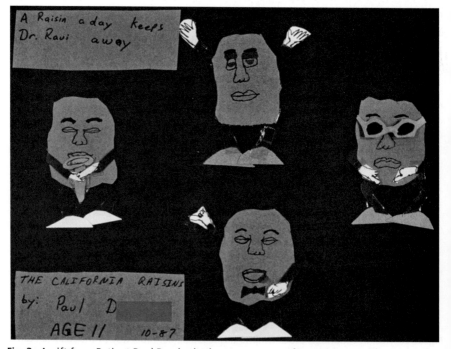

Fig. 3. A gift from Patient Paul D, who had osteosarcoma, after a visit to California for limb salvage. (*Courtesy of* Paul D, now 27 years posttherapy; with permission.)

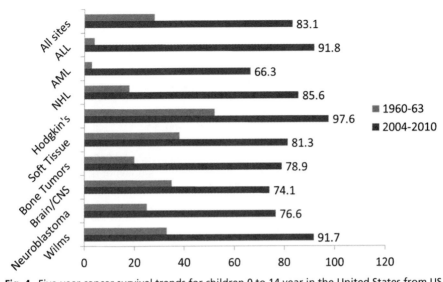

Fig. 4. Five-year cancer survival trends for children 0 to 14 year in the United States from US SEER registry.

obviating the need for external beam radiation with a high risk for secondary osteosarcoma or enucleation of both eyes resulting in blindness.[56]

Concurrent with these improvements in chemotherapy, supportive care measures to prevent pneumocystis carinii pneumonia in ALL and febrile illnesses associated with prolonged neutropenia have significantly contributed to the improved the cure rates. Use of modern day antiemetics made chemotherapy more tolerable, and it is no longer necessary for patients to send whimsical postcards (**Fig. 3**).

Yes, it has been an adventure, or, more accurately, a series of adventures. In an era with limited resources (no oncology nurses, no dedicated pharmacists, and no social workers) the treatment results were beyond expectation. New frontiers were explored and new supportive disciplines were established, which paved the way for the current molecular era, which promises to discover new targets for therapy so that we can achieve high cure rates with low morbidity in children with cancer. It has been an exhilarating experience for me and my contemporaries to be part of such a dynamically changing process and to see the cure rates go from less than 15% to ≥80% (**Fig. 4**) for all children with cancer in one's own career lifetime.

ACKNOWLEDGMENTS

The author thanks patient GB for allowing him to write his story and patient PD for allowing him to publish his art work. This article is dedicated to all of the patients seen by the author over the years and their courageous battles with cancer.

REFERENCES

1. Leikin SI. Leukemia: current concepts in therapy. Pediatr Clin North Am 1962;9: 753–68.
2. Burchenal JH, Murphy ML. Long-term survivors in acute leukemia. Cancer Res 1965;25:1491–4.
3. Zuelzer WW, Flatz G. Acute childhood leukemia: a ten-year study. Am J Dis Child 1960;100:886–907.

4. Zuelzer WW. Implications of Long-Term Survival in Acute Stem Cell Leukemia of Childhood Treated with Composite Cyclic Therapy. Blood 1964;24:477–94.
5. Oleson JJ, Hutchings BL, Subbarow Y. Studies on the inhibitory nature of 4-aminopteroylglutamic acid. J Biol Chem 1948;175:359–65.
6. Farber S, Diamond LK. Temporary remissions in acute leukemia in children produced by folic acid antagonist, 4-aminopteroyl-glutamic acid. N Engl J Med 1948;238:787–93.
7. Ravindranath Y. Forty-five-year follow-up of a childhood leukemia survivor: serendipity or karma? Med Pediatr Oncol 1999;33:409–10.
8. Pinkel D, Simone J, Hustu HO, et al. Nine years' experience with "total therapy" of childhood acute lymphocytic leukemia. Pediatrics 1972;50:246–51.
9. Simone J, Aur RJ, Hustu HO, et al. "Total therapy" studies of acute lymphocytic leukemia in children. Current results and prospects for cure. Cancer 1972;30:1488–94.
10. Aur RJ, Simone J, Hustu HO, et al. Central nervous system therapy and combination chemotherapy of childhood lymphocytic leukemia. Blood 1971;37:272–81.
11. Zeulzer WW, Ravindranath Y, Lusher JM, et al. IMFRA (intermittent intrathecal methotrexate and fractional radiation) plus chemotherapy in childhood leukemia. Am J Hematol 1976;1:191–9.
12. Wang JJ, Freeman AI, Sinks LF. Treatment of acute lymphocytic leukemia by high-dose intravenous methotrexate. Cancer Res 1976;36:1441–4.
13. Djerassi I, Rominger CJ, Kim JS, et al. Phase I study of high doses of methotrexate with citrovorum factor in patients with lung cancer. Cancer 1972;30:22–30.
14. Jaffe N, Paed D, Farber S, et al. Favorable response of metastatic osteogenic sarcoma to pulse high-dose methotrexate with citrovorum rescue and radiation therapy. Cancer 1973;31:1367–73.
15. Freeman AI, Weinberg V, Brecher ML, et al. Comparison of intermediate-dose methotrexate with cranial irradiation for the post-induction treatment of acute lymphocytic leukemia in children. N Engl J Med 1983;308:477–84.
16. Balis FM, Savitch JL, Bleyer WA, et al. Remission induction of meningeal leukemia with high-dose intravenous methotrexate. J Clin Oncol 1985;3:485–9.
17. Nathan PC, Whitcomb T, Wolters PL, et al. Very high-dose methotrexate (33.6 g/m(2)) as central nervous system preventive therapy for childhood acute lymphoblastic leukemia: results of National Cancer Institute/Children's Cancer Group trials CCG-191P, CCG-134P and CCG-144P. Leuk Lymphoma 2006;47:2488–504.
18. Zuelzer WW. Current trends Hematology. Pediatrics 1949;4:269–76.
19. Coccia PS, Sather H, Nesbit M, et al. Interrelationship of initial WBC, age, and sex in predicting prognosis in childhood Acute Lymphoblastic Leukemia (ALL). American Society of Hematology; 1976. p. 214 [abstract: # 125].
20. Bleyer WA, Sather HN, Nickerson HJ, et al. Monthly pulses of vincristine and prednisone prevent bone marrow and testicular relapse in low-risk childhood acute lymphoblastic leukemia: a report of the CCG-161 study by the Childrens Cancer Study Group. J Clin Oncol 1991;9:1012–21.
21. Hardisty RM, Till MM. Acute leukaemia 1959–64: factors affecting prognosis. Arch Dis Child 1968;43:107–15.
22. Kersey JH, Sabad A, Gajl-Peczalska K, et al. Acute lymphoblastic leukemic cells with T (thymus-derived) lymphocyte markers. Science 1973;182:1355–6.
23. Sen L, Borella L. Clinical importance of lymphoblasts with T markers in childhood acute leukemia. N Engl J Med 1975;292:828–32.
24. Ravindranath Y, Kaplan J, Zuelzer WW. Significance of mediastinal mass in acute lymphoblastic leukemia. Pediatrics 1975;55:889–93.

25. Kaplan J, Ravindranath Y, Peterson WD Jr. T and B lymphocyte antigen-positive null cell leukemias. Blood 1977;49:371–8.
26. Greaves M, Janossy G. Patterns of gene expression and the cellular origins of human leukaemias. Biochim Biophys Acta 1978;516:193–230.
27. Greaves MF, Janossy G, Peto J, et al. Immunologically defined subclasses of acute lymphoblastic leukaemia in children: their relationship to presentation features and prognosis. Br J Haematol 1981;48:179–97.
28. Greaves MF, Hariri G, Newman RA, et al. Selective expression of the common acute lymphoblastic leukemia (gp 100) antigen on immature lymphoid cells and their malignant counterparts. Blood 1983;61:628–39.
29. Sallan SE, Ritz J, Pesando J, et al. Cell surface antigens: prognostic implications in childhood acute lymphoblastic leukemia. Blood 1980;55:395–402.
30. Civin CI, Banquerigo ML, Strauss LC, et al. Antigenic analysis of hematopoiesis. VI. Flow cytometric characterization of My-10-positive progenitor cells in normal human bone marrow. Exp Hematol 1987;15:10–7.
31. Secker-Walker LM, Lawler SD, Hardisty RM. Prognostic implications of chromosomal findings in acute lymphoblastic leukaemia at diagnosis. Br Med J 1978; 2:1529–30.
32. Borowitz MJ, Hunger SP, Carroll AJ, et al. Predictability of the t(1;19)(q23;p13) from surface antigen phenotype: implications for screening cases of childhood acute lymphoblastic leukemia for molecular analysis: a Pediatric Oncology Group study. Blood 1993;82:1086–91.
33. Ludwig WD, Bartram CR, Harbott J, et al. Phenotypic and genotypic heterogeneity in infant acute leukemia. I. Acute lymphoblastic leukemia. Leukemia 1989;3:431–9.
34. Pui CH, Rubnitz JE, Hancock ML, et al. Reappraisal of the clinical and biologic significance of myeloid-associated antigen expression in childhood acute lymphoblastic leukemia. J Clin Oncol 1998;16:3768–73.
35. Biondi A, Rossi V, di Celle PF, et al. Unique genotypic features of infant acute lymphoblastic leukaemia at presentation and at relapse. Br J Haematol 1992; 80:472–9.
36. Harris MB, Shuster JJ, Pullen J, et al. Treatment of children with early pre-B and pre-B acute lymphocytic leukemia with antimetabolite-based intensification regimens: a pediatric oncology group study. Leukemia 2000;14:1570–6.
37. Moe PJ, Seip M, Finne PH. Intermediate dose methotrexate (IDM) in childhood acute lymphocytic leukemia in Norway. Preliminary results of a national treatment program. Acta Paediatr Scand 1981;70:73–9.
38. Borsi JD, Schuler D, Moe PJ. Methotrexate administered by 6-h and 24-h infusion: a pharmacokinetic comparison. Cancer Chemother Pharmacol 1988;22:33–5.
39. Borsi JD, Moe PJ. A comparative study on the pharmacokinetics of methotrexate in a dose range of 0.5 g to 33.6 g/m2 in children with acute lymphoblastic leukemia. Cancer 1987;60:5–13.
40. Matherly LH, Taub JW, Wong SC, et al. Increased frequency of expression of elevated dihydrofolate reductase in T-cell versus B-precursor acute lymphoblastic leukemia in children. Blood 1997;90:578–89.
41. Galpin AJ, Schuetz JD, Masson E, et al. Differences in folylpolyglutamate synthetase and dihydrofolate reductase expression in human B-lineage versus T-lineage leukemic lymphoblasts: mechanisms for lineage differences in methotrexate polyglutamylation and cytotoxicity. Mol Pharmacol 1997;52:155–63.
42. Djerassi I, Kim JS. Methotrexate and citrovorum factor rescue in the management of childhood lymphosarcoma and reticulum cell sarcoma (non-Hodgkin's lymphomas): parolonged unmaintained remissions. Cancer 1976;38:1043–51.

43. Bleyer WA, Dedrick RL. Clinical pharmacology of intrathecal methotrexate. I. Pharmacokinetics in nontoxic patients after lumbar injection. Cancer Treat Rep 1977;61:703–8.

44. Poplack DG, Bleyer WA, Wood JH, et al. A primate model for study of methotrexate pharmacokinetics in the central nervous system. Cancer Res 1977;37:1982–5.

45. Pullen J, Boyett J, Shuster J, et al. Extended triple intrathecal chemotherapy trial for prevention of CNS relapse in good-risk and poor-risk patients with B-progenitor acute lymphoblastic leukemia: a pediatric oncology group study. J Clin Oncol 1993;11:839–49.

46. Ortega JA, Nesbit ME Jr, Donaldson MH, et al. L-Asparaginase, vincristine, and prednisone for induction of first remission in acute lymphocytic leukemia. Cancer Res 1977;37:535–40.

47. Henze G, Langermann HJ, Ritter J, et al. Treatment strategy for different risk groups in childhood acute lymphoblastic leukemia: a report from the BFM study group. Haematol Blood Transfus 1981;26:87–93.

48. Henze G, Langermann HJ, Bramswig J, et al. The BFM 76/79 acute lymphoblastic leukemia therapy study (author's transl). Klin Padiatr 1981;193:145–54 [in German].

49. Clavell LA, Gelber RD, Cohen HJ, et al. Four-agent induction and intensive asparaginase therapy for treatment of childhood acute lymphoblastic leukemia. N Engl J Med 1986;315:657–63.

50. Sallan SE, Hitchcock-Bryan S, Gelber R, et al. Influence of intensive asparaginase in the treatment of childhood non-T-cell acute lymphoblastic leukemia. Cancer Res 1983;43:5601–7.

51. Matherly LH, Taub JW, Ravindranath Y, et al. Elevated dihydrofolate reductase and impaired methotrexate transport as elements in methotrexate resistance in childhood acute lymphoblastic leukemia. Blood 1995;85:500–9.

52. Patte C, Philip T, Rodary C, et al. Improved survival rate in children with stage III and IV B cell non-Hodgkin's lymphoma and leukemia using multi-agent chemotherapy: results of a study of 114 children from the French Pediatric Oncology Society. J Clin Oncol 1986;4:1219–26.

53. Bowman WP, Shuster JJ, Cook B, et al. Improved survival for children with B-cell acute lymphoblastic leukemia and stage IV small noncleaved-cell lymphoma: a pediatric oncology group study. J Clin Oncol 1996;14:1252–61.

54. Little PA, Sampath A, Subbarow Y. The use of antagonists of pteroylglutamic acid in controlling Rous chicken sarcoma. J Lab Clin Med 1948;33:1144–9.

55. Link MP, Goorin AM, Miser AW, et al. The effect of adjuvant chemotherapy on relapse-free survival in patients with osteosarcoma of the extremity. N Engl J Med 1986;314:1600–6.

56. Taub JW, Roarty J, DeCamillo D, et al. Platinum based chemotherapy protocols are an effective upfront therapy for newly diagnosed bilateral retinoblastoma. Poster presentation at the XXVIIth meeting of the International Society of Paediatric Oncology (SIOP), Oct. 10-15, 1995, Montevideo, Uruguay. Med Ped Oncol 1995;25:320, abstract # P-168.

Genetic and Nongenetic Risk Factors for Childhood Cancer

Logan G. Spector, PhD[a],*, Nathan Pankratz, PhD[b],
Erin L. Marcotte, PhD[a]

KEYWORDS

- Epidemiology • Etiology • Genome-wide association studies • Case-control studies
- Pediatric cancer

KEY POINTS

- Apart from high-dose radiation and prior chemotherapy there are few or no strong external risk factors with relative risks greater than 2.
- Inherent risk factors including birth weight, parental age, and congenital anomalies are consistently associated with most types of pediatric cancer.
- Common genetic variation has been associated with several childhood cancers in genome-wide association studies, often with subtype specificity, and explains a larger proportion of childhood than adult cancers.

INTRODUCTION

The causes of childhood cancer have been systematically studied for several decades. The incidence of all cancers occurring in children younger than 20 years of age is about 175 cases per million in the United States,[1] with the incidence of many individual types (typically grouped by the International Classification of Childhood Cancer schema[2]), in the low dozens (**Fig. 1**). Rarity is thus a central fact that dictates the quality and quantity of evidence for causal associations between putative risk factors and childhood cancers. Most etiologic investigations of childhood cancer have thus of necessity used the case-control study design[3] where the characteristics of patients with a disease are compared with those of a carefully selected group of disease-free control subjects. When they require participant involvement, as in the many studies of childhood cancer that have collected exposure information through parental interview, case-control studies are susceptible to recall and selection biases.

[a] Division of Epidemiology/Clinical Research, Department of Pediatrics, University of Minnesota, 420 Delaware Street, Southeast, Minneapolis, MN 55455, USA; [b] Department of Lab Medicine and Pathology, University of Minnesota, 515 Delaware Street SE, Minneapolis, MN 55455, USA
* Corresponding author. 420 Delaware Street, Southeast, MMC 715, Minneapolis, MN 55455.
E-mail address: spector@umn.edu

Pediatr Clin N Am 62 (2015) 11–25
http://dx.doi.org/10.1016/j.pcl.2014.09.013
pediatric.theclinics.com

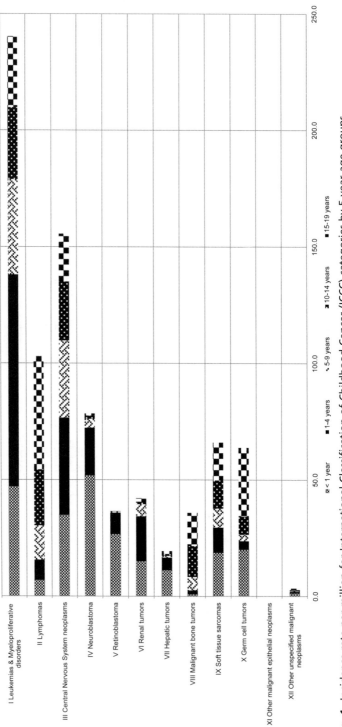

Fig. 1. Incidence rate per million for International Classification of Childhood Cancer (ICCC) categories by 5-year age groups.

Given the milieu for childhood cancer epidemiology, evidence regarding causal associations has accumulated slowly. However, for the most common types of cancer, particularly acute lymphoblastic leukemia (ALL), the body of literature is now sufficiently large to allow data synthesis through meta-analyses and data pooling. This article discusses such analyses of external, or environmental, risk factors because they have mainly demonstrated weak or null associations. In contrast, intrinsic characteristics or conditions of patients with childhood cancer have shown stronger, more consistent associations and in the last half-decade the application of genome-wide single nucleotide variant (SNV) arrays to several childhood cancers has generated surprising insights into their biology. Hence, most of this article for the general pediatrician covers these topics in a broad overview to reflect their increased importance in the current understanding of causes of childhood cancer.

DEMOGRAPHIC RISK FACTORS

Childhood cancer incidence has long been noted to vary by age, sex, and race and ethnicity. Overall incidence is highest in infancy at about 240 cases per million per year. This rate drops to a nadir of 128 cases per million at 5 to 9 years of age before rising to 220 cases per million at 15 to 19 years of age.[1] Grouped incidence, however, obscures interesting patterns among individual cancers (see **Fig. 1**). For instance, all the embryonal tumors (neuroblastoma, Wilms tumor, retinoblastoma, and so forth) share a downward sloping incidence, which starts high at birth and dissipates after about 5 years of age. ALL is notable for the incidence peak that occurs between 2 to 5 years of age, whereas bone sarcoma incidence peaks sharply around the time of the pubertal growth spurt in early-to-mid adolescence.

For most childhood cancers there is a slight male preponderance (**Fig. 2**). The male-to-female ratio ranges from 1.04 to 1.64 in neuroblastoma and germ cell tumors, respectively, in cases 0 to 19 years of age but varies considerably by age group and more specific diagnosis. Wilms tumor is notable for being the one major childhood cancer that is more common in females.

Childhood cancer risk also differs by race and ethnicity (**Fig. 3**). Relative to white children in the United States the incidence of most types of cancer is lower in black, Asian, and Hispanic children. In some cases, such as the near complete lack of Ewing sarcoma among black and Asian children, the disparity is dramatic. In a few notable instances cancer incidence is higher in other groups compared with white children. That acute leukemia incidence is about 10% higher in Hispanic children compared with white children is particularly notable. The extent that racial and ethnic differences are attributable to genetic versus environmental differences has yet to be determined but will surely come into focus as the genetic architecture of childhood cancer continues to be elucidated.

ENVIRONMENTAL RISK FACTORS

High-dose ionizing radiation and prior chemotherapy are accepted causes of childhood cancers, each raising risk several fold.[4–7] No other environmental risk factors, by which is meant any exposure that originates outside the body, have emerged as definitively causal for childhood cancer.

Measurement of environmental exposures poses a challenge in elucidating their effects on childhood cancer risk. Prospective studies would require hundreds of thousands, if not millions, of children to identify enough cases to generate statistically meaningful results. Thus most childhood cancer studies must rely on the case-control design, which is particularly problematic for evaluating certain types of

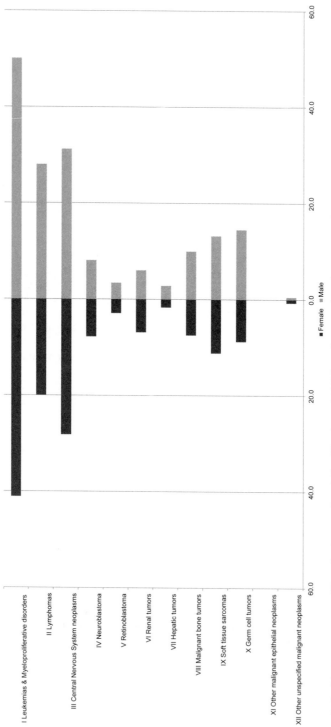

Fig. 2. Incidence rates per million for International Classification of Childhood Cancer (ICCC) categories by sex.

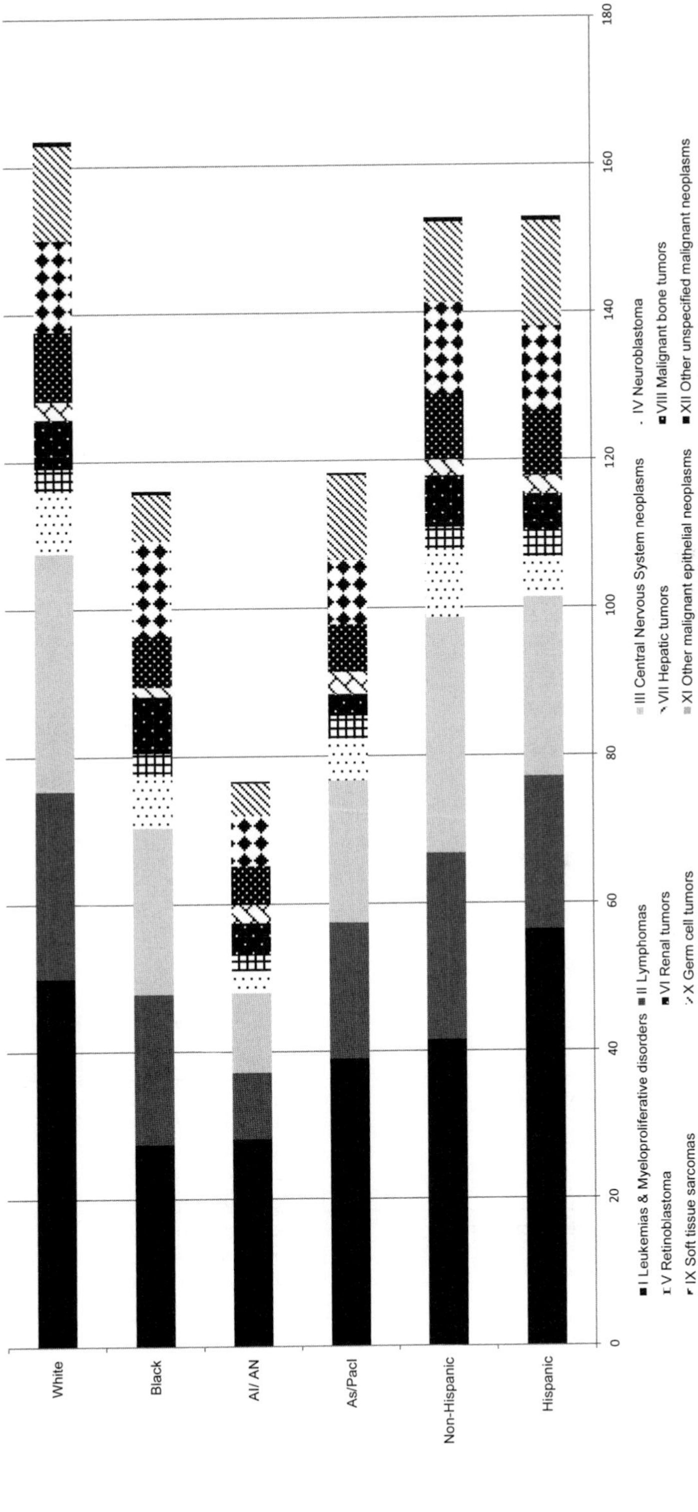

Fig. 3. Incidence rates per million for International Classification of Childhood Cancer (ICCC) categories by race/ethnicity. AI/AN, American Indian/Alaska Native; As/PacI, Asian/Pacific Islander.

exposures. Demographic and intrinsic factors are unambiguous; easy to obtain via questionnaire; and in such cases as parental age, race and ethnicity, and birth defects, generally not subject to recall error. In contrast, environmental factors, such as parental diet, maternal medication, caffeine, and alcohol use, and pesticide and air pollution exposure are difficult to measure accurately in a retrospective design. Although use of registries, birth and medical records, and other data sources reduces some sources of bias, accurate exposure assessment remains a major barrier to determining the causal impact of environmental factors on childhood cancer risk.

For many childhood cancers findings are inconsistent or studies too few to conduct meta-analysis; moreover, synthesis is hampered by the need to separately examine exposures during the preconceptional, pregnancy, and postnatal periods and the progressively finer classifications of tumors. ALL, being the most common childhood cancer, has been the subject of several meta-analyses of putative environmental risk factors (**Table 1**).[8–15]

Table 1				
Results of selected meta-analyses of environmental risk factors and childhood ALL				
Exposure	**Time Period**	**N Studies**	**Findings**	**Reference**
Maternal alcohol use	Pregnancy	10	No association of any alcohol use during pregnancy with ALL (mOR = 1.10 [0.93–1.29])	[11]
Maternal coffee use	Pregnancy	5	Small association of any coffee consumption during pregnancy with ALL (mOR = 1.16 [1.00–1.34])	[8]
Daycare attendance	Postnatal	14	Small reduced risk of ALL associated with daycare attendance (mOR = 0.76 [0.67–0.87])	[13]
Electromagnetic field exposure	Postnatal	9	No association of electromagnetic field exposure ≥ 0.2 µT with ALL (mOR = 1.25 [0.97–1.60])	[15]
Occupational pesticide exposure	Pregnancy	5	Strong association of maternal occupational exposure to pesticides during pregnancy and ALL (mOR = 2.64 [1.40–5.00])	[14]
Maternal prenatal vitamins	Pregnancy	3	Small reduced risk of ALL associated with maternal prenatal vitamin consumption (mOR = 0.61 [0.50–0.74])	[9]
Paternal smoking	Preconception	10	Small association of any paternal preconceptional smoking with ALL (mOR = 1.15 [1.06–1.24])	[12]
Maternal smoking	Pregnancy	20	No association of any maternal smoking during pregnancy with ALL (mOR = 1.03 [0.95–1.12])	[10]

Abbreviation: mOR, meta-analytic odds ratio.

Exposure to infections has been one of the most commonly examined environmental exposures in relation to ALL risk, and there are two main hypotheses regarding the nature of this relationship. Kinlen[16] proposes that previously isolated, and therefore immunologically naive, populations are susceptible when exposed to specific infectious agents because of population mixing. A recent meta-analysis estimated an increased risk of ALL in rural settings of population mixing.[17] Greaves[18,19] hypothesized that an immature and unchallenged immune system, resulting from delayed exposure to common infections, produces an unregulated immune response and leads to ALL in the presence of susceptible cells. Although direct measurement of exposure to infections and the resulting immune response is generally not feasible, several proxies have been used including birth order,[20–22] daycare attendance,[23,24] breastfeeding,[25] infectious illness histories,[26] and vaccinations.[27] Meta-analyses have shown protective effects for breastfeeding[28] and daycare attendance,[13] although because these are indirect exposure measures, it is unclear whether infection exposure or some other factor is driving these associations.

Several recent meta-analyses have identified increased risk for residential[29,30] and maternal occupational[14] exposure to pesticides. Studies of residential pesticide exposure have generally relied on self-report, which is subject to recall bias that may inflate risk estimates. Some recent studies have used residential proximity to pesticide applications,[31–33] a method that is less prone to bias but still prone to measurement error, which may attenuate risk estimates.[34] Occupational studies typically rely on either self-report or record data. Although an association between pesticide exposure and ALL is supported by the available meta-analytic data, it is difficult to estimate the true magnitude of effect, if there is indeed a causal relationship, given the varying exposure assessment methods and the inherent biases and measurement errors therein.

Associations for other exposures examined using meta-analyses, including maternal alcohol,[11] coffee,[8] and vitamin use,[9] and paternal[12] and maternal[10] smoking have yielded mostly null[10,11] or slightly elevated[8,12] results. Maternal prenatal vitamin use was associated with a decreased risk of ALL in offspring, although the meta-analysis was based on only three studies.[9] Although a causal role for these risk factors is possible, observational epidemiology is not conclusive in these circumstances. High-quality studies with a focus on accurate exposure assessment are necessary to evaluate environmental risk factors for childhood cancer.

INTRINSIC RISK FACTORS

Several intrinsic characteristics of children or their parents have been consistently associated with childhood cancers. Risk of ALL,[35] central nervous system tumors,[36] neuroblastoma,[37] and Wilms tumor[38] rises as a linear function of birth weight, to varying degrees, and recent analyses that have used alternate measures of birth size (eg, size for gestational age, percent of optimal birth weight) have found similar results.[39] Risk of acute myeloid leukemia is elevated with low and high birth weight,[40] whereas risk of hepatoblastoma is inversely related to birth weight and strikingly elevated among the smallest infants.[41] The reasons behind the association of higher birth weight with childhood cancers have not been explored in detail, but may include prenatal growth hormone exposure,[42] the underlying genetics of birth weight,[43] and the greater number of cells at risk for carcinogenic transformation. The strong inverse association of hepatoblastoma with birth weight has been thought to be related to neonatal treatment, but no culprit exposure has been identified to date.[44]

Advanced parental age has also been associated with most childhood cancers. A large pooled analysis of population-based record-linkage studies found significant positive linear trends in leukemia, lymphoma, brain tumor, neuroblastoma, Wilms tumor, bone tumors, and soft tissue sarcomas with 6% to 15% increased risk per 5 years of maternal age.[45] Paternal age was not associated with these cancers after adjustment for maternal age; however, because the two are highly correlated it is not clear that maternal age was solely responsible. As with birth weight, the reasons behind these findings are unclear, but may include genetic or epigenetic mutations associated with advanced parental age.[46]

Structural birth defects have consistently been found to increase the risk of childhood cancers as a group about three-fold,[47–49] although because of the rarity of individual birth defects and individual childhood cancers more specific associations have not been reported to date. Undoubtedly some of this association is explained by underlying genetic causes, but because most birth defects seem sporadic[50] genetics are likely not the sole explanation for co-occurrence.

GENETIC RISK FACTORS

Inherited syndromes caused by high-penetrance germline DNA mutations,[51,52] chromosomal aneuploidy,[53] or epigenetic disorders[54] are known to cause a minority of childhood cancers. Although the proportion attributable to syndromes has rarely been precisely quantified for common childhood cancers the estimate is typically 5% to 10%. For especially rare cancers, such as pediatric adrenocortical carcinoma, the proportion can be much higher.[55] Specific syndromes predisposing to particular childhood cancers are covered elsewhere in this issue.

Genome-wide association studies (GWAS) compare the frequency of hundreds of thousands of common SNVs in those with a disease with those without.[56] Because of the large number of comparisons made in GWAS a SNV-disease association must reach a high degree of statistical significance (generally $P < 5 \times 10^{-8}$) to be convincing. This requires large sample sizes not readily achievable for rare diseases. Yet, despite the a priori presumption that the GWAS design could not be successfully applied to childhood cancers investigations of ALL,[57–63] neuroblastoma,[64–73] Wilms tumor,[74] osteosarcoma,[75] and Ewing sarcoma,[76] each have identified multiple variants associated with each disease (**Table 2**). The unexpected success of GWAS to studies of these rare cancers seems to be caused by the larger magnitude of SNV-disease association among young-onset cancers compared with those with adult-onset, which was recently formally quantified (**Fig. 4**).[77] An implication of this finding, besides reaffirming the applicability of GWAS to other childhood cancers not yet studied thusly, is that common genetic variation explains a greater proportion of the population-attributable risk for childhood than adult cancers.

The GWAS and replication studies of ALL and neuroblastoma include diverse populations and subtype-specific analyses, giving a more mature picture of the genetic architecture of each disease than is available for those with a single GWAS to date. Two recent GWAS of ALL conducted with African-American and Hispanic cases and control subjects replicated many of the SNVs first identified in studies of subjects with European ancestry; SNVs in ARID5B, IKZF1, and PIP4K2A were associated with ALL in both ethnicities, and CEBPE in Hispanics.[59] Odds ratios per allele were similar in each group, in line with the generally high transethnic replicability of GWAS results.[78] However, frequencies varied in directions that suggest several SNVs may explain a substantial proportion of lower incidence of ALL in African-Americans and the higher one in Hispanics compared with Europeans. ARID5B rs10821936 was

Table 2
SNVs identified by GWAS of childhood cancers

Cancer	Gene	SNV	Population	Subtype	OR	95% CI	P Value	Reference
ALL	ARID5B	rs10821936	European	Total	1.91	1.6–2.2	1.4×10^{-15}	38
ALL	ARID5B	rs10740055	European	Total	1.53	1.4–1.6	5.35×10^{-14}	37
ALL	ARID5B	rs10821936	African-American	Total	1.52	1.1–2.0	.004	39
ALL	ARID5B	rs10821936	Hispanic	Total	1.95	1.6–2.4	3.78×10^{-11}	39
ALL	ARID5B	rs10821936	European	B-hyperdiploid	2.17	1.5–3.1	1.62×10^{-5}	38
ALL	CDK2NA	rs3731217	European	Total	0.71	0.6–0.8	3.01×10^{-11}	40
ALL	CDK2NA	rs17756311	European	Total	1.43	1.2–1.7	3.25×10^{-5}	39
ALL	CEBPE	rs2239633	European	Total	1.34	1.2–1.5	2.88×10^{-7}	37
ALL	CEBPE	rs4982731	Hispanic	Total	1.58	1.3–1.9	2.32×10^{-6}	39
ALL	COMMD3/BMI1	rs4266962	European	Total	1.41	1.2–1.7	4.35×10^{-8}	39
ALL	GATA3	rs3824662	European	Total	1.31	1.2–1.4	8.62×10^{-12}	43
ALL	GATA3	rs3824662	European	Philadelphia-like	3.85	2.7–5.47	2.17×10^{-14}	42
ALL	IKZF1	rs11978267	European	Total	1.69	1.4–1.9	8.8×10^{-11}	38
ALL	IKZF1	rs4132601	European	Total	1.69	1.6–1.8	1.2×10^{-19}	37
ALL	PIP4K2A	rs10828317	European	Total	1.23	1.2–1.3	2.3×10^{-9}	43
Ewing sarcoma	TARDBP	rs9430161	European	Total	2.20	1.8–2.7	1.4×10^{-20}	56
Ewing sarcoma	EGR2	rs224278	European	Total	1.66	1.4–1.9	4×10^{-17}	56
Neuroblastoma	FLJ22536	rs6939340	European	Total	1.40	1.3–1.6	5.82×10^{-8}	51
Neuroblastoma	BARD1	rs6435862	European	Total	1.64	1.4–1.9	3.19×10^{-9}	45
Neuroblastoma	BARD1	rs6435862	African-American	Total	1.44	1.2–1.7	1.8×10^{-5}	45
Neuroblastoma	HACE1	rs4336470	European	Total	1.26	1.2–1.4	2.7×10^{-11}	48
Neuroblastoma	LIN28B	rs17065417	European	Total	1.38	1.2–1.5	1.2×10^{-8}	48
Neuroblastoma	LMO1	rs110419	European	Total	1.34	1.3–1.4	5.2×10^{-16}	53
Osteosarcoma	GRM4	rs1906953	European	Total	1.57	1.4–1.8	8.0×10^{-9}	55
Osteosarcoma	Intergenic at 2p25.2	rs7591996	European	Total	1.39	1.2–1.5	1.0×10^{-8}	55
Wilms tumor	Intergenic at 2p24	rs3755132	European	Total	1.48	1.3–1.7	1.03×10^{-14}	54
Wilms tumor	Intergenic at 11q14	rs790356	European	Total	1.43	1.3–1.6	4.25×10^{-15}	54

Abbreviations: CI, confidence interval; OR, odds ratio.

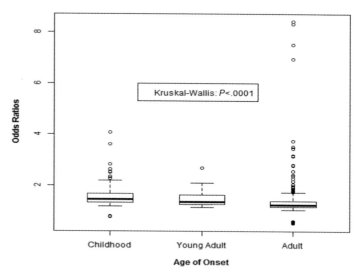

Fig. 4. Boxplot of SNV odds ratios from GWAS of cancer by age group. *Dark horizontal lines* represent the median and the *box* represents the 25th and 75th percentiles. (*From* Raynor LA, Pankratz N, Spector LG, et al. An analysis of measures of effect size by age of onset in cancer genomewide association studies. Genes Chromosomes Cancer 2013;52(9): 857; with permission.)

present in 33% of Europeans, 24% of African-Americans, and 47% of Hispanics; the equivalent numbers for IKZF1 rs11978267 were 28%, 19%, and 26%. CEBP rs4982731 was present in 28% of Europeans and 39% of Hispanics, and 38% of African-Americans in which this SNV did not replicate. Similarly, SNVs in BARD1 replicated in a GWAS of neuroblastoma among African-Americans, whereas no others did, possibly because of small sample size.[70]

Several SNVs in both diseases show far stronger odds ratios with specific subtypes, demonstrating that lumping disparate cases can dilute associations. In ALL, *ARID5B* SNVs have been more strongly associated with hyperdiploid disease[58,79,80] and *GATA3* SNVs with leukemias displaying a Philadelphia chromosome–like expression pattern[62]; the latter is an especially dramatic instance, with subtype-specific odds ratios per allele of about 3.5 versus 1.3 in total ALL. *BARD1* and *LMO1* SNVs are associated with aggressive disease in neuroblastoma[65,66,72] and SNVs in or near *DUSP12*, *DDX4*, *IL31RA*, and *HSD17B12* with low-risk disease.[72] It seems reasonable to speculate that similarly specific associations with subtypes of other childhood cancers will emerge as the GWAS literature expands.

Although the progress in identifying common variants associated with several childhood cancers in the past several years has been remarkable, a large portion of heritability remains unexplained. For instance, estimates indicate that about 25% of genetic variation in ALL risk was caused by common variants identified by GWAS available in 2012.[81] The remainder of genetic risk may be attributable to several other plausible mechanisms that will more often be evaluated as next-generation sequencing and the inclusion of parental samples are adopted by the field. Rare variation is generally defined as that with a population allele frequency of less than 0.01. A recent exome-sequencing study of infant leukemia, among the first of its kind, identified compound heterozygosity for rare pathogenic variants in the *MLL3* gene as risk factors.[82] Sequencing of parents and children and comparing exomes or genomes can identify de novo mutations that will not be apparent by other technologies.[46] Lastly, because many childhood cancers are presumed to initiate in utero,[83] maternal genetic effects may be relevant,[84] but have only been examined in a candidate gene rather than genome-wide context to date.[85,86]

SUMMARY

The rarity of childhood cancer slows the search for their causes, but the accumulation of case-control studies and advancement of genomic technology have improved clinicians' knowledge in recent years. Few environmental risk factors for childhood cancer have been identified that exceed the capacity of observational epidemiology to distinguish causal associations from those caused by bias. Inherent risk factors, such as birth weight, parental age, and birth defects, and common genetic variation, are consistently associated with childhood cancers.

REFERENCES

1. Howlader N, Noone AM, Krapcho M, et al. SEER cancer statistics review, 1975-2011. Bethesda (MD): National Cancer Institute; 2014.
2. Steliarova-Foucher E, Stiller C, Lacour B, et al. International Classification of Childhood Cancer, third edition. Cancer 2005;103(7):1457–67.
3. Wacholder S. Design issues in case-control studies. Stat Methods Med Res 1995; 4(4):293–309.
4. Hawkins MM, Wilson LM, Stovall MA, et al. Epipodophyllotoxins, alkylating agents, and radiation and risk of secondary leukaemia after childhood cancer. BMJ 1992;304(6832):951–8.
5. Pui CH, Relling MV. Topoisomerase II inhibitor-related acute myeloid leukaemia. Br J Haematol 2000;109(1):13–23.
6. Tucker MA, Meadows AT, Boice JD Jr, et al. Leukemia after therapy with alkylating agents for childhood cancer. J Natl Cancer Inst 1987;78(3):459–64.
7. Ron E, Modan B, Boice JD Jr, et al. Tumors of the brain and nervous system after radiotherapy in childhood. N Engl J Med 1988;319(16):1033–9.
8. Cheng J, Su H, Zhu R, et al. Maternal coffee consumption during pregnancy and risk of childhood acute leukemia: a metaanalysis. Am J Obstet Gynecol 2014; 210(2):151.e1–10.
9. Goh YI, Bollano E, Einarson TR, et al. Prenatal multivitamin supplementation and rates of pediatric cancers: a meta-analysis. Clin Pharmacol Ther 2007;81(5): 685–91.
10. Klimentopoulou A, Antonopoulos CN, Papadopoulou C, et al. Maternal smoking during pregnancy and risk for childhood leukemia: a nationwide case-control study in Greece and meta-analysis. Pediatr Blood Cancer 2012;58(3):344–51.
11. Latino-Martel P, Chan DS, Druesne-Pecollo N, et al. Maternal alcohol consumption during pregnancy and risk of childhood leukemia: systematic review and meta-analysis. Cancer Epidemiol Biomarkers Prev 2010;19(5):1238–60.
12. Milne E, Greenop KR, Scott RJ, et al. Parental prenatal smoking and risk of childhood acute lymphoblastic leukemia. Am J Epidemiol 2012;175(1):43–53.
13. Urayama KY, Buffler PA, Gallagher ER, et al. A meta-analysis of the association between day-care attendance and childhood acute lymphoblastic leukaemia. Int J Epidemiol 2010;39(3):718–32.
14. Wigle DT, Turner MC, Krewski D. A systematic review and meta-analysis of childhood leukemia and parental occupational pesticide exposure. Environ Health Perspect 2009;117(10):1505–13.

15. Zhao L, Liu X, Wang C, et al. Magnetic fields exposure and childhood leukemia risk: a meta-analysis based on 11,699 cases and 13,194 controls. Leuk Res 2014;38(3):269–74.
16. Kinlen L. Evidence for an infective cause of childhood leukaemia: comparison of a Scottish new town with nuclear reprocessing sites in Britain. Lancet 1988; 2(8624):1323–7.
17. Kinlen LJ. An examination, with a meta-analysis, of studies of childhood leukaemia in relation to population mixing. Br J Cancer 2012;107(7):1163–8.
18. Greaves MF. Aetiology of acute leukaemia. Lancet 1997;349(9048):344–9.
19. Greaves MF. Speculations on the cause of childhood acute lymphoblastic leukemia. Leukemia 1988;2(2):120–5.
20. Roman E, Simpson J, Ansell P, et al. Perinatal and reproductive factors: a report on haematological malignancies from the UKCCS. Eur J Cancer 2005;41(5):749–59.
21. Jourdan-Da Silva N, Perel Y, Mechinaud F, et al. Infectious diseases in the first year of life, perinatal characteristics and childhood acute leukaemia. Br J Cancer 2004;90(1):139–45.
22. Dockerty JD, Draper G, Vincent T, et al. Case-control study of parental age, parity and socioeconomic level in relation to childhood cancers. Int J Epidemiol 2001; 30(6):1428–37.
23. Gilham C, Peto J, Simpson J, et al. Day care in infancy and risk of childhood acute lymphoblastic leukaemia: findings from UK case-control study. BMJ 2005;330(7503):1294.
24. Neglia JP, Linet MS, Shu XO, et al. Patterns of infection and day care utilization and risk of childhood acute lymphoblastic leukaemia. Br J Cancer 2000;82(1): 234–40.
25. Infante-Rivard C, Fortier I, Olson E. Markers of infection, breast-feeding and childhood acute lymphoblastic leukaemia. Br J Cancer 2000;83(11):1559–64.
26. van Steensel-Moll HA, Valkenburg HA, van Zanen GE. Childhood leukemia and infectious diseases in the first year of life: a register-based case-control study. Am J Epidemiol 1986;124(4):590–4.
27. Dockerty JD, Skegg DC, Elwood JM, et al. Infections, vaccinations, and the risk of childhood leukaemia. Br J Cancer 1999;80(9):1483–9.
28. Kwan ML, Buffler PA, Abrams B, et al. Breastfeeding and the risk of childhood leukemia: a meta-analysis. Public Health Rep 2004;119(6):521–35.
29. Van Maele-Fabry G, Lantin AC, Hoet P, et al. Residential exposure to pesticides and childhood leukaemia: a systematic review and meta-analysis. Environ Int 2011;37(1):280–91.
30. Turner MC, Wigle DT, Krewski D. Residential pesticides and childhood leukemia: a systematic review and meta-analysis. Environ Health Perspect 2010;118(1):33–41.
31. Rull RP, Gunier R, Von Behren J, et al. Residential proximity to agricultural pesticide applications and childhood acute lymphoblastic leukemia. Environ Res 2009;109(7):891–9.
32. Reynolds P, Von Behren J, Gunier RB, et al. Agricultural pesticide use and childhood cancer in California. Epidemiology 2005;16(1):93–100.
33. Reynolds P, Von Behren J, Gunier RB, et al. Childhood cancer and agricultural pesticide use: an ecologic study in California. Environ Health Perspect 2002; 110(3):319–24.
34. Rull RP, Ritz B. Historical pesticide exposure in California using pesticide use reports and land-use surveys: an assessment of misclassification error and bias. Environ Health Perspect 2003;111(13):1582–9.

35. Hjalgrim LL, Westergaard T, Rostgaard K, et al. Birth weight as a risk factor for childhood leukemia: a meta-analysis of 18 epidemiologic studies. Am J Epidemiol 2003;158(8):724–35.
36. Harder T, Plagemann A, Harder A. Birth weight and subsequent risk of childhood primary brain tumors: a meta-analysis. Am J Epidemiol 2008;168(4):366–73.
37. Harder T, Plagemann A, Harder A. Birth weight and risk of neuroblastoma: a meta-analysis. Int J Epidemiol 2010;39(3):746–56.
38. Chu A, Heck JE, Ribeiro KB, et al. Wilms' tumour: a systematic review of risk factors and meta-analysis. Paediatr Perinat Epidemiol 2010;24(5):449–69.
39. Milne E, Greenop KR, Metayer C, et al. Fetal growth and childhood acute lymphoblastic leukemia: findings from the childhood leukemia international consortium. Int J Cancer 2013;133(12):2968–79.
40. Caughey RW, Michels KB. Birth weight and childhood leukemia: a meta-analysis and review of the current evidence. Int J Cancer 2009;124(11):2658–70.
41. Spector LG, Puumala SE, Carozza SE, et al. Cancer risk among children with very low birth weights. Pediatrics 2009;124(1):96–104.
42. Ross JA, Perentesis JP, Robison LL, et al. Big babies and infant leukemia: a role for insulin-like growth factor-1? Cancer Causes Control 1996;7(5):553–9.
43. Lunde A, Melve KK, Gjessing HK, et al. Genetic and environmental influences on birth weight, birth length, head circumference, and gestational age by use of population-based parent-offspring data. Am J Epidemiol 2007;165(7):734–41.
44. Turcotte LM, Georgieff MK, Ross JA, et al. Neonatal medical exposures and characteristics of low birth weight hepatoblastoma cases: A report from the Children's Oncology Group. Pediatr Blood Cancer 2014;61:2018–23.
45. Johnson KJ, Carozza SE, Chow EJ, et al. Parental age and risk of childhood cancer: a pooled analysis. Epidemiology 2009;20(4):475–83.
46. Veltman JA, Brunner HG. De novo mutations in human genetic disease. Nat Rev Genet 2012;13(8):565–75.
47. Botto LD, Flood T, Little J, et al. Cancer risk in children and adolescents with birth defects: a population-based cohort study. PLoS One 2013;8(7):e69077.
48. Carozza SE, Langlois PH, Miller EA, et al. Are children with birth defects at higher risk of childhood cancers? Am J Epidemiol 2012;175(12):1217–24.
49. Fisher PG, Reynolds P, Von Behren J, et al. Cancer in children with nonchromosomal birth defects. J Pediatr 2012;160(6):978–83.
50. Hobbs CA, Chowdhury S, Cleves MA, et al. Genetic epidemiology and nonsyndromic structural birth defects: from candidate genes to epigenetics. JAMA Pediatr 2014;168(4):371–7.
51. Malkin D. Li-Fraumeni syndrome. Genes Cancer 2011;2(4):475–84.
52. Seif AE. Pediatric leukemia predisposition syndromes: clues to understanding leukemogenesis. Cancer Genet 2011;204(5):227–44.
53. Ross JA, Spector LG, Robison LL, et al. Epidemiology of leukemia in children with Down syndrome. Pediatr Blood Cancer 2005;44(1):8–12.
54. DeBaun MR, Tucker MA. Risk of cancer during the first four years of life in children from The Beckwith-Wiedemann Syndrome Registry. J Pediatr 1998;132(3 Pt 1): 398–400.
55. Choong SS, Latiff ZA, Mohamed M, et al. Childhood adrenocortical carcinoma as a sentinel cancer for detecting families with germline TP53 mutations. Clin Genet 2012;82(6):564–8.
56. Christensen K, Murray JC. What genome-wide association studies can do for medicine. N Engl J Med 2007;356(11):1094–7.

57. Papaemmanuil E, Hosking FJ, Vijayakrishnan J, et al. Loci on 7p12.2, 10q21.2 and 14q11.2 are associated with risk of childhood acute lymphoblastic leukemia. Nat Genet 2009;41(9):1006–10.

58. Trevino LR, Yang W, French D, et al. Germline genomic variants associated with childhood acute lymphoblastic leukemia. Nat Genet 2009;41(9):1001–5.

59. Xu H, Yang W, Perez-Andreu V, et al. Novel susceptibility variants at 10p12.31-12.2 for childhood acute lymphoblastic leukemia in ethnically diverse populations. J Natl Cancer Inst 2013;105(10):733–42.

60. Sherborne AL, Hosking FJ, Prasad RB, et al. Variation in CDKN2A at 9p21.3 influences childhood acute lymphoblastic leukemia risk. Nat Genet 2010;42(6):492–4.

61. Ellinghaus E, Stanulla M, Richter G, et al. Identification of germline susceptibility loci in ETV6-RUNX1-rearranged childhood acute lymphoblastic leukemia. Leukemia 2012;26(5):902–9.

62. Perez-Andreu V, Roberts KG, Harvey RC, et al. Inherited GATA3 variants are associated with Ph-like childhood acute lymphoblastic leukemia and risk of relapse. Nat Genet 2013;45(12):1494–8.

63. Migliorini G, Fiege B, Hosking FJ, et al. Variation at 10p12.2 and 10p14 influences risk of childhood B-cell acute lymphoblastic leukemia and phenotype. Blood 2013;122(19):3298–307.

64. Bosse KR, Diskin SJ, Cole KA, et al. Common variation at BARD1 results in the expression of an oncogenic isoform that influences neuroblastoma susceptibility and oncogenicity. Cancer Res 2012;72(8):2068–78.

65. Capasso M, Devoto M, Hou C, et al. Common variations in BARD1 influence susceptibility to high-risk neuroblastoma. Nat Genet 2009;41(6):718–23.

66. Capasso M, Diskin SJ, Totaro F, et al. Replication of GWAS-identified neuroblastoma risk loci strengthens the role of BARD1 and affirms the cumulative effect of genetic variations on disease susceptibility. Carcinogenesis 2013;34(3):605–11.

67. Diskin SJ, Capasso M, Diamond M, et al. Rare variants in TP53 and susceptibility to neuroblastoma. J Natl Cancer Inst 2014;106(4):dju047.

68. Diskin SJ, Capasso M, Schnepp RW, et al. Common variation at 6q16 within HACE1 and LIN28B influences susceptibility to neuroblastoma. Nat Genet 2012;44(10):1126–30.

69. Diskin SJ, Hou C, Glessner JT, et al. Copy number variation at 1q21.1 associated with neuroblastoma. Nature 2009;459(7249):987–91.

70. Latorre V, Diskin SJ, Diamond MA, et al. Replication of neuroblastoma SNP association at the BARD1 locus in African-Americans. Cancer Epidemiol Biomarkers Prev 2012;21(4):658–63.

71. Maris JM, Mosse YP, Bradfield JP, et al. Chromosome 6p22 locus associated with clinically aggressive neuroblastoma. N Engl J Med 2008;358(24):2585–93.

72. Nguyen le B, Diskin SJ, Capasso M, et al. Phenotype restricted genome-wide association study using a gene-centric approach identifies three low-risk neuroblastoma susceptibility loci. PLoS Genet 2011;7(3):e1002026.

73. Wang K, Diskin SJ, Zhang H, et al. Integrative genomics identifies LMO1 as a neuroblastoma oncogene. Nature 2011;469(7329):216–20.

74. Turnbull C, Perdeaux ER, Pernet D, et al. A genome-wide association study identifies susceptibility loci for Wilms tumor. Nat Genet 2012;44(6):681–4.

75. Savage SA, Mirabello L, Wang Z, et al. Genome-wide association study identifies two susceptibility loci for osteosarcoma. Nat Genet 2013;45(7):799–803.

76. Postel-Vinay S, Veron AS, Tirode F, et al. Common variants near TARDBP and EGR2 are associated with susceptibility to Ewing sarcoma. Nat Genet 2012; 44(3):323–7.

77. Raynor LA, Pankratz N, Spector LG. An analysis of measures of effect size by age of onset in cancer genomewide association studies. Genes Chromosomes Cancer 2013;52(9):855–9.
78. Marigorta UM, Navarro A. High trans-ethnic replicability of GWAS results implies common causal variants. PLoS Genet 2013;9(6):e1003566.
79. Chokkalingam AP, Hsu LI, Metayer C, et al. Genetic variants in ARID5B and CEBPE are childhood ALL susceptibility loci in Hispanics. Cancer Causes Control 2013;24(10):1789–95.
80. Linabery AM, Blommer CN, Spector LG, et al. ARID5B and IKZF1 variants, selected demographic factors, and childhood acute lymphoblastic leukemia: a report from the Children's Oncology Group. Leuk Res 2013;37(8):936–42.
81. Enciso-Mora V, Hosking FJ, Sheridan E, et al. Common genetic variation contributes significantly to the risk of childhood B-cell precursor acute lymphoblastic leukemia. Leukemia 2012;26(10):2212–5.
82. Valentine MC, Linabery AM, Chasnoff S, et al. Excess congenital non-synonymous variation in leukemia-associated genes in MLL-infant leukemia: a Children's Oncology Group report. Leukemia 2014;28(6):1235–41.
83. Spector LG, Hooten AJ, Ross JA. Ontogeny of gene expression: a changing environment for malignancy. Cancer Epidemiol Biomarkers Prev 2008;17(5):1021–3.
84. Santure AW, Spencer HG. Influence of mom and dad: quantitative genetic models for maternal effects and genomic imprinting. Genetics 2006;173(4):2297–316.
85. Nousome D, Lupo PJ, Okcu MF, et al. Maternal and offspring xenobiotic metabolism haplotypes and the risk of childhood acute lymphoblastic leukemia. Leuk Res 2013;37(5):531–5.
86. Lupo PJ, Nousome D, Kamdar KY, et al. A case-parent triad assessment of folate metabolic genes and the risk of childhood acute lymphoblastic leukemia. Cancer Causes Control 2012;23(11):1797–803.

Supportive Care in Pediatric Oncology

Oncologic Emergencies and Management of Fever and Neutropenia

Meret Henry, MD, MS[a],*, Lillian Sung, MD, PhD[b]

KEYWORDS

- Oncologic emergencies • Fever • Neutropenia • Infection • Cancer
- Early signs of childhood cancer

KEY POINTS

- Children with fever and neutropenia are not a homogenous group. They can be stratified and therapy altered according to risk classification.
- Initial broad-spectrum monotherapy is recommended for children with fever and neutropenia. Therapy can then be tailored to each child based on culture results and clinical status.
- Hyperleukocytosis, tumor lysis syndrome, superior mediastinal syndrome, and spinal cord compression are among the most common oncologic emergencies seen at the time of diagnosis in children with cancer. Prompt recognition and management of these conditions is paramount to decreasing associated morbidity and mortality.

INTRODUCTION

Supportive Care in Pediatric Oncology

By current estimates greater than or equal to 80% of all children with cancer become long-term survivors. Thus, it is all the more important that the diagnosis of cancer should occur early in the course of the disease so that appropriate treatment can be initiated promptly. Delays in diagnosis may result in increased morbidity and mortality. However, such delays continue to occur in the present era of sophisticated laboratory and imaging studies. The most common reason for the delay in diagnosis is the continued stigma attached to the diagnosis of cancer/leukemia. Given current cure rates, pediatricians should not be reluctant to entertain cancer in the differential

[a] Division of Hematology/Oncology, Children's Hospital of Michigan/Wayne State University, 3901 Beaubien, Detroit, MI 48201, USA; [b] Division of Haematology/Oncology, The Hospital for Sick Children, 555 University Avenue, Toronto, Ontario M5G1X8, Canada
* Corresponding author.
E-mail address: mhenry@med.wayne.edu

Pediatr Clin N Am 62 (2015) 27–46
http://dx.doi.org/10.1016/j.pcl.2014.09.016   pediatric.theclinics.com
0031-3955/15/$ – see front matter © 2015 Elsevier Inc. All rights reserved.

diagnosis of an ill child. Symptoms and signs specific to each cancer are discussed separately in this article. **Box 1** lists some presenting symptoms of leukemias and common solid tumors in children.

When leukemia and cancer are suspected, an orderly set of investigations helps in confirming or excluding the diagnosis of malignancy. Aside from a complete blood count, laboratory studies should include uric acid and lactate dehydrogenase levels along with electrolytes, creatinine, and blood urea nitrogen (BUN). A lactate dehydrogenase level coupled with high uric acid level requires exclusion of leukemia/lymphoma. Plain radiographs of the chest are invaluable for separating benign cervical adenopathy from mediastinal lymphoma with minimal cervical adenopathy. Plain films of the abdomen in children presenting with an abdominal mass might provide important clues of a possible neoplasm even if a mass is not easily noted (eg, punctate calcification in renal fossa may suggest neuroblastoma). An abnormal bowel pattern and signs of intestinal obstruction may indicate the presence of intestinal lymphoma (Burkitt lymphoma) and distinguish such cases from constipation from impacted feces in the colon. Advanced imaging studies such as MRI or computed tomography (CT) can then be used. For most tumors, other than anterior mediastinal masses, MRI is preferred rather than CT imaging because of better delineation of the anatomy and ability to combine imaging of the arterial system and venous invasion of the tumor. In children with neuroblastoma, MRI has the added benefit of imaging of dumbbell tumors with tumor extension into the vertebral canal. MRI is the preferred imaging study for bone tumors. For anterior mediastinal tumors, CT scans provide better estimates of the degree of compression of trachea and superior vena cava.

Improvements in supportive care over the last 2 decades have been among the contributors to the current high cure rates in childhood cancer. Further improvement in overall survival requires close attention to the prevention of disease-related early

---

Box 1
Common chief complaints in children with cancer

Chief Complaints	Possible Cancer
Petechiae, bruising/bleeding	Leukemia
Pallor and fatigue	Leukemia, NHL
Recurrent fever with bone pain	Leukemia, Ewing sarcoma
Bone pain	Leukemia, Ewing sarcoma, osteosarcoma, neuroblastoma
Limping	Bone tumors, leukemia, neuroblastoma
Proptosis	Leukemia, rhabdomyosarcoma, LCH, neuroblastoma
White dot in eye	Retinoblastoma
Swollen face and neck	T-ALL, NHL, Hodgkin lymphoma
Persistent adenopathy	Hodgkin lymphoma, NHL
Wheezing/orthopnea	T-ALL, Hodgkin lymphoma, NHL
Morning headache with vomiting	Brain tumors
Unsteadiness of gait	Brain tumors
Distended abdomen/with or without constipation	Neuroblastoma, Wilms tumor, Burkitt lymphoma, ovarian tumor, tumors arising from bladder, retroperitoneal tumors
Hematuria (painless)	Wilms tumor
Bleeding from vagina	Yolk sac tumor, rhabdomyosarcoma
Weight loss	Hodgkin lymphoma
Chronic ear drainage	LCH, rhabdomyosarcoma

Abbreviations: LCH, Langerhans cell histiocytosis; NHL, non-Hodgkin lymphoma; T-ALL, T-cell acute lymphoblastic leukemia.

deaths before initiation of specific treatment, as well as optimal management of infectious complications that result from current intensified treatment strategies. This article first reviews emergencies at presentation, followed by management of infectious complications.

Emergencies in childhood cancer

Emergencies in the care of children with cancer can arise at any time in the course of their care. They can occur as the first manifestation of cancer, as a result of therapy, or at the time of recurrence. Some of the most commonly seen pediatric oncologic emergencies seen at the time of presentation are discussed here: hyperleukocytosis, tumor lysis syndrome, superior mediastinal syndrome, and spinal cord compression.

HYPERLEUKOCYTOSIS

Hyperleukocytosis occurs in 10% to 20% of children newly diagnosed with acute leukemia.[1–4] It is defined as a white blood cell (WBC) count greater than 100,000/mm^3. Leukostasis is the sludging that develops in the microcirculation of the central nervous system (CNS) and lungs in the setting of hyperleukocytosis, which can lead to life-threatening complications.[5] Blood viscosity increases logarithmically as the leukocyte fractional volume (leukocrit) increases. In part, this is caused by the poor deformability of lymphoblasts and myeloblasts, compared with erythrocytes.[6] Lymphoblasts have a volume of 250 to 350 μm^3 and myeloblasts 350 to 450 μm^3, therefore nearly double the number of lymphoblasts (compared with myeloblasts) is required to result in the same increase in leukocrit,[6] which accounts, in part, for the lower incidence of leukostasis in lymphoid leukemia compared with myeloid leukemia at any given leukocyte count.[6] Leukemic blast-endothelial cell interaction has also been shown to contribute to the development of luekostasis.[5,7] Stucki and colleagues[8] showed that myeloblasts secrete cytokines and activate endothelial cells, promoting their own adhesion to the endothelium.

The clinical manifestations of leukostasis involve the lungs and CNS and include pulmonary hemorrhage and hypoxia, as well as CNS hemorrhage and infarct.[2,9,10] Children with hyperleukocytosis are also at risk for metabolic derangements.

Studies have shown that most children with chronic myeloid leukemia (CML) present with WBC counts greater than 100,000/mm^3, occurring in 80% of children with CML.[11–13] The reported incidence of leukostasis in these children has varied widely, ranging from less than 10%[11,12] to 60%.[13] Papilledema and visual disturbances, neurologic deficits, respiratory insufficiency, and priapism have been described.[11–13]

The incidence of hyperleukocytosis in acute myeloid leukemia (AML) has been reported as 18% to 23%.[1,3,14] Inaba and colleagues[1] reported that 21.7% of their patients with AML and hyperleukocytosis presented with complications related to leukostasis. In another study, 33% of children with AML and hyperleukocytosis had metabolic, respiratory, or hemorrhagic complications before or within the first 2 weeks of induction therapy.[15] The risk of complications related to leukostasis increases with increasing WBC count.[3] Risk factors associated with symptomatic leukostasis include French-American-British classification of M_4 or M_5 and age less than 1 year.[3]

Among children diagnosed with acute lymphoblastic leukemia (ALL) the incidence of hyperleukocytosis is 13% to 18%.[4,15] Those with T-cell ALL (T-ALL) have a higher incidence of hyperleukocytosis.[4] Among those with ALL and hyperleukocytosis, metabolic derangements are more common than other complications. Pulmonary leukostasis is seen much less frequently, in 0% to 6% of patients.[2,15,16] The risk of CNS changes, particularly hemorrhage, or early death is also significantly less than in patients with AML.[2,15] In those with ALL, these complications are more likely to be seen with an initial WBC of greater than 400,000/mm^3.[2]

Leukapheresis and exchange transfusion have been used to treat hyperleukocytosis. Both are fairly safe procedures and are effective in decreasing the WBC count.[17,18] However, their roles in the prevention and management of complications related to leukostasis remain in question. Among children presenting with hyperleukocytosis, numerous recent studies have shown that the use of leukapheresis does not decrease the risk of leukostasis-related complications, or induction deaths, compared with patients managed without the use of leukapheresis.[1,3,9,14,19,20] Therefore, prompt initiation of chemotherapy is the most effective approach to treatment of hyperleukocytosis. Red blood cell transfusion should be limited until the WBC count is reduced in order to avoid further increase in viscosity.[6] Dexamethasone may be helpful in management of pulmonary leukostasis in AML and differentiation syndrome in acute promyelocytic leukemia.[21,22]

Although remission rates do not seem to differ compared with patients without hyperleukocytosis, the long-term outcome of patients with hyperleukocytosis has been shown to be inferior.[1,3,4,9] Therefore, future studies evaluating novel therapies for this subgroup of patients are warranted.

TUMOR LYSIS SYNDROME

Tumor lysis syndrome is one of the most commonly encountered complications for clinicians treating children with lymphoid malignancies. It is characterized by metabolic disturbances, including hyperkalemia, hyperphosphatemia, hyperuricemia, and hypocalcemia. Potassium, phosphorus, and nucleic acids are released into the circulation when malignant cells lyse. If their release is greater than the kidneys' ability to clear them, metabolic derangement and acute kidney injury can occur. Acute kidney injury occurs when calcium phosphate, uric acid, and xanthine precipitate in renal tubules, causing obstruction and inflammation.[23] Metabolic derangement and cytokine release can result in fatal cardiac dysrhythmias, seizures, and multiorgan failure.[23–25]

The definitions of laboratory and clinical tumor lysis syndrome are discussed by Cairo and Bishop.[23,24] Risk factors for the development of tumor lysis syndrome include large tumor burden (bulky tumor, organomegaly, or bone marrow replacement), rapid cell proliferation, and chemosensitivity.[23] Preexisting hyperuricemia, renal insufficiency, and dehydration are also risk factors.[23,25,26] Those at highest risk in the pediatric population include those with Burkitt lymphoma/leukemia, T-lymphoblastic lymphoma, and acute leukemia with WBC greater than 100,000/mm^3.[23–25] The reported incidence varies, and has been reported as 4% to 23% of children with hematologic malignancies.[23]

The mainstay of management is aggressive hydration, allopurinol, and rasburicase.[27] In recent years, risk classification algorithms have been developed, and recommendations for management made based on risk group.[25,26,28] Hyperhydration (3000 mL/m^2/d or greater) should be instituted.[23] Management of hyperkalemia and hyperphosphatemia is key to the prevention of cardiac dysrhythmias. Allopurinol is effective; however, decrease in uric acid levels occurs slowly over several days, and, because of buildup of xanthine, there is risk of xanthine nephropathy and urolithiasis. Therefore, it is recommended for patients classified as intermediate risk for the development of tumor lysis syndrome.[23,25,26]

Recombinant urate oxidase (rasburicase) catalyzes the oxidation of uric acid to allantoin, which is 5 to 10 times more urine soluble than uric acid.[29] It is recommended for those with hyperuricemia or high risk of tumor lysis syndrome.[23,25,26] Because rasburicase has been widely used, the incidence of clinical tumor lysis has decreased significantly, and has prevented the need for dialysis in most cases.[30] It has also obviated urinary alkalinization.[23] Rasburicase should not be used in patients with known glucose-6-phosphate dehydrogenase deficiency, because it may result in methemoglobinemia and hemolysis in these patients.[31] The dose recommended in children is 0.1 to 0.2 mg/kg. Recent studies have been published evaluating the necessary dose of rasburicase in the adult population. There is some evidence that prevention of tumor lysis syndrome can be achieved with lower doses of rasburicase than were originally recommended.[32–34]

SUPERIOR VENA CAVA AND SUPERIOR MEDIASTINAL SYNDROME

Superior vena cava (SVC) syndrome is a constellation of symptoms caused by compression of venous drainage in the mediastinum. When associated with tracheal compression, it is referred to as superior mediastinal syndrome. In children, the two occur together. Among children with cancer it is seen in those with anterior mediastinal masses.[35] The most common cause in the pediatric population is non-Hodgkin lymphoma, specifically T-lymphoblastic lymphoma, but is also seen in T-ALL and Hodgkin lymphoma. The incidence of SVC syndrome in these subtypes of pediatric cancer ranges from 2% to 5%.[36] Other causes include neuroblastoma, germ cell tumors, and sarcomas.[37] Compression of the SVC leads to dilation of vessels proximal to the obstruction and development of collateral vessels. This process leads to symptoms such as facial and neck edema, plethora, dyspnea, cough, stridor, chest pain, and headache.[37,38] Pleural and pericardial effusions are also commonly associated, occurring in 50% and 20%, respectively, of children with anterior mediastinal masses in one study.[36]

Establishing a diagnosis in these patients can be challenging. Chest radiographs should be performed and, if the patient is stable, chest CT should also be performed, for better evaluation of distorted anatomy and more accurate delineation of tracheal compression.[37] Echocardiography should be used to assess for pericardial effusion and SVC obstruction. There is risk in biopsy of these masses, because of anesthetic complications. The least invasive diagnostic procedure should be performed first, and can be performed with the child in an upright position. In children with pleural or pericardial effusion, a tap may be diagnostic. Bone marrow aspiration may also be diagnostic in patients with marrow involvement, which may be present even in those with normal blood counts. Peripheral adenopathy should be biopsied when found, and can be performed using local anesthesia alone.

In cases in which biopsy of the mediastinal mass is necessary, a discussion between oncology, surgical, and anesthesia teams should take place to determine the best approach.[39,40] In a supine position, passing an endotracheal tube may be difficult, or impossible, because of tracheal compression. Patients who are intubated may not be easily extubated after anesthesia and require steroid treatment at that point.

In patients with cardiovascular or respiratory compromise, emergency steroid therapy may be necessary before a diagnosis is established. Careful consideration should be paid in these cases, because the administration of corticosteroids or radiotherapy for as short a time as 24 hours may make a subsequent tissue biopsy uninterpretable.[41] Corticosteroids are an appropriate initial treatment choice, because the most common causes of anterior mediastinal masses in children are responsive. For tumors that are unresponsive to steroids and for which a diagnosis cannot be established, radiation therapy may be used.[42]

SPINAL CORD COMPRESSION

Spinal cord compression occurs in 3% to 5% of children with cancer, often at presentation.[37] The most common cause is a tumor that involves the epidural or subarachnoid space. Symptoms include motor deficits, diplegia or quadriplegia, sensory deficits, or sphincteric abnormalities. Back pain is also a common symptom.[37] The childhood tumors most commonly implicated are neural tumors (neuroblastoma), sarcomas (Ewing, osteosarcoma, rhabdomyosarcoma), non-Hodgkin lymphoma, and germ cell tumors.[43,44] Spinal cord compression has also been reported in patients with acute leukemia, Hodgkin lymphoma, and Wilms tumor.[45–49]

When spinal cord dysfunction is suspected based on history and physical examination findings, dexamethasone should be given immediately. A dose of 1 to 2 mg/kg, followed by 0.25 mg/kg every 6 hours, has been suggested,[37] but doses as high as 100 mg have been used in adults.[50] MRI should then be performed emergently. Therapeutic options for spinal cord compression include laminectomy with decompression, radiation therapy, and chemotherapy.[51–53] The most appropriate initial treatment varies by diagnosis.

When evaluated in children diagnosed with neuroblastoma, all 3 modalities were effective. De Bernardi and colleagues[51] reported an incidence of spinal cord compression of 5.2% among children with neuroblastoma. Of these patients, 64% with a resectable primary tumor underwent laminectomy first, whereas chemotherapy was preferred in those with unresectable primary tumors (53%) or disseminated disease (43%). Chemotherapy was also used initially for most patients with mild to moderate motor deficits (46% and 55%, respectively), and laminectomy was performed in 80% of those who presented with a grade 3 motor deficit. Almost 62% of all patients had significant improvement or achieved full neurologic recovery. Those who received chemotherapy as initial treatment were unlikely to require surgical or radiotherapy for further treatment of spinal cord compression.[51] A significant proportion of children have persistent neurologic deficits after treatment, with proportions of 44% to 72% reported in previous studies.[51,54,55] Neurologic sequelae include motor and sphincteric deficits, scoliosis, and spinal deformities. Severity of deficits at the time of presentation is the most predictive parameter. In the De Bernardi and colleagues[51] study, of the group who received chemotherapy, 59% did not have sequelae, compared with 38% treated with laminectomy and 40% treated with radiotherapy. Spine deformities, such as scoliosis, occurred more frequently in those who received laminectomy.[51,54] Therefore, chemotherapy should be the initial treatment choice for children with neuroblastoma and spinal cord compression who do not require emergent laminectomy, because late sequelae related to radiation or laminectomy can be avoided in these patients (**Box 2**).

Fever and Neutropenia in Pediatric Patients

Fever and neutropenia (FN) is one of the most common complications of cancer therapy in children. FN is important because it is associated with morbidity, hospitalization, reduced quality of life (QoL), costs, and rarely mortality.[56,57] A large body of research has been conducted in both adult and pediatric FN over the last several decades, which has allowed different therapeutic approaches to evolve while reducing mortality and improving other clinical end points.[58,59] Development of clinical practice guidelines for pediatric patients is important because children have unique issues compared with adults. In 2012, an international group of experts in pediatric FN developed recommendations using the GRADE (Grades of Recommendation, Assessment, Development and Evaluation) approach to evidence synthesis and recommendation generation.[60] Recommendations are presented here that reflect the content of these guidelines.

Box 2
Definitions of laboratory and clinical tumor lysis syndrome

	Hyperuricemia	Hyperkalemia	Hyperphosphatemia	Hypocalcemia	Acute Kidney Injury
Laboratory tumor lysis syndrome[a]	Uric acid level >8 mg/dL or more than the upper limit of normal for children	Potassium level >6 mmol/L	Phosphorus level >4.5 mg/dL in adults or 6.5 mg/dL in children	Corrected calcium level <7.0 mg/dL or ionized calcium level <1.12	None
Clinical tumor lysis syndrome	—	Cardiac dysrhythmia or sudden death related to hyperkalemia	—	Cardiac dysrhythmia, sudden death, seizure related to hypocalcemia	Increase in serum creatinine level to >1.5 times the upper limit of normal for age

[a] Laboratory tumor lysis syndrome is defined by the presence of 2 or more metabolic abnormalities within 3 days before or 7 days after starting chemotherapy.

Adapted from Howard SC, Jones DP, Pui CH. The tumor lysis syndrome. N Engl J Med 2011;364(19):1844–54.

Initial risk stratification

Children with FN are not a homogenous group and much effort has been devoted to risk stratification. Determining which children are at lower risk of complications can allow a reduction in the intensity of therapy and monitoring. In contrast, identifying children at higher risk of complications can allow prophylactic approaches, rapid escalation of therapy, and/or close observation.

In adults with FN, the risk stratification schema from the Multinational Association of Supportive Care in Cancer (MASCC) has been validated and is widely accepted as the standard approach. However, the MASCC score cannot be applied to children because age less than 60 years and absence of chronic obstructive pulmonary disease are items in the score and these are not applicable to pediatric patients.[61] At least 25 studies of risk prediction have been conducted in pediatric cancer.[62] These studies have been highly variable using different pediatric cancer populations and different end points (such as bacteremia, serious infection, death, and intensive care unit admission), reducing the ability to generalize from the results.

Six low-risk stratification schemas have been validated in children.[63–68] Selection of a single schema to be applied across all clinical scenarios has not been feasible, likely owing to divergence in clinical settings. Therefore, clinicians should review the 6 validated low-risk stratification schemas, choose the schema that matches the clinical setting, and determine whether the application of that schema is feasible for the center. Some rules may not be feasible to implement universally. For example, some rules use biomarkers such as C-reactive protein and require expeditious analysis and return of results to be useful. Others require clinician judgment and thus require that trained health care professionals are readily available. Whichever schema is chosen, centers should have a mechanism to routinely review their own results to ensure that the rule continues to have local applicability.

Initial investigations

At initial presentation, an evaluation for the cause of fever should be conducted. The evaluation should include a careful history and physical examination with the assessment focusing on potential sites of infection. Sites that warrant particular attention are the mouth to search for viral and candidal infection, central venous line (CVL) exit site and tunnel, chest, abdomen, and perianal area.

The standard evaluation should include blood cultures from each lumen of the CVL, if present. Peripheral blood culture at the initial evaluation of FN is controversial. There are 2 primary reasons why a peripheral culture may be useful. First, a peripheral culture can help to identify central line–associated bloodstream infection (CLABSI). However, because the diagnosis of CLABSI does not influence the management of the bacteremia, many clinicians argue that this reason does not justify obtaining a peripheral culture. Second, the addition of a peripheral blood culture may detect more bacteremia than a central culture alone. There are 7 studies that evaluated the contribution of peripheral blood cultures in addition to CVL cultures in adults and children with cancer or who were undergoing HSCT.[69–75] Thirteen percent (95% confidence interval [CI], 8%–18%) of all bacteremias were identified only by the peripheral blood culture. This result is likely explained by false-negative CVL blood cultures when obtained culture volumes are small.[76] It is not known whether this problem can be overcome by increasing the central line culture volumes or whether failure to identify these episodes of bacteremia affects patient outcomes. The role of peripheral blood culture therefore remains uncertain.

Urinalysis and urine culture for the detection of urinary tract infections (UTIs) is also controversial in the evaluation of FN. A UTI is typically suspected from pyuria on urinalysis and nitrate positivity. However, in this population, neutropenia limits the ability to use pyuria as a diagnostic criterion[77] and reliance on nitrite testing is not ideal because the test may be negative in young children with UTI.[78] Therefore, urinalysis testing has limited utility in the setting of FN. It may be reasonable to obtain a sterile urine culture and define the presence of a UTI on the culture results alone. However, sterile urine collection can be difficult in young children and infants, and often requires urinary catheterization, a procedure that is often discouraged in a neutropenic and often thrombocytopenic patients. Therefore, where a clean-catch or midstream urine can be collected, urinalysis and urine culture should be included in the initial FN investigations. Antibiotic administration should not be delayed to obtain a urine sample.

Another controversial evaluation is routine chest radiograph (CXR) for the detection of occult pneumonia at the onset of FN. There have been 4 studies,[79–82] including 540 episodes of FN, that investigated CXR as a component of the initial FN evaluation. These studies showed that pneumonia is detected in less than 5% of children without respiratory symptoms and that the omission of routine CXR does not lead to adverse outcomes.[79,83] Thus, routine CXR should not be performed in asymptomatic children with FN.

Initial antibiotic therapy

Empiric broad-spectrum antibiotic therapy at the onset of FN has been the standard of care for many decades because of the risk of life-threatening infections in neutropenic patients. In general, empiric antimicrobial therapy choices should provide good coverage for gram-negative organisms. For high-risk patients with FN, antibiotic therapy should include coverage for viridans group streptococci and *Pseudomonas aeruginosa*. Various factors need to be considered in determining empiric antibiotic regimen, route of administration, and location of therapy. One of the most important factors to consider is local hospital resistance patterns and sites should have a mechanism to review these patterns on a regular basis. Other factors include patient and family social factors, clinical presentation, ability of the hospital to support an ambulatory approach, and availability and cost of drugs.

The original empiric antibiotic regimens for FN consisted of parental administration of 2 agents with antipseudomonal coverage. Since then, the role of combination antibiotic therapy versus monotherapy for FN has been debated. Monotherapy was supported by 2 meta-analyses that compared monotherapy with an aminoglycoside-containing regimen in FN[84] and in immunocompromised patients with sepsis.[85] These analyses showed that monotherapy is not inferior to, and is less toxic than, combination therapy. The analysis in FN observed fewer treatment failures with monotherapy (odds ratio, 0.88; 95% CI, 0.78–0.99) but only included 4 trials that enrolled patients younger than 14 years of age.[84] In the pediatric setting, monotherapy was supported by a meta-analysis that found similar clinical outcomes when antipseudomonal penicillin monotherapy was compared with antipseudomonal penicillin plus an aminoglycoside.[86] Therefore, monotherapy is strongly recommended for pediatric FN in patients who are clinically stable and who are treated at centers with a low rate of resistant pathogens.

Published monotherapy regimens that have been evaluated in children include antipseudomonal penicillins such as piperacillin-tazobactam and ticarcillin-clavulanic acid, antipseudomonal cephalosporins such as cefepime, and carbapenems such as meropenem or imipenem. Two pediatric-specific evaluations found that treatment failure, mortality, and adverse effects were similar when antipseudomonal penicillins were compared with antipseudomonal cephalosporins or carbapenems.[87,88] There are potential disadvantages of carbapenems and cefepime. Carbapenems were associated with an increased risk of pseudomembranous colitis compared with other β-lactam antibiotics in a large meta-analysis.[87] Cefepime was associated with increased all-cause mortality in another large meta-analysis compared with other patients treated with β-lactam.[87] However, these findings were not replicated in other studies.[79,89] As a result, cefepime remains an option for empiric therapy. Ceftazidime monotherapy lacks adequate coverage against viridans group streptococci and resistant gram-negative organisms and thus should not be used if these organisms are of concern.[90]

Routine empiric glycopeptides (such as vancomycin) are not recommended. A meta-analysis of 14 randomized controlled trials (RCTs) showed that inclusion of a glycopeptide did not lead to a difference in success (if addition of glycopeptide in the control arm was not considered failure) but was associated with more adverse effects.[91] Empiric glycopeptides should be reserved for patients who are clinically unstable or who have a signs or symptoms that suggest a gram-positive infection.

Considerations for low-risk patients with fever and neutropenia

Patients with FN at low risk of adverse outcomes may be appropriate for a reduction in therapy intensity. Although there has been some effort to identify a group of patients with FN who do not require any empiric antibiotics,[92] this approach has not had widespread adoption. The 2 strategies commonly considered are outpatient management and oral antibiotic administration. These two strategies are often used together and, in adults with low-risk FN, outpatient management with oral antibiotics is recommended for selected patients.[61,93] There has been a concern that it may not be possible for these recommendations to be generalized to children.[94] However, over the last several years, data have emerged related to efficacy and safety, costs, and QoL/preference considerations for different management strategies in pediatric FN.

Efficacy and safety of outpatient management and oral antibiotic administration There are several advantages of outpatient management, including better QoL for children,[95] and a reduction in costs,[96] nosocomial infection,[97] and acquisition of resistant microorganisms.[98] Outpatient management can be instituted at the onset of FN or after a brief period of hospitalization, also termed step-down management. A meta-analysis synthesized the results of 6 RCTs, 2 of which were pediatric.[99] No difference in treatment failure with outpatient versus inpatient management was observed (rate ratio [RR], 0.81; 95% CI, 0.55–1.28). This analysis was biased against outpatient care because readmission was a criterion for failure and this end point is only applicable to outpatients. No difference in mortality was shown (RR, 1.11; 95% CI, 0.41–3.05). Results stratified by the 2 pediatric studies showed similar findings to the overall analysis. However, only 2 pediatric studies enrolling 278 children were included. In order to address this concern, a subsequent systematic review combined all prospective randomized and nonrandomized pediatric trials that evaluated ambulatory or inpatient management within 24 hours of FN.[100] Among the 16 included studies, treatment failure was significantly less frequent with outpatient (15%) compared with inpatient management (27%; $P = .04$). A critically important finding was that there were no infection-related deaths among the 953 children treated as outpatients. As a result, outpatient management seems to be a safe approach as long as appropriate steps can be implemented. In order to institute outpatient management of FN, the institution must be able to identify low-risk patients, and must develop a program to monitor patients and expeditiously admit them in the case of deterioration. Social circumstances and travel considerations dictate the feasibility of an ambulatory approach in specific patients. The optimal frequency and nature of follow-up evaluations for children treated as outpatients for FN has not been determined, although daily clinic visits are rarely feasible.

The second approach to reduced intensity of therapy for low-risk FN is oral antibiotic treatment. Oral antibiotic administration may be advantageous because it facilitates outpatient management, is usually less expensive, and does not require intravenous access. However, specific considerations unique to children include the requirement for suspension formulation in young children and refusal of oral medication by some children, particularly when they are unwell. Two meta-analyses of RCTs compared oral and parenteral antibiotic administration for FN; both did not restrict their review to low-risk patients. One included inpatients and outpatients (N = 2770),[101] whereas the other only evaluated outpatients (N = 1595).[99] Results were similar in both analyses with no difference in treatment failure, mortality, or adverse effects of antibiotics by mode of antibiotic administration. Results were similar when restricted to pediatric studies except for a trend toward lower risk of readmission for outpatient episodes treated with intravenous antibiotics compared with oral antibiotics (RR, 0.52; 95% CI, 0.24–1.09).[99] To augment these data, more information about the safety of oral administration was obtained from a meta-analysis of prospective pediatric trials in which oral antibiotics were instituted within 24 hours of FN onset.[100] No difference in treatment failure among subjects who received oral versus intravenous antibiotics was observed (20% vs 22%; $P = .68$). There was also no difference in the rate of antibiotic discontinuation caused by adverse events (2% vs 1%; $P = .73$). Note that no infection-related deaths were observed among the 676 children given oral antibiotics. In summary, more readmissions were observed among children treated with oral antibiotics in the outpatient setting, although no difference in treatment failure or adverse events occurred and no child treated with oral antibiotics within 24 hours of FN onset died. Thus, oral antibiotic administration may be appropriate if the health care team is confident that the child can tolerate oral medications reliably. Oral antibiotic regimens that have been used in pediatric FN include fluoroquinolone monotherapy, fluoroquinolone and amoxicillin-clavulanate, and cefixime.[100] One practical approach is to provide the first oral dose in the emergency or outpatient department to ensure that the child can tolerate oral administration of the planned empiric antibiotic. Discharge home would be contingent on successful administration. Even for children with low-risk FN managed as inpatients, oral administration may be advantageous because needs fewer nursing resources and may facilitate early discharge depending on the reason for admission.

Costs A pediatric cost-utility model showed that outpatient management was the most cost-effective approach for children with low-risk FN.[96] Outpatient parenteral management was more cost-effective compared with outpatient oral management because of the higher rate of readmission among patients who receive oral antibiotics. However, in sensitivity analyses, outpatient oral management may be more cost-effective depending on model assumptions. Inpatient management with intravenous antibiotic administration was always the least cost-effective approach irrespective of model assumptions. These data suggest that outpatient management with intravenous or oral antibiotics are better strategies for pediatric low-risk FN when probabilities, costs, and QoL are considered.

Preferences and quality of life In implementing ambulatory and oral antibiotic approaches for low-risk FN, consideration of patient and family preferences may facilitate program development. When asked which approach they preferred, approximately 50% of parents chose inpatient intravenous management.[102,103] Both parents and children typically ranked inpatient intravenous management ahead of early discharge or ambulatory approaches.[102] A discrete choice experiment was used to assess how attributes contributed to preferences toward FN management.[104] Discrete choice experiment is an emerging approach for the measurement of preferences if there are multiple trade-offs in health care. Parents were only willing to tolerate 2.1 (95% CI, 1.1–3.2) clinic visits weekly to accept outpatient oral management. If a program were developed with clinic visits 3 times weekly and a 7.5% chance of readmission, the probability of parental acceptance of such an ambulatory program was 43% (95% CI, 39%–48%).[104]

Evaluation of QoL is also important to help with decision making and to conduct cost-utility analyses. In one study in which parents and health care professionals compared inpatient intravenous and outpatient oral management,[103] respondents rated child QoL as higher at home compared with at hospital. Compared with parents, health care professionals overestimated QoL for children at home and underestimated QoL for parents in hospital. In another study in which parents rated child QoL with different FN management options, early discharge and outpatient intravenous therapy were associated with the highest anticipated QoL.[102]

These data suggest that parents may have reservations with an ambulatory oral antibiotic approach. In a qualitative study, the identified major themes when parents make decisions regarding site of care and route of drug administration were convenience/disruptiveness for the family, child physical and emotional health, and modifiers of parental decision making.[105] Reasons for preferring an inpatient approach included the inconvenience of clinic visits, apprehension regarding whether they could adequately monitor their child, and concerns related to child acceptance of oral antibiotic administration. In summary, although child QoL is anticipated to be better with outpatient management, many parents voice a preference for inpatient management.

Modification of empiric antibacterial therapy

After empiric antibiotics for FN have been initiated, the initial empiric regimen should be adjusted to provide appropriate coverage for any positive microbiology results or identified clinical focus of infection. The spectrum of antibiotics should not be narrowed until criteria for discontinuation of empiric antibiotics are met.[106] In patients in whom empiric glycopeptides or dual gram-negative coverage was initiated, reassessment at 24 to 72 hours should be conducted. In the absence of a specific microbiological reason to continue these agents, they should be discontinued. For children with persistent fever, careful evaluation for an undetected source of infection is important. In this setting, modification of antibiotics, including addition of empiric vancomycin, is not warranted in children who remain clinically stable.[107] Children who clinically deteriorate warrant broadening of empiric antibacterial therapy to include coverage for resistant gram-positive, gram-negative, and anaerobic organisms.

Empiric antibiotics should be discontinued if cultures are negative, the child is clinically well, fever has resolved, and there is evidence of neutrophil recovery.[60] One randomized trial of pediatric low-risk patients found that cessation of antibiotics on day 3 irrespective of count recovery versus continuation of antibiotics was associated with similar outcomes.[108] However, enterobacter bacteremia occurred in 1 child in the early cessation study arm. It may therefore be reasonable to discontinue antibiotics on day 3 in low-risk children with FN who have become afebrile with negative cultures as long as careful monitoring is in place. In high-risk patients, the optimal duration of antibiotic therapy is unknown in the setting of persistent profound neutropenia. A small study of 33 high-risk patients suggested that cessation of empiric antibiotics on day 7 is associated with bacteremia and poor infection outcomes compared with continuation for 14 days.[109] However, this study was conducted many decades ago and it is not known whether these results can be generalized to the current era. Thus, continuation of empiric antibiotics for at least 14 days for high-risk FN in the absence of evidence of neutrophil recovery is a reasonable strategy.

Evaluation for invasive fungal infection and empiric antifungal therapy
Children with FN and persistent or recurrent fever 96 hours or more after initiation of broad-spectrum antibiotics who are at higher risk of invasive fungal infection (IFI) should undergo an evaluation for fungal infection including careful physical examination, blood and urine cultures, and CT of the chest.[110–113] The roles of routine CT sinuses and imaging of the abdomen have not been defined in the standard investigation of IFI, although routine CT sinuses should not be conducted in children 2 years of age or younger because of insufficient pneumatization of the sinus cavities.[60] In children with demonstrated pulmonary lesions, investigations may include bronchoalveolar lavage and lung biopsy, although fatal bleeding may occur with biopsy of angioinvasive mold lesions. Thus, the decision to biopsy requires careful consideration. Better understanding of the risks and yields of these procedures is required in pediatric patients.

Empiric antifungal therapy should consist of either caspofungin or liposomal amphotericin B (L-AmB) because these two therapies are similarly effective and L-AmB is slightly better and less nephrotoxic than amphotericin B deoxycholate.[114–116] Empiric antifungal therapy may be discontinued at resolution of severe neutropenia if the patient is clinically well and without evidence of an IFI.

SUMMARY

In summary, the prompt recognition and initiation of the proper management of cancer and treatment-related complications are paramount to further improvement in the overall survival of children with cancer.

REFERENCES

1. Inaba H, Fan Y, Pounds S, et al. Clinical and biologic features and treatment outcome of children with newly diagnosed acute myeloid leukemia and hyperleukocytosis. Cancer 2008;113(3):522–9.
2. Lowe EJ, Pui CH, Hancock ML, et al. Early complications in children with acute lymphoblastic leukemia presenting with hyperleukocytosis. Pediatr Blood Cancer 2005;45(1):10–5.
3. Sung L, Aplenc R, Alonzo TA, et al. Predictors and short-term outcomes of hyperleukocytosis in children with acute myeloid leukemia: a report from the Children's Oncology Group. Haematologica 2012;97(11):1770–3.
4. Eguiguren JM, Schell MJ, Crist WM, et al. Complications and outcome in childhood acute lymphoblastic leukemia with hyperleukocytosis. Blood 1992;79(4):871–5.
5. Porcu P, Farag S, Marcucci G, et al. Leukocytoreduction for acute leukemia. Ther Apher 2002;6(1):15–23.
6. Lichtman MA, Rowe JM. Hyperleukocytic leukemias: rheological, clinical, and therapeutic considerations. Blood 1982;60(2):279–83.
7. Porcu P, Cripe LD, Ng EW, et al. Hyperleukocytic leukemias and leukostasis: a review of pathophysiology, clinical presentation and management. Leuk Lymphoma 2000;39(1–2):1–18.

8. Stucki A, Rivier AS, Gikic M, et al. Endothelial cell activation by myeloblasts: molecular mechanisms of leukostasis and leukemic cell dissemination. Blood 2001;97(7):2121–9.

9. Kong SG, Seo JH, Jun SE, et al. Childhood acute lymphoblastic leukemia with hyperleukocytosis at presentation. Blood Res 2014;49(1):29–35.

10. Tryka AF, Godleski JJ, Fanta CH. Leukemic cell lysis pneumonopathy. A complication of treated myeloblastic leukemia. Cancer 1982;50(12):2763–70.

11. Castro-Malaspina H, Schaison G, Briere J, et al. Philadelphia chromosome-positive chronic myelocytic leukemia in children. Survival and prognostic factors. Cancer 1983;52(4):721–7.

12. Millot F, Traore P, Guilhot J, et al. Clinical and biological features at diagnosis in 40 children with chronic myeloid leukemia. Pediatrics 2005;116(1):140–3.

13. Rowe JM, Lichtman MA. Hyperleukocytosis and leukostasis: common features of childhood chronic myelogenous leukemia. Blood 1984;63(5):1230–4.

14. Chen KH, Liu HC, Liang DC, et al. Minimally early morbidity in children with acute myeloid leukemia and hyperleukocytosis treated with prompt chemotherapy without leukapheresis. J Formos Med Assoc 2014. [Epub ahead of print].

15. Bunin NJ, Pui CH. Differing complications of hyperleukocytosis in children with acute lymphoblastic or acute nonlymphoblastic leukemia. J Clin Oncol 1985; 3(12):1590–5.

16. Maurer HS, Steinherz PG, Gaynon PS, et al. The effect of initial management of hyperleukocytosis on early complications and outcome of children with acute lymphoblastic leukemia. J Clin Oncol 1988;6(9):1425–32.

17. Ganzel C, Becker J, Mintz PD, et al. Hyperleukocytosis, leukostasis and leukapheresis: practice management. Blood Rev 2012;26(3):117–22.

18. Greze V, Chambon F, Merlin E, et al. Leukapheresis in management of hyperleukocytosis in children's leukemias. J Pediatr Hematol Oncol 2014. [Epub ahead of print].

19. Oberoi S, Lehrnbecher T, Phillips B, et al. Leukapheresis and low-dose chemotherapy do not reduce early mortality in acute myeloid leukemia hyperleukocytosis: a systematic review and meta-analysis. Leuk Res 2014;38(4):460–8.

20. Pastore F, Pastore A, Wittmann G, et al. The role of therapeutic leukapheresis in hyperleukocytotic AML. PLoS One 2014;9(4):e95062.

21. Azoulay E, Canet E, Raffoux E, et al. Dexamethasone in patients with acute lung injury from acute monocytic leukaemia. Eur Respir J 2012;39(3):648–53.

22. Moreau AS, Lengline E, Seguin A, et al. Respiratory events at the earliest phase of acute myeloid leukemia. Leuk Lymphoma 2014. [Epub ahead of print].

23. Howard SC, Jones DP, Pui CH. The tumor lysis syndrome. N Engl J Med 2011; 364(19):1844–54.

24. Cairo MS, Bishop M. Tumour lysis syndrome: new therapeutic strategies and classification. Br J Haematol 2004;127(1):3–11.

25. Cairo MS, Coiffier B, Reiter A, et al, TLS Expert Panel. Recommendations for the evaluation of risk and prophylaxis of tumour lysis syndrome (TLS) in adults and children with malignant diseases: an expert TLS panel consensus. Br J Haematol 2010;149(4):578–86.

26. Coiffier B, Altman A, Pui CH, et al. Guidelines for the management of pediatric and adult tumor lysis syndrome: an evidence-based review. J Clin Oncol 2008; 26(16):2767–78.

27. Galardy PJ, Hochberg J, Perkins SL, et al. Rasburicase in the prevention of laboratory/clinical tumour lysis syndrome in children with advanced mature B-NHL: a Children's Oncology Group Report. Br J Haematol 2013;163(3):365–72.

28. Pession A, Masetti R, Gaidano G, et al. Risk evaluation, prophylaxis, and treatment of tumor lysis syndrome: consensus of an Italian expert panel. Adv Ther 2011; 28(8):684–97.
29. Pui CH, Mahmoud HH, Wiley JM, et al. Recombinant urate oxidase for the prophylaxis or treatment of hyperuricemia in patients with leukemia or lymphoma. J Clin Oncol 2001;19(3):697–704.
30. Cairo MS, Gerrard M, Sposto R, et al. Results of a randomized international study of high-risk central nervous system B non-Hodgkin lymphoma and B acute lymphoblastic leukemia in children and adolescents. Blood 2007; 109(7):2736–43.
31. Sonbol MB, Yadav H, Vaidya R, et al. Methemoglobinemia and hemolysis in a patient with G6PD deficiency treated with rasburicase. Am J Hematol 2013; 88(2):152–4.
32. Agrawal AK, Feusner JH. Management of tumour lysis syndrome in children: what is the evidence for prophylactic rasburicase in non-hyperleucocytic leukaemia? Br J Haematol 2011;153(2):275–7.
33. Coutsouvelis J, Wiseman M, Hui L, et al. Effectiveness of a single fixed dose of rasburicase 3 mg in the management of tumour lysis syndrome. Br J Clin Pharmacol 2013;75(2):550–3.
34. Knoebel RW, Lo M, Crank CW. Evaluation of a low, weight-based dose of rasburicase in adult patients for the treatment or prophylaxis of tumor lysis syndrome. J Oncol Pharm Pract 2011;17(3):147–54.
35. Janin Y, Becker J, Wise L, et al. Superior vena cava syndrome in childhood and adolescence: a review of the literature and report of three cases. J Pediatr Surg 1982;17(3):290–5.
36. Ingram L, Rivera GK, Shapiro DN. Superior vena cava syndrome associated with childhood malignancy: analysis of 24 cases. Med Pediatr Oncol 1990; 18(6):476–81.
37. Pizzo P, Poplack D. Principles and practice of pediatric oncology. 6th edition. Philadelphia: Lippincott, Williams & Wilkins; 2011.
38. Wilson LD, Detterbeck FC, Yahalom J. Clinical practice. Superior vena cava syndrome with malignant causes. N Engl J Med 2007;356(18):1862–9.
39. Stricker PA, Gurnaney HG, Litman RS. Anesthetic management of children with an anterior mediastinal mass. J Clin Anesth 2010;22(3):159–63.
40. Sola C, Choquet O, Prodhomme O, et al. Management of mediastinal syndromes in pediatrics: a new challenge of ultrasound guidance to avoid high-risk general anesthesia. Paediatr Anaesth 2014;24(5):534–7.
41. Borenstein SH, Gerstle T, Malkin D, et al. The effects of prebiopsy corticosteroid treatment on the diagnosis of mediastinal lymphoma. J Pediatr Surg 2000;35(6): 973–6.
42. Issa PY, Brihi ER, Janin Y, et al. Superior vena cava syndrome in childhood: report of ten cases and review of the literature. Pediatrics 1983;71(3): 337–41.
43. Klein SL, Sanford RA, Muhlbauer MS. Pediatric spinal epidural metastases. J Neurosurg 1991;74(1):70–5.
44. Tantawy AA, Ebeid FS, Mahmoud MA, et al. Spinal cord compression in childhood pediatric malignancies: multicenter Egyptian study. J Pediatr Hematol Oncol 2013;35(3):232–6.
45. Mora J, Wollner N. Primary epidural non-Hodgkin lymphoma: spinal cord compression syndrome as the initial form of presentation in childhood non-Hodgkin lymphoma. Med Pediatr Oncol 1999;32(2):102–5.

46. Pashankar FD, Steinbok P, Blair G, et al. Successful chemotherapeutic decompression of primary endodermal sinus tumor presenting with severe spinal cord compression. J Pediatr Hematol Oncol 2001;23(3):170–3.
47. Daley MF, Partington MD, Kadan-Lottick N, et al. Primary epidural Burkitt lymphoma in a child: case presentation and literature review. Pediatr Hematol Oncol 2003;20(4):333–8.
48. Meltzer JA, Jubinsky PT. Acute myeloid leukemia presenting as spinal cord compression. Pediatr Emerg Care 2005;21(10):670–2.
49. Gupta V, Srivastava A, Bhatia B. Hodgkin disease with spinal cord compression. J Pediatr Hematol Oncol 2009;31(10):771–3.
50. Cole JS, Patchell RA. Metastatic epidural spinal cord compression. Lancet Neurol 2008;7(5):459–66.
51. De Bernardi B, Pianca C, Pistamiglio P, et al. Neuroblastoma with symptomatic spinal cord compression at diagnosis: treatment and results with 76 cases. J Clin Oncol 2001;19(1):183–90.
52. Walter KN, Kratz C, Uhl M, et al. Chemotherapy as a therapeutic option for congenital neuroblastoma complicated by paraplegia. Klin Padiatr 2008;220(3):175–7.
53. Capasso M, Cinalli G, Nastro A, et al. Symptomatic epidural compression in infants with neuroblastoma: a single-center experience with 5 cases. J Pediatr Hematol Oncol 2013;35(4):260–6.
54. Angelini P, Plantaz D, De Bernardi B, et al. Late sequelae of symptomatic epidural compression in children with localized neuroblastoma. Pediatr Blood Cancer 2011;57(3):473–80.
55. Simon T, Niemann CA, Hero B, et al. Short- and long-term outcome of patients with symptoms of spinal cord compression by neuroblastoma. Dev Med Child Neurol 2012;54(4):347–52.
56. Bodey GP, Buckley M, Sathe YS, et al. Quantitative relationships between circulating leukocytes and infection in patients with acute leukemia. Ann Intern Med 1966;64(2):328–40.
57. Santolaya ME, Alvarez AM, Aviles CL, et al. Predictors of severe sepsis not clinically apparent during the first twenty-four hours of hospitalization in children with cancer, neutropenia, and fever: a prospective, multicenter trial. Pediatr Infect Dis J 2008;27(6):538–43.
58. Schimpff S, Satterlee W, Young VM, et al. Empiric therapy with carbenicillin and gentamicin for febrile patients with cancer and granulocytopenia. N Engl J Med 1971;284(19):1061–5.
59. Pizzo PA. Management of fever in patients with cancer and treatment-induced neutropenia. N Engl J Med 1993;328(18):1323–32.
60. Lehrnbecher T, Phillips R, Alexander S, et al. Guideline for the Management of Fever and Neutropenia in Children With Cancer and/or Undergoing Hematopoietic Stem-Cell Transplantation. J Clin Oncol 2012;30(35):4427–38.
61. Klastersky J, Paesmans M, Rubenstein EB, et al. The Multinational Association for Supportive Care in Cancer risk index: a multinational scoring system for identifying low-risk febrile neutropenic cancer patients. J Clin Oncol 2000;18(16):3038–51.
62. Phillips RS, Lehrnbecher T, Alexander S, et al. Updated systematic review and meta-analysis of the performance of risk prediction rules in children and young people with febrile neutropenia. PLoS One 2012;7(5):e38300.
63. Alexander SW, Wade KC, Hibberd PL, et al. Evaluation of risk prediction criteria for episodes of febrile neutropenia in children with cancer. J Pediatr Hematol Oncol 2002;24(1):38–42.

64. Ammann RA, Bodmer N, Hirt A, et al. Predicting adverse events in children with fever and chemotherapy-induced neutropenia: the prospective multicenter SPOG 2003 FN study. J Clin Oncol 2010;28(12):2008–14.
65. Ammann RA, Hirt A, Luthy AR, et al. Identification of children presenting with fever in chemotherapy-induced neutropenia at low risk for severe bacterial infection. Med Pediatr Oncol 2003;41(5):436–43.
66. Rackoff WR, Gonin R, Robinson C, et al. Predicting the risk of bacteremia in children with fever and neutropenia. J Clin Oncol 1996;14(3):919–24.
67. Rondinelli PI, Ribeiro Kde C, de Camargo B. A proposed score for predicting severe infection complications in children with chemotherapy-induced febrile neutropenia. J Pediatr Hematol Oncol 2006;28(10):665–70.
68. Santolaya ME, Alvarez AM, Becker A, et al. Prospective, multicenter evaluation of risk factors associated with invasive bacterial infection in children with cancer, neutropenia, and fever. J Clin Oncol 2001;19(14):3415–21.
69. Barriga FJ, Varas M, Potin M, et al. Efficacy of a vancomycin solution to prevent bacteremia associated with an indwelling central venous catheter in neutropenic and non-neutropenic cancer patients. Med Pediatr Oncol 1997;28(3): 196–200.
70. Handrup MM, Moller JK, Schroder H. Catheter-related bloodstream infections in children with cancer admitted with fever. 42nd Congress of the International Society of Pediatric Oncology (SIOP). Boston: Pediatr Blood Cancer; 2010.
71. Raad I, Hanna HA, Alakech B, et al. Differential time to positivity: a useful method for diagnosing catheter-related bloodstream infections. Ann Intern Med 2004;140(1):18–25.
72. Adamkiewicz TV, Lorenzana A, Doyle J, et al. Peripheral vs. central blood cultures in patients admitted to a pediatric oncology ward. Pediatr Infect Dis J 1999;18(6):556–8.
73. DesJardin JA, Falagas ME, Ruthazer R, et al. Clinical utility of blood cultures drawn from indwelling central venous catheters in hospitalized patients with cancer. Ann Intern Med 1999;131(9):641–7.
74. Scheinemann K, Ethier MC, Dupuis LL, et al. Utility of peripheral blood cultures in bacteremic pediatric cancer patients with a central line. Support Care Cancer 2010;18(8):913–9.
75. Chen WT, Liu TM, Wu SH, et al. Improving diagnosis of central venous catheter-related bloodstream infection by using differential time to positivity as a hospital-wide approach at a cancer hospital. J Infect 2009;59(5):317–23.
76. Wilson ML, Mitchell M, Morris AJ, et al. Principles and procedures for blood cultures; Approved guideline. CLSI document M47-A, vol. 27. Wayne (PA): Clinical and Laboratory Standards Institute; 2007 (17).
77. Klaassen IL, de Haas V, van Wijk JA, et al. Pyuria is absent during urinary tract infections in neutropenic patients. Pediatr Blood Cancer 2011;56(5):868–70.
78. Mori R, Yonemoto N, Fitzgerald A, et al. Diagnostic performance of urine dipstick testing in children with suspected UTI: a systematic review of relationship with age and comparison with microscopy. Acta Paediatr 2010;99(4): 581–4.
79. Renoult E, Buteau C, Turgeon N, et al. Is routine chest radiography necessary for the initial evaluation of fever in neutropenic children with cancer? Pediatr Blood Cancer 2004;43(3):224–8.
80. Korones DN, Hussong MR, Gullace MA. Routine chest radiography of children with cancer hospitalized for fever and neutropenia: is it really necessary? Cancer 1997;80(6):1160–4.

81. Feusner J, Cohen R, O'Leary M, et al. Use of routine chest radiography in the evaluation of fever in neutropenic pediatric oncology patients. J Clin Oncol 1988;6(11):1699–702.

82. Katz JA, Bash R, Rollins N, et al. The yield of routine chest radiography in children with cancer hospitalized for fever and neutropenia. Cancer 1991; 68(5):940–3.

83. Phillips B, Wade R, Westwood M, et al. Systematic review and meta-analysis of the value of clinical features to exclude radiographic pneumonia in febrile neutropenic episodes in children and young people. J Paediatr Child Health 2012;48(8):641–8.

84. Furno P, Bucaneve G, Del Favero A. Monotherapy or aminoglycoside-containing combinations for empirical antibiotic treatment of febrile neutropenic patients: a meta-analysis. Lancet Infect Dis 2002;2(4):231–42.

85. Paul M, Soares-Weiser K, Leibovici L. Beta lactam monotherapy versus beta lactam-aminoglycoside combination therapy for fever with neutropenia: systematic review and meta-analysis. BMJ 2003;326(7399):1111.

86. Manji A, Lehrnbecher T, Dupuis LL, et al. A systematic review and meta-analysis of anti-pseudomonal penicillins and carbapenems in pediatric febrile neutropenia. Support Care Cancer 2012;20(10):2295–304.

87. Paul M, Yahav D, Bivas A, et al. Anti-pseudomonal beta-lactams for the initial, empirical, treatment of febrile neutropenia: comparison of beta-lactams. Cochrane Database Syst Rev 2010;(11):CD005197.

88. Manji A, Lehrnbecher T, Dupuis LL, et al. A meta-analysis of anti-pseudomonal penicillins and cephalosporins in pediatric patients with fever and neutropenia. Pediatr Infect Dis J 2012;31(4):353–8.

89. Kim PW, Wu YT, Cooper C, et al. Meta-analysis of a possible signal of increased mortality associated with cefepime use. Clin Infect Dis 2010; 51(4):381–9.

90. Marron A, Carratala J, Alcaide F, et al. High rates of resistance to cephalosporins among viridans-group streptococci causing bacteraemia in neutropenic cancer patients. J Antimicrob Chemother 2001;47(1):87–91.

91. Vardakas KZ, Samonis G, Chrysanthopoulou SA, et al. Role of glycopeptides as part of initial empirical treatment of febrile neutropenic patients: a meta-analysis of randomised controlled trials. Lancet Infect Dis 2005;5(7):431–9.

92. Oude Nijhuis C, Kamps WA, Daenen SM, et al. Feasibility of withholding antibiotics in selected febrile neutropenic cancer patients. J Clin Oncol 2005; 23(30):7437–44.

93. Freifeld AG, Bow EJ, Sepkowitz KA, et al. Clinical practice guideline for the use of antimicrobial agents in neutropenic patients with cancer: 2010 update by the Infectious Diseases Society of America. Clin Infect Dis 2011;52(4): e56–93.

94. Ammann RA, Simon A, de Bont ES. Low risk episodes of fever and neutropenia in pediatric oncology: Is outpatient oral antibiotic therapy the new gold standard of care? Pediatr Blood Cancer 2005;45(3):244–7.

95. Speyer E, Herbinet A, Vuillemin A, et al. Agreement between children with cancer and their parents in reporting the child's health-related quality of life during a stay at the hospital and at home. Child Care Health Dev 2009;35(4): 489–95.

96. Teuffel O, Amir E, Alibhai SM, et al. Cost-effectiveness of outpatient management for febrile neutropenia in children with cancer. Pediatrics 2011;127(2): e279–86.

97. Kamboj M, Sepkowitz KA. Nosocomial infections in patients with cancer. Lancet Oncol 2009;10(6):589–97.

98. El-Mahallawy HA, El-Wakil M, Moneer MM, et al. Antibiotic resistance is associated with longer bacteremic episodes and worse outcome in febrile neutropenic children with cancer. Pediatr Blood Cancer 2011;57(2):283–8.

99. Teuffel O, Ethier MC, Alibhai SM, et al. Outpatient management of cancer patients with febrile neutropenia: a systematic review and meta-analysis. Ann Oncol 2011;22(11):2358–65.

100. Manji A, Beyene J, Dupuis LL, et al. Outpatient and oral antibiotic management of low-risk febrile neutropenia are effective in children–a systematic review of prospective trials. Support Care Cancer 2012;20(6):1135–45.

101. Vidal L, Paul M, Ben-Dor I, et al. Oral versus intravenous antibiotic treatment for febrile neutropenia in cancer patients. Cochrane Database Syst Rev 2004;(4):CD003992.

102. Cheng S, Teuffel O, Ethier MC, et al. Health-related quality of life anticipated with different management strategies for paediatric febrile neutropaenia. Br J Cancer 2011;105(5):606–11.

103. Sung L, Feldman BM, Schwamborn G, et al. Inpatient versus outpatient management of low-risk pediatric febrile neutropenia: measuring parents' and healthcare professionals' preferences. J Clin Oncol 2004;22(19):3922–9.

104. Sung L, Alibhai SM, Ethier MC, et al. Discrete choice experiment produced estimates of acceptable risks of therapeutic options in cancer patients with febrile neutropenia. J Clin Epidemiol 2012;65(6):627–34.

105. Diorio C, Martino J, Boydell KM, et al. Parental perspectives on inpatient versus outpatient management of pediatric febrile neutropenia. J Pediatr Oncol Nurs 2011;28(6):355–62.

106. Tran TH, Mitchell D, Dix D, et al. Infections in children with Down syndrome and acute myeloid leukemia: a report from the Canadian Infections in AML Research Group. Infect Agent Cancer 2013;8(1):47.

107. Cometta A, Kern WV, De Bock R, et al. Vancomycin versus placebo for treating persistent fever in patients with neutropenic cancer receiving piperacillin-tazobactam monotherapy. Clin Infect Dis 2003;37(3):382–9.

108. Santolaya ME, Villarroel M, Avendano LF, et al. Discontinuation of antimicrobial therapy for febrile, neutropenic children with cancer: a prospective study. Clin Infect Dis 1997;25(1):92–7.

109. Pizzo PA, Robichaud KJ, Gill FA, et al. Duration of empiric antibiotic therapy in granulocytopenic patients with cancer. Am J Med 1979;67(2):194–200.

110. Agrawal AK, Saini N, Gildengorin G, et al. Is routine computed tomographic scanning justified in the first week of persistent febrile neutropenia in children with malignancies? Pediatr Blood Cancer 2011;57(4):620–4.

111. Burgos A, Zaoutis TE, Dvorak CC, et al. Pediatric invasive aspergillosis: a multicenter retrospective analysis of 139 contemporary cases. Pediatrics 2008; 121(5):e1286–94.

112. Taccone A, Occhi M, Garaventa A, et al. CT of invasive pulmonary aspergillosis in children with cancer. Pediatr Radiol 1993;23(3):177–80.

113. Archibald S, Park J, Geyer JR, et al. Computed tomography in the evaluation of febrile neutropenic pediatric oncology patients. Pediatr Infect Dis J 2001; 20(1):5–10.

114. Prentice HG, Hann IM, Herbrecht R, et al. A randomized comparison of liposomal versus conventional amphotericin B for the treatment of pyrexia of unknown origin in neutropenic patients. Br J Haematol 1997;98(3):711–8.

115. Maertens JA, Madero L, Reilly AF, et al. A randomized, double-blind, multicenter study of caspofungin versus liposomal amphotericin B for empiric antifungal therapy in pediatric patients with persistent fever and neutropenia. Pediatr Infect Dis J 2010;29(5):415–20.
116. Sandler ES, Mustafa MM, Tkaczewski I, et al. Use of amphotericin B colloidal dispersion in children. J Pediatr Hematol Oncol 2000;22(3):242–6.

Biology of Childhood Acute Lymphoblastic Leukemia

Deepa Bhojwani, MD[a,b,*], Jun J. Yang, PhD[b,c],
Ching-Hon Pui, MD[a,b]

KEYWORDS

- Childhood acute lymphoblastic leukemia • Chromosomal alterations • Genomics
- Host germline polymorphisms

KEY POINTS

- Childhood acute lymphoblastic leukemia (ALL) is a heterogeneous disease with multiple distinct biological subtypes.
- High-throughput genomic profiling and next-generation sequencing technologies have identified submicroscopic genomic lesions and sequence mutations that define novel subtypes of ALL.
- The discovery of various oncogenic pathways and candidate genes has led to the development of biologically based targeted therapy.
- Host germline polymorphisms influence susceptibility to ALL, chemotherapy-related toxicities, and response to therapy.

INTRODUCTION

Acute lymphoblastic leukemia (ALL) is the most common childhood malignancy, accounting for 25% of all childhood cancers. In the United States, approximately 3000 children aged 1 to 19 years are diagnosed with ALL annually.[1] Giant strides have been made in the management of childhood ALL over the past 50 years, which has resulted in improvement in cure rates from approximately 10% to approximately 90%.[2,3] The rational use of multiagent systemic chemotherapy over a prolonged

Funding: National Institutes of Health grant P30-CA021765 and the American Lebanese Syrian Associated Charities.
[a] Department of Oncology, St. Jude Children's Research Hospital, 262 Danny Thomas Place, Memphis, TN 38105, USA; [b] Department of Pharmaceutical Sciences, St. Jude Children's Research Hospital, 262 Danny Thomas Place, Memphis, TN 38105, USA; [c] Department of Pediatrics, University of Tennessee Health Sciences Center, 920 Madison Avenue, Memphis, TN 38163, USA
* Corresponding author. Department of Oncology, St. Jude Children's Research Hospital, 262 Danny Thomas Place, MS 260, Memphis, TN 38105.
E-mail address: deepa.bhojwani@stjude.org

duration (2–3 years) and adequate central nervous system (CNS)-directed therapy, in addition to improved antibiotic and blood product support in the 1960s and 1970s were responsible for the early improvements in outcome. However, insights into the heterogenic biology of ALL and monitoring of minimal residual disease (MRD) have helped to refine therapy based on risk of relapse to maximize cure and minimize toxicities. For example, identification of the Philadelphia chromosome in a subset of patients with ALL has made it possible to incorporate ABL tyrosine kinase inhibitors into chemotherapy regimens. This targeted-therapy approach has improved the cure rate of patients with Philadelphia chromosome–positive ALL from 35% to approximately 70% over the last 10 years, even without stem cell transplantation.[4]

Leukemic cells have, and are being thoroughly investigated by methods ranging from karyotyping, which identifies large chromosomal alterations, to whole-genome sequencing, which identifies cryptic changes in the entire genome. ALL is particularly amenable to biological studies because of the relative ease of obtaining samples, which in most cases is an enriched population of blasts. Moreover, because most children with ALL are treated uniformly on large clinical trials, well-annotated clinical information is available to correlate with biological findings. Extensive collaborative efforts among various study groups internationally have played a vital role in the remarkable progress made in not only improving therapeutic outcomes but also deciphering the complex biology of childhood ALL.[5]

This review summarizes various insights gained from biological studies of childhood ALL, with a focus on recent studies, and also discusses genomic lesions and epigenetic regulatory mechanisms associated with leukemic transformation. Finally, the importance of studying the biology of the host so as to understand additional heterogeneity in treatment response and toxicities is highlighted.

B-CELL ACUTE LYMPHOBLASTIC LEUKEMIA

Eighty-five percent of the cases of childhood ALL are of the B-cell lineage (B-ALL). To keep pace with the growing impact of biological findings on treatment outcomes, in 2008 the World Health Organization revised the nomenclature from solitary precursor B-ALL to a classification based on 7 specific, recurring genetic lesions (eg, B-ALL with ETV6-RUNX1, B-ALL with hyperdiploidy).[6] Of note, the term B-ALL is not used for Burkitt leukemia/lymphoma, which is a mature B-cell malignancy. As newer subtypes are identified, biology-centered classifications need to be continually reviewed and updated (**Fig. 1**).

Conventional Chromosomal Alterations

ALL commonly arises from a series of genetic alterations and, in most ALL subtypes, the interplay of these alterations. For the last 3 decades, several conventional cytogenetic studies of genetic aberrations that include chromosomal translocations and alterations in chromosome number have provided information on the pathogenesis of ALL. Common translocations in children with B-ALL include t(12;21) [ETV6-RUNX1] (25%), t(1;19) [TCF3-PBX1] (5%), t(9;11) [BCR-ABL1] (3%), and translocations involving the MLL gene with various partner fusion genes (5%). Gains in whole chromosomes, or high hyperdiploidy (>50 chromosomes), accounts for 25% of childhood ALL, whereas hypodiploidy (<44 chromosomes) accounts for approximately 1% of cases. Several of these genetic changes have prognostic and therapeutic implications and are important in risk-stratification schemes.[7] The overall survival (OS) of patients with ETV6-RUNX1 or high-hyperdiploid ALL is more than 93%[8,9]; therefore these patients are treated on less intensive regimens, provided that they have an adequate

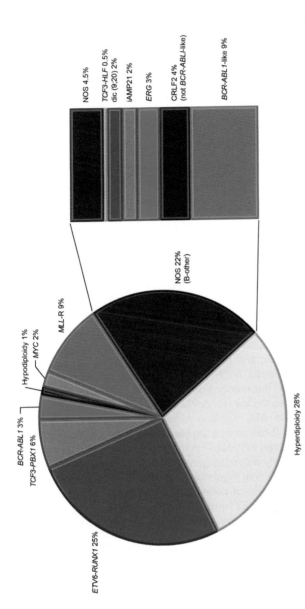

Fig. 1. Distribution of molecular subtypes of childhood B-cell acute lymphoblastic leukemia. The pie chart on the left depicts molecular subtypes that were identified before 2004, incorporated in the 2008 World Health Organization classification, and are currently used for risk stratification. Subtype was unknown in 22% of patients (termed B-other). Since then, various novel molecular subtypes have been characterized, shown in the bar graph on the right. NOS, not otherwise specified. (*Modified from* Pui CH, Relling MV, Downing JR. Acute lymphoblastic leukemia. N Engl J Med 2004;350:1535–48; and Pui CH, Mullighan CG, Evans WE, et al. Pediatric acute lymphoblastic leukemia: where are we going and how do we get there? Blood 2012;120:1165–74.)

early response to remission induction therapy (as currently assessed by the measurement of MRD). Contemporary therapy has abolished the previously unfavorable prognostic impact of *TCF3-PBX1* (t[1;19]). However, because bone marrow and CNS relapse could be competitive events, patients with *TCF3-PBX1* may need more intensive intrathecal therapy to reduce the risk of CNS relapse with improved systemic therapy.[10] Similarly, the addition of tyrosine kinase inhibitors has dramatically improved the bone marrow control of patients with *BCR-ABL1*–positive ALL,[4] and attention should be paid to optimal intrathecal therapy in this genetic subtype of ALL. Hypodiploidy continues to be a high-risk feature,[11] necessitating further understanding of oncogenic mechanisms and the rational use of targeted therapy (eg, for RAS pathway inhibition).[12] The frequency and prognostic impact of *MLL* rearrangements differ by age. Approximately 80% of infants younger than 1 year harbor *MLL* rearrangements, and their overall outcome is poor (5-year survival 50%) despite receiving very intensive therapy.[13]

Fusion gene products that result from chromosomal translocations provide the lymphoid progenitor or stem cell with leukemogenic potential, such as constitutional activation of tyrosine kinases (eg, *ABL1*) or disruption of genes that regulate normal lymphoid development (eg, *ETV6*, *PAX5*). Additional genetic hits are often required for the ultimate development of leukemia, and include loss of the tumor-suppressor gene *CDKN2A* and deletion of the nontranslocated *ETV6* allele in *ETV6-RUNX1*–positive ALL.[14] High-resolution genomic studies are revealing the entire range of cooperating genetic changes and pathogenic mechanisms.[12,15–20]

Submicroscopic Alterations

The advent of genome-wide profiling of RNA and DNA and next-generation sequencing (NGS) technologies has greatly increased our ability to identify and catalog submicroscopic genetic alterations and sequence mutations in ALL, which in turn help define new molecular subtypes. Some novel genomic lesions have prognostic and therapeutic significance, and may be used to refine risk-stratification schemes in the near future; for example, *IKZF1* deletion predicts poor prognosis in children with B-ALL.[18] In addition, the recognition of specific molecular lesions and critical oncogenic pathways paves the way for developing novel targeted approaches to therapy (eg, inhibition of the ABL tyrosine kinase or JAK-STAT pathways). Single-nucleotide polymorphism (SNP) array analyses revealed that gross genomic instability is not present in most children with ALL.[17] A mean of 6.4 genomic lesions were present per case, with wide variability within the genetic subtypes of ALL. Structural alterations in genes encoding transcriptional regulators of B-lymphoid development and differentiation occur in more than 40% of patients with B-ALL. *PAX5* is the most common target; other targets include *IKZF1* and *EBF1*. Several additional lesions have also been identified in lymphoid signaling, transcription factors, and tumor suppressors. Several of these alterations cooperate in leukemogenesis. For example, the deletion of *IKZF1* accelerates the onset of ALL in murine models of *BCR-ABL1* ALL.[20] The assortment and accumulation of "driver" and "passenger" mutations, and the sequence of events in leukemia development and progression, continue to be investigated.

HIGH-RISK SUBTYPES OF B-CELL ACUTE LYMPHOBLASTIC LEUKEMIA
BCR-ABL–Like Acute Lymphoblastic Leukemia

IKZF1 deletions are a hallmark of *BCR-ABL1*–positive ALL, but these deletions also occur in a subset of patients with poor-response, high-risk ALL without any known chromosomal rearrangement.[18] Using genome-wide analyses, 2 groups of investigators independently identified a subgroup of B-ALL, which has a gene-expression profile similar to that of BCR-ABL1–positive ALL including a high frequency of IKZF1 alterations, but lacks the BCR-ABL1 fusion protein; they termed this genetic subtypes BCR-ABL1–like or Philadelphia chromosome–like ALL.[18,21] This subtype comprises 10% of the cases of B-ALL in children and 25% of the cases of ALL in adolescents and young adults.[22] NGS techniques and downstream functional experiments show that BCR-ABL1–like ALL is characterized by genetic changes that result in constitutive activation of cytokine receptor and/or tyrosine kinase signaling.[19,22] The spectrum of genetic alterations is extremely diverse; however, several rearrangements involve tyrosine kinases such as ABL and PDGFR, which respond to imatinib and dasatinib in vitro and in vivo.[22,23] Even though risk-directed therapy including intensive chemotherapy, with or without transplant based on MRD level during remission induction therapy may abolish the poor prognosis of this group of patients, it is important to look for genetic lesions responsive to ABL tyrosine kinase inhibitor so that some patients can be spared transplantation.[24] Several other rearrangements target JAK and EPOR, which are sensitive to JAK inhibitors in preclinical models.[25] In addition, rearrangements involving the cytokine receptor gene CRLF2 have been identified in 50% of patients with BCR-ABL1–like ALL, with frequent coexisting JAK mutations, also potentially sensitive to JAK inhibition.[19,25] In view of the therapeutic implications for this high-risk subset of patients, array-based and sequencing-based methodologies are being developed for rapid classification of patients with BCR-ABL1–like ALL and identification of targetable lesions; the incorporation of tyrosine kinase inhibitors in frontline therapy is also planned.[26]

Acute Lymphoblastic Leukemia with Intrachromosomal Amplification of Chromosome 21

ALL with intrachromosomal amplification of chromosome 21 (iAMP21) was originally discovered by the observation of multiple copies of the RUNX1 gene during routine screening for ETV6-RUNX1 by fluorescent in situ hybridization. This particular ALL subtype is characterized by the instability of chromosome 21.[27] The incidence of iAMP21 is approximately 2%, and the median age of patients is 9 to 11 years. Intensification of chemotherapy has abolished the poor prognosis once associated with this ALL subtype.[28]

Down Syndrome Acute Lymphoblastic Leukemia

Patients with Down syndrome are at an approximately 20-fold increased risk of developing ALL, although the precise role of the extra chromosome 21 in leukemogenesis is unknown.[29] These patients have low frequencies of T-cell ALL (T-ALL) and common ALL translocations such as ETV6-RUNX1. Patients with Down syndrome ALL have inferior outcome owing to their increased risk of relapse and high rate of treatment-related mortality.[30] High-resolution SNP profiling has identified a submicroscopic deletion of the pseudoautosomal regions of chromosomes X and Y, which leads to the P2RY8-CRLF2 fusion in approximately 50% of patients with Down syndrome ALL.[31] These fusions and other CRLF2 alterations were associated with JAK mutations. Together, these lesions activate the JAK-STAT pathway and promote cytokine-independent growth. Therefore, the inhibition of JAK tyrosine kinase is a potentially useful therapeutic strategy in patients with Down syndrome ALL.

T-CELL ACUTE LYMPHOBLASTIC LEUKEMIA

T-ALL accounts for 10% to 15% of the cases of childhood ALL. The outcome of children with T-ALL, which has been historically poor, has improved gradually with the use of intensified therapy, including dexamethasone, asparaginase, and high-dose methotrexate.[3,8] However, children who relapse have a dismal outcome even with hematopoietic stem cell transplantation.[32] Therefore, it is critical to identify aberrant molecular pathways and targets for therapeutic intervention for T-ALL. Genetic lesions in T-ALL are diverse and complex, and a multitude of alterations contribute in the pathogenesis of various subtypes of T-ALL.[33,34] Chromosomal translocations are present in approximately 50% of patients with T-ALL cases, but unlike in B-ALL their prognostic impact is not well defined and they are not used for risk stratification. Some translocations result in the juxtaposition of oncogenes to T-cell receptor (TCR) genes, leading to overexpression of the oncogene in T-cell progenitor cells (eg, *TLX1-TCRδ*), whereas others result in the fusion of 2 transcription factor oncogenes (eg, *STIL-TAL1*). In addition, rearrangements of the *MLL* gene occur in 5% to 10% of patients with T-ALL. Gene-expression profiling studies have identified 4 major subtypes of T-ALL on the basis of the predominant oncogenic pathway activation (*TLX1, LYL1, TAL/LMO2*, and *TLX3*).[35]

NOTCH Activation in T-Cell Acute Lymphoblastic Leukemia

Constitutive activation of *NOTCH* signaling, primarily via somatic mutations, is seen in more than 50% of patients with T-ALL, a finding that is not restricted to specific subtypes of T-ALL.[36] In general, the presence of *NOTCH1* mutations indicates a favorable prognosis. NOTCH1 is a transmembrane receptor crucial for T-cell development, lineage commitment, cell growth, and survival. Activation of *NOTCH1* and the presence of cooperating lesions, such as deletion of the tumor suppressor *CDKN2A* (found in 70% of patients with T-ALL), can lead to leukemic transformation. In addition, mutations in *FBXW7*, which encodes a ubiquitin protein ligase (found in 8%–10% of patients with T-ALL), attenuate the degradation of activated *NOTCH1*, further enhancing its downstream signaling.[37] Thus, the inhibition of *NOTCH1*, either by small-molecule inhibitors of γ-secretase (which impede the release of activated *NOTCH1*) or by anti-*NOTCH1* antibodies, is being actively pursued as a therapeutic strategy for T-ALL.[38,39]

Early T-Cell Precursor Acute Lymphoblastic Leukemia

Early T-cell precursors (ETPs) are a subset of immature thymocytes that retain stem cell–like features and can differentiate into multiple lineages, including lymphoid and myeloid lineage. Complementary studies of flow cytometry, gene expression, and DNA copy number showed that the genetic profile of approximately 12% of patients with T-ALL is similar to that of these immature thymocytes.[40] A whole-genome study showed that ETP ALL has frequent mutations of genes involved in hematopoietic development, cytokine receptor and RAS signaling, and chromatin modification.[41] The incidence of activating *NOTCH1* mutations is low in ETP ALL, which also lacks a unifying chromosomal abnormality. In general, the outcome of patients with ETP ALL is poor, but myeloid-directed and epigenetic therapies may be beneficial for these patients.[41] A recent, small study suggested that patients with ETP ALL have an intermediate outcome when treated with intensive chemotherapy that includes pegylated asparaginase and dexamethasone (5-year event-free survival of 76.7%),[42] a finding that requires confirmation.

EPIGENETICS IN ACUTE LYMPHOBLASTIC LEUKEMIA

In recent years, the importance of epigenetic regulatory mechanisms in normal and malignant hematopoiesis has become increasingly evident. Alterations in the methylation of DNA promoters and the modification of histones can significantly perturb transcriptional regulation and modify gene expression. Different subtypes of ALL are characterized by distinct DNA methylation signatures, which in turn correlate with gene expression profiles.[15] Several genes related to lymphoid development that are targets of somatic mutations in ALL are also inactivated by aberrant methylation, suggesting that multiple mechanisms of silencing of critical genes may contribute to leukemic transformation. Mutations in histone writers, erasers, and readers are more frequent in T-ALL than in most other pediatric cancers.[43] Moreover, several studies show that various *MLL* fusion proteins characteristically modulate chromatin structure through histone modifications; thus, *MLL*-rearranged leukemia is considered an epigenetic malignancy.[13,44] Epigenetics can also influence chemoresistance in ALL, as manifested by increased global promoter methylation at relapse.[16] Therapy with demethylating agents led to reexpression of hypermethylated genes and restored chemosensitivity in an experimental model.[45] The interplay among the altered epigenetic landscape and structural changes in the genome, along with the development of epigenetic therapies such as histone deacetylase inhibitors and demethylating agents, provides exciting opportunities for therapeutic interventions.

BIOLOGY OF RELAPSED ACUTE LYMPHOBLASTIC LEUKEMIA

Studies of matched diagnosis-relapse samples have shed light on the clonal evolution leading to relapse, pathways associated with chemoresistance, and potential targets for therapy. In one study, 86% of the patients at relapse had outgrowth of a minor subclone present at diagnosis, which had genetic alterations both similar to and different from the major clone at diagnosis.[46] In some patients, relapse may have genetic alterations either identical to or entirely different from those seen at diagnosis. The latter scenario likely represents a second malignancy. Preclinical studies and clinical experience show that leukemic blasts are more resistant to various chemotherapeutic agents at relapse than at initial diagnosis.[47,48] Mechanisms of resistance may include selection of a preexisting resistant subclone or the acquisition of additional genomic lesions under the selective pressure of chemotherapy. In a recent study, gain-of-function mutations in *NT5C2* were identified in leukemic blasts of approximately 20% of patients at relapse.[49,50] *NT5C2* encodes a 5'-nucleotidase enzyme that catalyzes the inactivation of nucleoside analogues such as mercaptopurine and thioguanine. As mercaptopurine and methotrexate represent the mainstay of maintenance therapy for ALL, acquisition of the *NT5C2* mutation can lead to emergence of drug-resistant clones and early relapse. Other genomic lesions at relapse include mutations in *CREBBP* (which mediates glucocorticoid response and histone acetylation),[51] and focal deletions in the mismatch repair gene *MSH6*[52] and the glucocorticoid receptor *NR3C1*.[53]

BIOLOGY OF THE HOST
Acute Lymphoblastic Leukemia Susceptibility

Besides constitutional trisomy 21 (Down syndrome) and rare DNA damage repair defects (eg, ataxia-telangiectasia and Bloom syndrome), little is known about the genetic predisposition to ALL.[54] The frequency of hematologic malignancies is 4% in patients with common cancer predisposition syndromes such as Li-Fraumeni syndrome (caused by inherited mutations in *TP53*), approximately half of which are ALL.[55] However, a study of hypodiploid ALL with whole-genome and whole-exome sequencing revealed that 91% of patients with low-hypodiploid ALL (32-39 chromosomes) harbored somatic *TP53* alterations.[12] In 43% of these patients, *TP53* mutations were also present in nontumor DNA, indicating a previously unrecognized link between Li-Fraumeni syndrome and low-hypodiploid ALL, with implications for genetic counseling. Recently, whole-exome sequencing identified a new familial leukemia syndrome in kindreds harboring a novel germline variant in *PAX5* on chromosome 9.[56] PAX5 is a lymphoid transcription factor that plays a crucial role in B-cell development, and is a common target for submicroscopic deletion in B-ALL blasts. Leukemic samples from family members with ALL showed 9p deletion with loss of heterozygosity and retention of the mutant *PAX5* allele, leading to significantly reduced transcriptional activity and, perhaps, leukemic transformation.

In the search for common inherited ALL susceptibility variants, several large genome-wide association studies (GWAS) have identified polymorphisms in *ARID5B*, *IKZF1*, *CEBPE*, *CDKN2A*, and *PIP4K2A-BMI1* were overrepresented in patients with ALL compared with non-ALL controls.[57–59] There were significant differences in the prevalence of these variants among patients of different ancestries, possibly contributing to racial differences in the incidence of ALL. Each of these variants accounts for a modest increase in the risk of developing ALL (odds ratio 1.5–2), but independently and cumulatively contribute to genetic susceptibility to ALL.[58] *CDKN2A* and *IKZF1* are also targeted by somatic alterations in ALL,[17] suggesting that both inherited and somatic genetic variations cooperate in the pathogenesis of ALL. It is interesting that the risk of developing various subtypes of ALL is also influenced by genetic inheritance. An intronic SNP in *TP63* (a member of the TP53 family of transcription factors) conferred susceptibility to *ETV6-RUNX1*–positive ALL,[60] and SNPs in *GATA3* conferred susceptibility to *BCR-ABL1*–like ALL and its underlying somatic lesions (*IKZF1* deletions, *CRLF2* rearrangements, and *JAK* mutations).[61]

Toxicity

An individual's genetic makeup can influence drug transport and metabolism and, subsequently, efficacy and toxicity. Thiopurine S-methyltransferase (TPMT) enzymatic activity is deficient in approximately 10% of individuals with polymorphisms in the *TPMT* gene. The reduced activity of TPMT leads to excessive cellular accumulation of active thiopurine metabolites and thereby excessive hematopoietic toxicity. In one study, the cumulative incidences of mercaptopurine-related myelosuppression were 100%, 35%, and 7% for patients with homozygous, heterozygous, and wild-type genotypes, respectively.[62] Tailoring the dose of mercaptopurine according to TPMT genotype results in equivalent systemic exposure, tolerance, and efficacy, and is an excellent example of widely used pharmacogenetic-guided therapy in clinical care. Germline variants associated with steroid-induced osteonecrosis,[63] vincristine-induced peripheral neuropathy,[64] anthracycline-induced cardiotoxicity,[65] and asparaginase allergy[66] have also been identified by candidate gene and genome-wide studies. Validation of these associations is warranted to determine their clinical relevance.

Response

Inherited genetic variation can contribute to interpatient variability in ALL treatment response, by influencing host disposition of antileukemic agents, interactions between tumor microenvironment and ALL, and tumor biology itself. At a genome-wide level, a

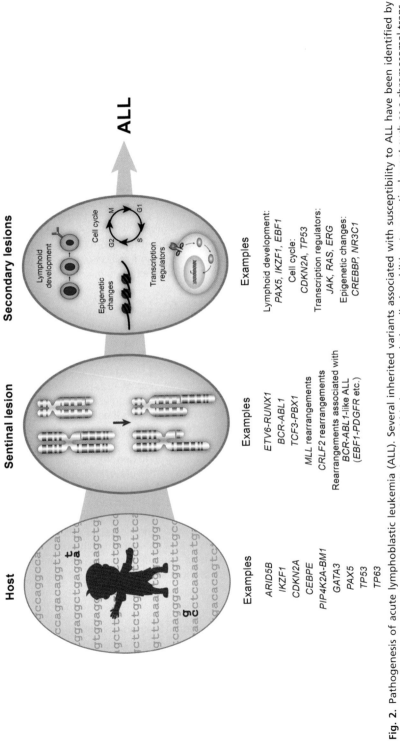

Fig. 2. Pathogenesis of acute lymphoblastic leukemia (ALL). Several inherited variants associated with susceptibility to ALL have been identified by genome-wide association studies and studies of familial ALL. Within hematopoietic cells, in addition to a sentinel event such as a chromosomal translocation, a multitude of secondary genetic events contribute to leukemic transformation.

study of more than 400,000 host germline polymorphisms in 487 children with ALL identified 102 SNPs (representing 71 unique genomic loci) that were significantly associated with MRD at the end of remission induction therapy.[67] Twenty percent of these SNP genotypes associated with high MRD were related to decreased exposure to methotrexate and etoposide, because of either increased clearance of these agents or decreased intracellular accumulation of active methotrexate polyglutamates. These findings underscore the effect of host genetic makeup on the response to multiple agents. A subsequent GWAS of 2535 children with ALL identified 134 SNPs consistently associated with outcome, most of which remained prognostic even after adjusting for known risk factors (eg, MRD, molecular subtype). In particular, risk variants in *PDE4B* predisposed patients to relapse, plausibly by affecting methotrexate pharmacodynamics and tumor sensitivity to steroids.[68]

The outcome of Hispanic children with ALL is historically inferior to that of patients of European descent. This racial disparity may in part be due to increased frequency of germline variants associated with Native American ancestry in Hispanic patients, which negatively influences MRD and relapse.[69] Patients with Hispanic ethnicity are also predisposed to developing high-risk subtypes of ALL (eg, *GATA3* germline polymorphism in *BCR-ABL1*–like ALL).[61] Of importance, the addition of an extra block of delayed intensification therapy for Hispanic children seemed to mitigate the ancestry-related difference in outcome.[69]

SUMMARY

Modern-day management of childhood ALL exemplifies the successful integration of biology into therapeutic decision making. In addition to the prognostic impact of conventional chromosomal translocations and aneuploidy, functional studies of key genetic alterations have contributed to our understanding of ALL pathogenesis. With the advent of high-throughput genomics and NGS technologies, knowledge of specific molecular lesions and critical pathways of leukemogenesis has exponentially increased. The incorporation of targeted therapy is expected to improve outcome for high-risk patients, particularly those with *BCR-ABL1*–positive ALL and those with the novel *BCR-ABL1*–like ALL subtype. In addition to genomic lesions, alterations in the epigenome modulate gene expression, and contribute significantly to leukemic transformation and resistance to therapy. Therefore, epigenetic therapy is another strategy being actively pursued in the clinic. A deeper understanding of the effect of inherited genetic variations can provide the opportunity to modify therapy to decrease toxicity without compromising efficacy. Furthermore, strong associations have been identified between inherited genetic variants and ALL susceptibility. Many of these polymorphisms are in genes that are targets of somatic lesions in ALL, highlighting plausible interactions between the biology of the disease and the host (**Fig. 2**).

ACKNOWLEDGMENTS

The authors thank Klo Spelshouse (Department of Biomedical Communications, St. Jude Children's Research Hospital) for assistance with illustrations, and Vani Shanker (Department of Scientific Editing, St. Jude Children's Research Hospital) for assistance with editing the article.

REFERENCES

1. Ward E, DeSantis C, Robbins A, et al. Childhood and adolescent cancer statistics, 2014. CA Cancer J Clin 2014;64:83–103.

2. Pui CH, Evans WE. A 50-year journey to cure childhood acute lymphoblastic leukemia. Semin Hematol 2013;50:185–96.
3. Hunger SP, Lu X, Devidas M, et al. Improved survival for children and adolescents with acute lymphoblastic leukemia between 1990 and 2005: a report from the children's oncology group. J Clin Oncol 2012;30:1663–9.
4. Schultz KR, Carroll A, Heerema NA, et al. Long-term follow-up of imatinib in pediatric Philadelphia chromosome-positive acute lymphoblastic leukemia: Children's Oncology Group study AALL0031. Leukemia 2014;28:1467–71.
5. Pui CH, Yang JJ, Hunger SP, et al. Childhood acute lymphoblastic leukemia: progress through collaboration. J Clin Oncol, in press.
6. Vardiman JW, Thiele J, Arber DA, et al. The 2008 revision of the World Health Organization (WHO) classification of myeloid neoplasms and acute leukemia: rationale and important changes. Blood 2009;114:937–51.
7. Schultz KR, Pullen DJ, Sather HN, et al. Risk- and response-based classification of childhood B-precursor acute lymphoblastic leukemia: a combined analysis of prognostic markers from the Pediatric Oncology Group (POG) and Children's Cancer Group (CCG). Blood 2007;109:926–35.
8. Pui CH, Campana D, Pei D, et al. Treating childhood acute lymphoblastic leukemia without cranial irradiation. N Engl J Med 2009;360:2730–41.
9. Moorman AV, Chilton L, Wilkinson J, et al. A population-based cytogenetic study of adults with acute lymphoblastic leukemia. Blood 2010;115:206–14.
10. Jeha S, Pei D, Raimondi SC, et al. Increased risk for CNS relapse in pre-B cell leukemia with the t(1;19)/TCF3-PBX1. Leukemia 2009;23:1406–9.
11. Nachman JB, Heerema NA, Sather H, et al. Outcome of treatment in children with hypodiploid acute lymphoblastic leukemia. Blood 2007;110:1112–5.
12. Holmfeldt L, Wei L, Diaz-Flores E, et al. The genomic landscape of hypodiploid acute lymphoblastic leukemia. Nat Genet 2013;45:242–52.
13. Pieters R. Infant acute lymphoblastic leukemia: lessons learned and future directions. Curr Hematol Malig Rep 2009;4:167–74.
14. Kim DH, Moldwin RL, Vignon C, et al. TEL-AML1 translocations with TEL and CDKN2 inactivation in acute lymphoblastic leukemia cell lines. Blood 1996;88: 785–94.
15. Figueroa ME, Chen SC, Andersson AK, et al. Integrated genetic and epigenetic analysis of childhood acute lymphoblastic leukemia. J Clin Invest 2013;123: 3099–111.
16. Hogan LE, Meyer JA, Yang J, et al. Integrated genomic analysis of relapsed childhood acute lymphoblastic leukemia reveals therapeutic strategies. Blood 2011;118:5218–26.
17. Mullighan CG, Goorha S, Radtke I, et al. Genome-wide analysis of genetic alterations in acute lymphoblastic leukaemia. Nature 2007;446:758–64.
18. Mullighan CG, Su X, Zhang J, et al. Deletion of IKZF1 and prognosis in acute lymphoblastic leukemia. N Engl J Med 2009;360:470–80.
19. Roberts KG, Morin RD, Zhang J, et al. Genetic alterations activating kinase and cytokine receptor signaling in high-risk acute lymphoblastic leukemia. Cancer Cell 2012;22:153–66.
20. Virely C, Moulin S, Cobaleda C, et al. Haploinsufficiency of the IKZF1 (IKAROS) tumor suppressor gene cooperates with BCR-ABL in a transgenic model of acute lymphoblastic leukemia. Leukemia 2010;24:1200–4.
21. Den Boer ML, van Slegtenhorst M, De Menezes RX, et al. A subtype of childhood acute lymphoblastic leukaemia with poor treatment outcome: a genome-wide classification study. Lancet Oncol 2009;10:125–34.

22. Roberts KG, Li Y, Payne-Turner D, et al. Targetable kinase-activating lesions in Ph-like acute lymphoblastic leukemia. N Engl J Med 2014;371(11):1005–15.
23. Weston BW, Hayden MA, Roberts KG, et al. Tyrosine kinase inhibitor therapy induces remission in a patient with refractory EBF1-PDGFRB-positive acute lymphoblastic leukemia. J Clin Oncol 2013;31:e413–6.
24. Roberts KG, Pei D, Campana D, et al. Outcomes of children with BCR-ABL1-like acute lymphoblastic leukemia treated with risk-directed therapy based on the levels of minimal residual disease. J Clin Oncol 2014. [Epub ahead of print].
25. Maude SL, Tasian SK, Vincent T, et al. Targeting JAK1/2 and mTOR in murine xenograft models of Ph-like acute lymphoblastic leukemia. Blood 2012;120: 3510–8.
26. Harvey RC, Kang H, Roberts AW, et al. Development and validation of a highly sensitive and specific gene expression classifier to prospectively screen and identify B-precursor acute lymphoblastic leukema patients with a Philadelphia Chromosome-like ("Ph-like" or "BCR-ABL1-like") signature for therapeutic targeting and clinical intervention. Blood 2013;122:826.
27. Rand V, Parker H, Russell LJ, et al. Genomic characterization implicates iAMP21 as a likely primary genetic event in childhood B-cell precursor acute lymphoblastic leukemia. Blood 2011;117:6848–55.
28. Moorman AV, Robinson H, Schwab C, et al. Risk-directed treatment intensification significantly reduces the risk of relapse among children and adolescents with acute lymphoblastic leukemia and intrachromosomal amplification of chromosome 21: a comparison of the MRC ALL97/99 and UKALL2003 trials. J Clin Oncol 2013;31:3389–96.
29. Hasle H, Clemmensen IH, Mikkelsen M. Risks of leukaemia and solid tumours in individuals with Down's syndrome. Lancet 2000;355:165–9.
30. Buitenkamp TD, Izraeli S, Zimmermann M, et al. Acute lymphoblastic leukemia in children with Down syndrome: a retrospective analysis from the Ponte di Legno study group. Blood 2014;123:70–7.
31. Mulligan CG, Collins-Underwood JR, Phillips LA, et al. Rearrangement of CRLF2 in B-progenitor- and Down syndrome-associated acute lymphoblastic leukemia. Nat Genet 2009;41:1243–6.
32. Nguyen K, Devidas M, Cheng SC, et al. Factors influencing survival after relapse from acute lymphoblastic leukemia: a Children's Oncology Group study. Leukemia 2008;22:2142–50.
33. Aifantis I, Raetz E, Buonamici S. Molecular pathogenesis of T-cell leukaemia and lymphoma. Nat Rev Immunol 2008;8:380–90.
34. Van Vlierberghe P, Ferrando A. The molecular basis of T cell acute lymphoblastic leukemia. J Clin Invest 2012;122:3398–406.
35. Ferrando AA, Neuberg DS, Staunton J, et al. Gene expression signatures define novel oncogenic pathways in T cell acute lymphoblastic leukemia. Cancer Cell 2002;1:75–87.
36. Weng AP, Ferrando AA, Lee W, et al. Activating mutations of NOTCH1 in human T cell acute lymphoblastic leukemia. Science 2004;306:269–71.
37. Thompson BJ, Buonamici S, Sulis ML, et al. The SCFFBW7 ubiquitin ligase complex as a tumor suppressor in T cell leukemia. J Exp Med 2007;204:1825–35.
38. Real PJ, Tosello V, Palomero T, et al. Gamma-secretase inhibitors reverse glucocorticoid resistance in T cell acute lymphoblastic leukemia. Nat Med 2009;15: 50–8.
39. Wu Y, Cain-Hom C, Choy L, et al. Therapeutic antibody targeting of individual Notch receptors. Nature 2010;464:1052–7.

40. Coustan-Smith E, Mullighan CG, Onciu M, et al. Early T-cell precursor leukaemia: a subtype of very high-risk acute lymphoblastic leukaemia. Lancet Oncol 2009; 10:147–56.

41. Zhang J, Ding L, Holmfeldt L, et al. The genetic basis of early T-cell precursor acute lymphoblastic leukaemia. Nature 2012;481:157–63.

42. Patrick K, Wade R, Goulden N, et al. Outcome for children and young people with Early T-cell precursor acute lymphoblastic leukaemia treated on a contemporary protocol, UKALL 2003. Br J Haematol 2014;166:421–4.

43. Huether R, Dong L, Chen X, et al. The landscape of somatic mutations in epigenetic regulators across 1,000 paediatric cancer genomes. Nat Commun 2014;5: 3630.

44. Krivtsov AV, Armstrong SA. MLL translocations, histone modifications and leukaemia stem-cell development. Nat Rev Cancer 2007;7:823–33.

45. Bhatla T, Wang J, Morrison DJ, et al. Epigenetic reprogramming reverses the relapse-specific gene expression signature and restores chemosensitivity in childhood B-lymphoblastic leukemia. Blood 2012;119:5201–10.

46. Mullighan CG, Phillips LA, Su X, et al. Genomic analysis of the clonal origins of relapsed acute lymphoblastic leukaemia. Science 2008;322:1377–80.

47. Klumper E, Pieters R, Veerman AJ, et al. In vitro cellular drug resistance in children with relapsed/refractory acute lymphoblastic leukemia. Blood 1995;86: 3861–8.

48. Bhojwani D, Pui CH. Relapsed childhood acute lymphoblastic leukaemia. Lancet Oncol 2013;14:e205–17.

49. Meyer JA, Wang J, Hogan LE, et al. Relapse-specific mutations in NT5C2 in childhood acute lymphoblastic leukemia. Nat Genet 2013;45:290–4.

50. Tzoneva G, Perez-Garcia A, Carpenter Z, et al. Activating mutations in the NT5C2 nucleotidase gene drive chemotherapy resistance in relapsed ALL. Nat Med 2013;19:368–71.

51. Mullighan CG, Zhang J, Kasper LH, et al. CREBBP mutations in relapsed acute lymphoblastic leukaemia. Nature 2011;471:235–9.

52. Yang JJ, Bhojwani D, Yang W, et al. Genome-wide copy number profiling reveals molecular evolution from diagnosis to relapse in childhood acute lymphoblastic leukemia. Blood 2008;112:4178–83.

53. Kuster L, Grausenburger R, Fuka G, et al. ETV6/RUNX1-positive relapses evolve from an ancestral clone and frequently acquire deletions of genes implicated in glucocorticoid signaling. Blood 2011;117:2658–67.

54. Seif AE. Pediatric leukemia predisposition syndromes: clues to understanding leukemogenesis. Cancer Genet 2011;204:227–44.

55. Kleihues P, Schauble B, zur Hausen A, et al. Tumors associated with p53 germline mutations: a synopsis of 91 families. Am J Pathol 1997;150:1–13.

56. Shah S, Schrader KA, Waanders E, et al. A recurrent germline PAX5 mutation confers susceptibility to pre-B cell acute lymphoblastic leukemia. Nat Genet 2013;45:1226–31.

57. Trevino LR, Yang W, French D, et al. Germline genomic variants associated with childhood acute lymphoblastic leukemia. Nat Genet 2009;41:1001–5.

58. Xu H, Yang W, Perez-Andreu V, et al. Novel susceptibility variants at 10p12.31-12.2 for childhood acute lymphoblastic leukemia in ethnically diverse populations. J Natl Cancer Inst 2013;105:733–42.

59. Papaemmanuil E, Hosking FJ, Vijayakrishnan J, et al. Loci on 7p12.2, 10q21.2 and 14q11.2 are associated with risk of childhood acute lymphoblastic leukemia. Nat Genet 2009;41:1006–10.

60. Ellinghaus E, Stanulla M, Richter G, et al. Identification of germline susceptibility loci in ETV6-RUNX1-rearranged childhood acute lymphoblastic leukemia. Leukemia 2012;26:902–9.
61. Perez-Andreu V, Roberts KG, Harvey RC, et al. Inherited GATA3 variants are associated with Ph-like childhood acute lymphoblastic leukemia and risk of relapse. Nat Genet 2013;45:1494–8.
62. Relling MV, Hancock ML, Rivera GK, et al. Mercaptopurine therapy intolerance and heterozygosity at the thiopurine S-methyltransferase gene locus. J Natl Cancer Inst 1999;91:2001–8.
63. French D, Hamilton LH, Mattano LA Jr, et al. A PAI-1 (SERPINE1) polymorphism predicts osteonecrosis in children with acute lymphoblastic leukemia: a report from the Children's Oncology Group. Blood 2008;111:4496–9.
64. Diouf B, Crews K, Lew G, et al. Genome-wide association analyses identify susceptibility loci for vincristine-induced peripheral neuropathy in children with acute lymphoblastic leukemia. Blood 2013;122:618.
65. Wang X, Liu W, Sun CL, et al. Hyaluronan synthase 3 variant and anthracycline-related cardiomyopathy: a report from the children's oncology group. J Clin Oncol 2014;32:647–53.
66. Fernandez CA, Smith C, Yang W, et al. HLA-DRB1*07:01 is associated with a higher risk of asparaginase allergies. Blood 2014;124:1266–76.
67. Yang JJ, Cheng C, Yang W, et al. Genome-wide interrogation of germline genetic variation associated with treatment response in childhood acute lymphoblastic leukemia. JAMA 2009;301:393–403.
68. Yang JJ, Cheng C, Devidas M, et al. Genome-wide association study identifies germline polymorphisms associated with relapse of childhood acute lymphoblastic leukemia. Blood 2012;120:4197–204.
69. Yang JJ, Cheng C, Devidas M, et al. Ancestry and pharmacogenomics of relapse in acute lymphoblastic leukemia. Nat Genet 2011;43:237–41.

Treatment of Pediatric Acute Lymphoblastic Leukemia

Stacy L. Cooper, MD[a], Patrick A. Brown, MD[b],*

KEYWORDS

- Acute lymphoblastic leukemia • Leukemia treatment • Risk-based stratification

KEY POINTS

- Pediatric acute lymphoblastic leukemia is the most common cancer diagnosed in children.
- Risk stratification allows treatment intensity to vary based on risk of treatment failure, and is based on age, initial leukocyte count, involvement of sanctuary sites, immunophenotype, cytogenetics, and response to treatment.
- The 4 main components of therapy are remission induction, consolidation, maintenance, and central nervous system–directed therapy, with an overall duration of therapy of 2 to 3 years.
- Prognosis after relapse depends on site of relapse and duration of initial remission.

INTRODUCTION

Acute lymphoblastic leukemia (ALL) is the most common cancer diagnosed in children. It has an overall survival of approximately 80%, with certain subsets experiencing greater than 98% cure rate.[1]

Incremental advances in therapy have led to marked improvements in survival since it was first treated, with these advances highlighting the importance of clinical trials through cooperative multicenter groups (**Table 1**). Childhood ALL also often serves as the paradigm for risk-based therapy, whereby stratification of treatment intensity is based on risk of treatment failure (**Fig. 1**).

RISK STRATIFICATION OF NEWLY DIAGNOSED ACUTE LYMPHOBLASTIC LEUKEMIA

One of the hallmarks of the treatment of childhood ALL is the reliance on risk-based stratification. By identifying the features that have been shown to affect prognosis,

[a] Pediatric Hematology/Oncology, Johns Hopkins/National Institutes of Health, Bloomberg 11379, 1800 Orleans Street, Baltimore, MD 21287, USA; [b] Pediatric Leukemia Program, Sidney Kimmel Comprehensive Cancer Center, Johns Hopkins University School of Medicine, 1650 Orleans Street, CRB1 Room 2M49, Baltimore, MD 21231, USA
* Corresponding author.
E-mail address: pbrown2@jhmi.edu

Table 1				
Outcomes for newly diagnosed childhood acute lymphoblastic leukemia				
Cooperative Group	Study	Years	Patients	5-y EFS (%)
Berlin-Frankfurt-Münster[52]	ALL-BFM-95	1995–2000	2169	79.6[a]
Children's Oncology Group[52]	Multiple	2000–2005	7153	90.4
Dana Farber Cancer Institute Consortium[52]	DFCI 95-01	1996–2001	491	82.0
Nordic Society of Pediatric Hematology and Oncology[52]	NOPHO	2002–2007	1023	79.0
St Jude Children's Research Hospital[52]	TOTXV	2000–2007	498	85.6
United Kingdom Acute Lymphoblastic Leukaemia[52]	UKALL 2003	2003–2011	3126	87.2

Abbreviation: EFS, event-free survival.
[a] 6-Year EFS used in ALL-BFM-95.

patients can be classified into groups based on risk of treatment failure. Those with favorable features can be treated with less toxic regimens, whereas more aggressive regimens are reserved for those with more high-risk disease.

It is therefore paramount to identify those features shown to consistently affect prognosis and, thus, influence treatment. Several clinical characteristics have been shown to aid in this classification, including age and white blood cell count (WBC) at presentation, together referred to as the National Cancer Institute (NCI) criteria. Age between 1 and 10 years is a standard risk feature, with more aggressive disease seen in infants and those older than 10 years. In part this is due to the higher rate of favorable cytogenetics in those aged 1 to 10 years.[2] The initial WBC at presentation also has been directly associated with increased risk, with high risk noted with WBC greater than 50,000/μL. Of importance is that this is a continuous function, but for practical purposes this threshold has been chosen as a useful categorical cut-off. The application of the NCI criteria results in those aged 1 to 10 years with initial

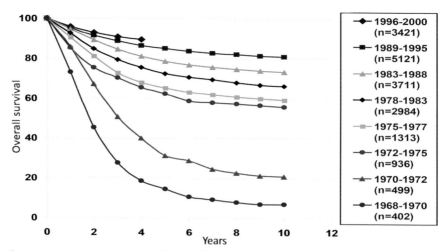

Fig. 1. Improved overall survival in childhood acute lymphoblastic leukemia (ALL). (From Hunger SP, Winick NJ, Sather HN et al. Therapy of low-risk subsets of childhood acute lymphoblastic leukemia: when do we say enough? Pediatr Blood Cancer 2005;45(7):876–80; with permission.)

WBC less than 50,000/μL classified as standard risk, with those not meeting those parameters classified as high risk.

Sanctuary sites are extramedullary anatomic locations that have historically been difficult to penetrate with systemic chemotherapy, and involvement of these sites at initial diagnosis has thus also been considered a high-risk feature. Approximately 3% of patients will demonstrate overt central nervous system (CNS) disease at diagnosis, defined either as a diagnostic lumbar puncture with the presence of leukemic blasts on cytospin and greater than 5 leukocytes/μL, or clinical evidence of CNS involvement (such as a cranial nerve palsy). Approximately 2% of boys with newly diagnosed ALL will present with testicular involvement, usually presenting with an enlarged, nonpainful testis. Leukemic involvement of the CNS or testis precludes a classification of standard risk in most treatment schemas.

Patients treated with corticosteroids before their complete diagnostic workup are also considered as high risk, as the tremendous efficacy of steroids to treat ALL may underestimate initial WBC and involvement of sanctuary sites, and limit confidence in staging.

The characteristics of the leukemia cells themselves can also be used to determine which patients are at higher risk. The immunophenotype describes the leukemic cells in terms of the proteins that are expressed, and whether these are more similar to cells that would eventually become B lymphocytes or T lymphocytes. This determination has also been shown to affect prognosis. At approximately 80%, most pediatric patients with ALL have B-precursor immunophenotype (Bp ALL), which encompasses a broad range of patients, including many of the lowest-risk patients with childhood ALL. Conversely, those with T-cell immunophenotype comprise approximately 10% to 15 % of pediatric ALL, and have historically been associated with a lower cure rate. However, identification of these patients and treatment with more aggressive regiments has led to survival rates that approach that of Bp ALL,[1,3] with the possible exception of early T-precursor (ETP) ALL, a particular subset of T-cell ALL that has been associated with a poor prognosis in some studies.[4] Additional rare immunophenotypic groups include those acute leukemias of mixed lineage, which occur in less than 5% of pediatric acute leukemias. These groups include undifferentiated acute leukemias that cannot be sufficiently characterized as either lymphoid or myeloid in origin, as well as those biphenotypic lineages that include markers of both myeloid and lymphoid origins and/or both B-cell and T-cell origins. These ambiguous immunophenotypes are often inconsistently defined but, regardless of exact classification, are associated with a poorer prognosis.[5]

Recurrent cytogenetic abnormalities in the leukemic blasts allow a molecular classification of risk, with certain markers shown to be associated with favorable or unfavorable outcomes. The 2 most well-established favorable cytogenetic aberrations include high hyperdiploidy and the ETV6/RUNX1 translocation. High hyperdiploidy is seen in 20% to 25% of cases of Bp ALL. It is defined as 51 to 65 chromosomes per cell or a DNA index of greater than 1.16, and is particularly favorable when associated with simultaneous trisomy 4 and 10.[6] The ETV6/RUNX1 translocation (due to t[12;21], formerly TEL/AML1) is also seen in approximately 20% to 25% of cases of Bp ALL, and is associated with improved survival, including improved survival even after relapse.[7] Both favorable subgroups occur in lower frequency in African Americans (sub-Saharan Africans), and in part accounts for the lower overall outcome in this population.[8,9] Several unfavorable cytogenetic changes have also been identified. One feature strongly associated with poor outcome is hypodiploidy, defined as fewer than 44 chromosomes or a DNA index of less than 0.81. Additional cytogenetic changes associated with higher-risk ALL include BCR-ABL fusion of t(9;22), known as the Philadelphia chromosome (seen in 3% of pediatric ALL), *MLL* rearrangements involving 11q23 (seen in 5% of pediatric ALL, often infants and adolescents), and, most recently identified, intrachromosomal amplification of chromosome 21 (iAMP21, seen in 1%–2% of Bp ALL).[10]

In addition to these features that are used to inform prognosis, the response to the initial therapy has emerged as a particularly powerful independent predictor. Traditionally a complete remission has been defined as less than 5% detectable blasts on microscopic morphology at the end of induction. Induction failure is seen in approximately 3% to 5% of children with newly diagnosed ALL and portends a very poor prognosis, with an overall survival of approximately 33%. It is most closely associated with patients with T-cell immunophenotype, Bp immunophenotype with a high presenting leukocyte count, *MLL* rearrangement, Philadelphia chromosome, or older age.[11]

Evaluation of the bone marrow by microscopy is often relatively insensitive, and has been shown to be complemented and, in part, displaced, by evaluation of minimum residual disease (MRD). This technique uses flow cytometry or the polymerase chain reaction (PCR) to assess for disease at a significantly lower limit of detection (1 leukemic blast in 10,000–100,000 cells). Evaluation of bone marrow MRD at the end of induction has proved to be an independent factor predicting outcome, and has also been shown to be useful in the peripheral blood as early as day 8 of therapy. End-induction MRD has been established in the risk stratification of Bp ALL patients[12] while studies using MRD to adjust the treatment of T-cell ALL are currently ongoing but also promising.

The application of these risk factors is operationalized in various methods by the different cooperative groups of pediatric oncology specialists. One group, the Children's Oncology Group (COG), utilizes a combination of the NCI criteria in addition to cytogenetics and response to therapy. Other groups, such as the Berlin-Franklin-Münster (BFM) Group, rely almost solely on response to initial therapy using MRD thresholds, although with certain cytogenetic changes treated as high risk regardless of response to therapy (**Box 1**).[13]

TREATMENT OF NEWLY DIAGNOSED ACUTE LYMPHOBLASTIC LEUKEMIA

There are 4 major components of treatment of newly diagnosed ALL, reflecting a reliance on multidrug regimens to avoid development of resistance. Different blocks of chemotherapy have varying intensity depending on the group of patients at risk, with increasingly intensive regimens corresponding to more aggressive disease categories.

Remission induction is the first block of chemotherapy, lasting 4 to 6 weeks. Patients are usually admitted to the hospital for their initial treatment and workup, but once any complications have stabilized the patient may be discharged before the completion of this phase with close outpatient follow-up. The goal of this block of

---

Box 1
High-risk features in pediatric acute lymphocytic leukemia (ALL)

- Age less than 1 year old or greater than 10 years old
- Initial white blood cell count greater than 50,000/μL
- Central nervous system involvement
- Testicular involvement
- Unfavorable cytogenetics (hypodiploidy, t(9;22), 11q23, iAMP21)
- Suboptimal induction response (induction failure or positive minimum residual disease)

therapy is to induce a complete remission by its completion, with approximately 95% of all patients achieving this benchmark. Of those that do not achieve completion remission by the end of induction, half suffer induction failure and the remainder succumb to treatment-related mortality. For those with induction failure, an allogeneic bone marrow transplant is usually pursued, although there is no consensus standard of care regarding the chemotherapy used to achieve remission before transplant.[11]

The agents used during induction include vincristine, corticosteroids, and asparaginase, with most regimens adding an anthracycline (usually doxorubicin or daunorubicin). Both anthracyclines have been shown to have similar efficacy and toxicity in randomized trials.[14] Certain groups spare the addition of anthracyclines to those lower-risk groups in an effort to decrease toxicity. The corticosteroid used is usually prednisone or dexamethasone, with dexamethasone demonstrating improved CNS penetration and decreased risk of relapse, but with increased incidence of toxicities, including avascular necrosis, infection, and reduction in linear growth.[15] Several different agents for asparagine depletion exist as well, including PEG asparaginase and Erwinia asparaginase. PEG asparaginase has been modified by covalently attaching polyethylene glycol, which has been demonstrated to result in a longer half-life and decreased immunogenicity in comparison with native *Escherichia coli* L-asparaginase. Randomized trials have also shown superior efficacy of the pegylated formulation.[16] Erwinia asparaginase is usually given to those patients who have experienced an allergic reaction to PEG asparaginase, and requires a more frequent administration schedule.

Remission induction is followed by consolidation, which aims to eradicate the submicroscopic residual disease that remains after a complete remission is obtained. Lasting approximately 6 to 9 months, it varies in length and intensity among different protocols, with those patients with higher-risk disease receiving longer and more intensive consolidation regimens.[17] Consolidation is usually administered on an outpatient basis, although there are protocols with more aggressive regimens that require inpatient care. This phase of chemotherapy involves combinations of different chemotherapeutic agents to maximize synergy and minimize drug resistance, often including agents not used in the initial remission induction, such as mercaptopurine, thioguanine, methotrexate, cyclophosphamide, etoposide, and cytarabine.

Maintenance chemotherapy is the final, and longest, stage of treatment in childhood ALL. A much less intensive regimen than the prior chemotherapy, the prolonged maintenance phase has been demonstrated to lower the risk of relapse once remission has been established. It usually lasts at least 2 years (extended to 3 years for boys in some protocols), is administered on an outpatient basis, and typically is associated with less disruptive toxicity. The cornerstone of maintenance therapy is antimetabolite therapy with methotrexate and mercaptopurine, both available in oral formulations, making strict adherence crucial.[18] Furthermore, emerging evidence regarding the pharmacogenomics of these drugs underscores the importance of interindividual differences in metabolism. For example, genotypic polymorphisms in the enzyme thiopurine methyltransferase are associated with increased myelosuppression and other toxicities, whereas other polymorphisms confer a "hypermetabolizer" state, with decreased levels of the active metabolite.[19] Understanding these differences in metabolism is particularly important because studies have shown that the degree of myelosuppression correlates with relapse risk.[20,21] Accordingly, many protocols include guidelines for dose adjustments to assist in achieving the goal of balancing the risks of inadequate myelosuppression with the risks of severe pancytopenia (infection, bleeding, and so forth). Some regimens also include monthly vincristine and steroids, although the evidence for additional benefit is unclear.[22]

The fourth component of the treatment of ALL is therapy directed against the CNS. This approach includes both treatment of patients with clinical CNS disease at diagnosis and prophylaxis for patients with subclinical disease. The importance of this component was clearly demonstrated before the 1970s, when treatment lacked this component. Although bone marrow remission could be achieved using systemic chemotherapy, most children eventually developed CNS relapse in the absence of specific therapy directed toward this sanctuary site.[23]

There are several methods of achieving the goal of eradication of disease from the CNS, including direct intrathecal administration of chemotherapy, systemic administration of chemotherapy able to penetrate the blood-brain barrier, and cranial radiation. All treatment plans include intrathecal administration of chemotherapy beginning during remission induction. Some protocols include intrathecal treatment throughout therapy, whereas others do not include it in maintenance. Options for intrathecal chemotherapy include including intrathecal methotrexate or a combination of intrathecal methotrexate, cytarabine, and hydrocortisone (known as triple intrathecal). Studies have shown no definitive difference in overall or event-free survival between the two, although some evidence points to decreased frequency of CNS relapse with the use of triple intrathecal therapy.[24] Systemically administered chemotherapy with CNS effects includes dexamethasone, high-dose methotrexate, cytarabine, and asparaginase.

Given the risk of toxicity of cranial radiation, manifesting primarily as intellectual disability (particularly with younger patients) and as second malignant neoplasms, its utilization has been progressively declining. Many protocols reserve its use for only those at highest risk of CNS relapse while some institutions defer its use altogether. For those patients with overt CNS disease at presentation, several small studies have shown that by increasing the intensity of the intrathecal and systemic chemotherapy, cranial irradiation can also be deferred for these patients. However, larger studies are needed to confirm this strategy.[25,26]

The role of allogeneic hematopoietic stem cell transplant (HSCT) in first remission of ALL is not yet well defined, and is a controversial topic. Broadly speaking, HSCT is considered for those patients with the very highest risk of relapse and/or treatment failure, which has been most closely associated with those patients demonstrating hypodiploidy or induction failure. General tenets of HSCT for ALL include the use of total body irradiation (TBI) in the preparative regimen, and improved outcomes for patients who undergo transplant after achieving MRD-negative disease status. The optimal donor has historically been a matched sibling, although advances with alternative donor sources are now also showing promise.[27]

CONSIDERATIONS FOR PARTICULAR SUBGROUPS OF ACUTE LYMPHOBLASTIC LEUKEMIA

Infants with ALL represent a particularly high-risk subclass, with higher risks of both treatment failure and treatment complications. The highest rates of treatment failure are seen in infants diagnosed before 6 months of age, those with high initial WBC count, or those with MLL gene rearrangements (which occur in 70%–80% of infants diagnosed with ALL). Infant regimens often contain intensive chemotherapy not typically administered on other ALL protocols. In cases with MLL rearrangement, the leukemic cells typically express high levels of FLT3, a tyrosine kinase oncogene; therefore, studies are currently ongoing to test the addition of a FLT3 inhibitor to conventional chemotherapy regimens. In addition, these patients have a high risk of treatment-related mortality,[28] and thus induction often includes a 1-week prophase of single-agent steroid to "debulk" the initial leukemic burden before initiation of multi-agent chemotherapy. Similar to MRD evaluation, response to this steroid prophase has been shown to correlate with risk of treatment failure.[29] Infants also have a particularly high rate of infectious complications and thus warrant aggressive supportive care, including broad-spectrum antimicrobial prophylaxis, use of growth factors, and inpatient management.

Adolescents have been shown to have lower rates of overall survival, in part owing to the association of an increased incidence of Philadelphia chromosome and T-cell immunophenotype. Therefore, most protocols will consider patients older than 10 years as high risk, with some protocols classifying those older than 13 years as "very high risk" based on age alone. Young adult patients also experience a higher rate of treatment-related morbidity and mortality, particularly secondary to infection, osteonecrosis, and thrombosis.[30,31] Multiple studies have demonstrated the benefit of treating adolescent and young adult patients with ALL on pediatric-based protocols.[32]

Patients with T-cell ALL comprise approximately 10% of pediatric ALL and, compared with those with Bp-ALL, have historically experienced a worse prognosis. With more aggressive modern regimens, however, many patients with T-ALL have survival approaching that of Bp-ALL. Unfortunately, T-ALL patients continue to experience a lower risk of survival after relapse. Studies are currently ongoing regarding the addition of nelarabine, a purine nucleoside analogue that appears to be particularly cytotoxic to T cells, with promising results in the relapsed setting.[33]

As discussed earlier, patients with mixed-lineage leukemia often represent a relatively recalcitrant subgroup. Although there is no well-defined consensus for the treatment of these patients, many groups recommend the combination of therapy directed at both lineages, and have shown that cure can potentially be achieved without the use of HSCT.[34]

Children with trisomy 21 (Down syndrome) have an increased risk of ALL, with a lower incidence of both favorable and unfavorable cytogenetics. These patients demonstrate a similar rate of relapse compared with patients without Down syndrome, but have an increased risk of treatment-related mortality, primarily secondary to infectious deaths. Therefore they are typically treated on specific protocols with enhanced supportive measures and more frequent use of leucovorin rescue to mitigate the toxic effects of methotrexate[35] (see the relevant article elsewhere in this issue for further details on Down syndrome and leukemia).

Chromosomal translocation of chromosomes 9 and 22, known as the Philadelphia chromosome and resulting in the fusion product BCR-ABL, occurs in approximately 3% of childhood ALL. Although these patients are classified as high risk, the introduction of imatinib, a tyrosine kinase inhibitor that targets the BCR-ABL fusion protein, has markedly improved the outcome of this disease. Addition of this agent to intensive, multidrug chemotherapy regimens has been shown to result in far superior event-free and overall survival in comparison with historical controls, and has rendered unclear the role of HSCT for these patients.[36] Newer generations of tyrosine kinase inhibitors (such as dasatinib, nilotinib, and ponatinib) have been recently introduced with evidence of improved efficacy in adults.

TREATMENT OF RELAPSED ACUTE LYMPHOBLASTIC LEUKEMIA

Despite significant advances in treatment, approximately 15% to 20% of patients with ALL will suffer relapsed disease, the most common cause of treatment failure. With intensive therapy that may include HSCT, overall survival from relapsed ALL is approximately 40%.[37] Similar to those patients with newly diagnosed ALL, those with relapsed disease can be risk stratified. Length of first complete remission (CR1) and site of relapse have consistently been demonstrated to be the 2 most important prognostic factors in these cases. For patients with Bp-ALL, relapses within 18 months of diagnosis fare the worst, those occurring between 18 and 36 months after diagnosis have an intermediate prognosis, and late relapses that occur more than 3 years from diagnosis have the best prognosis, with up to a 50% event-free survival.[38]

Site of relapse is the other salient risk feature to consider in relapsed disease, with isolated marrow relapses as the most common site, occurring in 50% to 60% of cases. The remainder comprises isolated CNS disease in approximately 20%, isolated testicular disease in approximately 5%, and a combination of marrow and extramedullary disease in the remainder. Isolated extramedullary relapses have the best prognosis, with the worst outcomes seen in isolated marrow relapses. Those with combined marrow and extramedullary involvement have an intermediate prognosis.[39]

The risk group at initial diagnosis has been shown to also play a role in the relapse setting, with increased survival in those initially classified as standard risk compared with those at high risk. This finding holds particularly true when considering those with T-cell immunophenotype, who experience a particularly poor prognosis after relapse. As with patients with newly diagnosed ALL, the response to reinduction chemotherapy has prognostic significance. Those with persistent morphologic disease after the first cycle of reinduction chemotherapy have an especially poor prognosis, and those with a morphologic remission but continued detectable minimal residual disease have a worse outcome than those with MRD-negative disease after reinduction.[40,41]

The application of cytogenetic abnormalities in the risk stratification of relapsed ALL has been limited, although a few have been shown to be informative. For example, those with relapsed disease who demonstrate ETV6-RUNX1 mutations have a relatively favorable prognosis, with an event-free survival of more than 80% if initial CR1 was at least 36 months.[42] Conversely, blasts demonstrating TP53 mutations show a particularly poor prognosis.[43]

Reinduction chemotherapy after first relapse is successful at inducing complete remission in 65% to 85%.[44] The chemotherapy regimens used vary by institution and protocol, but is often the same 4-drug induction used at initial diagnosis, consisting of vincristine, steroids, asparaginase, and an anthracycline. Clinical trials are currently ongoing to evaluate the addition of novel agents for reinduction chemotherapy but, given the lack of clear data, no consensus yet exists. Once a second complete remission (CR2) has been obtained, postremission treatment varies by risk. Those patients with T-cell immunophenotype (regardless of duration of CR1) or Bp-ALL early relapsed marrow disease are usually treated with HSCT. Those with Bp-ALL late marrow relapses can often be cured with chemotherapy alone, and this risk stratification in part relies on the use of detection of MRD at the end of reinduction.[45]

Patients with isolated CNS relapse usually receive a combination of chemotherapy and cranial radiation, with chemotherapy administered first to prevent an overt marrow relapse. Craniospinal radiation has not been shown to have increased efficacy, and therefore the addition of spinal radiation has largely been abandoned in contemporary trials. For those isolated CNS Bp-ALL relapses occurring more than 18 months from diagnosis, survival rates of 70% can be achieved with chemoradiation alone, and thus HSCT is usually not required. For those with early isolated CNS relapses and/or T-cell immunophenotype, prognosis is worse, and HSCT is often pursued, although no clear data exist regarding whether HSCT leads to superior outcomes. Treatment of isolated testicular relapse also depends on duration of CR1, with worse outcomes for those patients experiencing an isolated testicular relapse while still receiving upfront therapy. Therapy for testicular relapse usually consists of intensive reinduction chemotherapy (often including high-dose methotrexate) followed by testicular radiation or orchiectomy if complete remission is not achieved.[46]

Therapy for second and subsequent relapses is varied and without clear evidence-based guidance. Long-term survival is generally poor for these patients. For those receiving chemotherapy alone for their first relapse, HSCT once third remission (CR3) has been achieved is the standard therapy. For those who received HSCT in CR2, a select population of patients may be considered for a second HSCT. Donor leukocyte infusions are usually unsuccessful in achieving durable remissions in relapsed ALL after HSCT, particularly when used as monotherapy.[47]

NOVEL AGENTS IN THE TREATMENT OF ACUTE LYMPHOBLASTIC LEUKEMIA

Current efforts in advancing the treatment of ALL focus on unique mechanisms that contrast with the nonspecific targeting of conventional chemotherapy. Immunotherapy is a broad and promising field that seeks to harness the power of the immune system to allow for a more targeted approach. Chimeric antigen receptors are one example of modified adoptive cell transfer whereby the patient's own cytotoxic T cells are genetically engineered to express an antibody to target leukemic antigens (often CD19), often enhanced by the inclusion of costimulatory binding regions that allow for improved cytotoxicity and duration of cells.[48] Another example of immunotherapy is blinatumomab, a bispecific anti-CD19/CD3 molecule, which enhances cytotoxic killing by binding both a protein expressed on the leukemic blast (CD19) and one expressed on autologous T cells (CD3).[49] Finally, moxetumomab is an antibody conjugate wherein a monoclonal antibody recognizing CD22 is fused with a fragment of the *Pseudomonas* exotoxin, to allow for direct cell killing.[50] All 3 of these have shown promising results in early clinical trials, with larger studies under way. Another promising novel treatment strategy focuses on the epigenetic changes seen in leukemogenesis, with the use of histone deacetylase inhibitors (HDACi), such as vorinotstat.[51] Finally, bortezomib is a proteasome inhibitor that interferes with natural killer

---

Box 2
Effects of common chemotherapeutic agents used in the treatment of ALL

Agent	Effects
Asparaginase	Hypersensitivity reactions, pancreatitis, thrombosis
Clofarabine	Cardiotoxicity, cytokine release syndrome, hepatotoxicity (including sinusoidal obstruction syndrome), pancreatitis, nephrotoxicity
Corticosteroids	Hypertension, hyperglycemia, osteonecrosis, fluid retention, psychosis
Cyclophosphamide	Nephrotoxicity, hemorrhagic cystitis, hyponatremia, fluid retention
Cytarabine	Conjunctivitis, flu-like symptoms
Doxorubicin/ daunorubicin	Cardiotoxicity, benign red urine
Etoposide	Nephrotoxicity, hepatotoxicity, hypersensitivity reactions
Mercaptopurine	Hepatotoxicity
Methotrexate	Mucositis, nephrotoxicity, hepatotoxicity, encephalopathy
Thioguanine	Hepatotoxicity (including sinusoidal obstruction syndrome and portal hypertension)
Vincristine	Syndrome of inappropriate diuretic hormone, neuropathy (foot/wrist drop, paresthesias, constipation, ptosis, vocal cord paresis)

κB signaling and is able to enhance bcl-2 and bcl-x, rendering blasts more sensitive to apoptosis, particularly in combination with conventional chemotherapy agents.[52]

TOXICITIES IN THE TREATMENT OF ACUTE LYMPHOBLASTIC LEUKEMIA

Almost all chemotherapy agents cause myelosuppression, mucositis, and nausea/vomiting. Unique effects of common chemotherapeutic agents used in the treatment of ALL are listed in **Box 2**.

SUMMARY

Acute lymphoblastic leukemia is treated with a combination of chemotherapy drugs over the course of several years, with an overall survival of approximately 80% for all newly diagnosed patients. Those patients with higher risk of relapse receive more aggressive treatment, whereas those with more favorable features can be spared the more toxic effects. Treatment is progressively less intensive as the duration of therapy progresses, and must include central nervous system (CNS) directed therapy regardless of involvement of the CNS at diagnosis. Multi-center randomized clinical trials through international cooperative groups help to further improve survival through the investigation of novel therapeutic approaches.

REFERENCES

1. Gaynon PS, Angiolillo AL, Carroll WL, et al. Long-term results of the children's cancer group studies for childhood acute lymphoblastic leukemia 1983-2002: a Children's Oncology Group Report. Leukemia 2010;24(2):285–97.
2. Möricke A, Zimmermann M, Reiter A, et al. Prognostic impact of age in children and adolescents with acute lymphoblastic leukemia: data from the trials ALL-BFM 86, 90, and 95. Klin Padiatr 2005;217(6):310–20.
3. Reiter A, Schrappe M, Ludwig WD, et al. Chemotherapy in 998 unselected childhood acute lymphoblastic leukemia patients. Results and conclusions of the multicenter trial ALL-BFM 86. Blood 1994;84:3122–33.
4. Haydu JE, Ferrando AA. Early T-cell precursor acute lymphoblastic leukaemia. Curr Opin Hematol 2013;20(4):369–73.
5. Gerr H, Zimmermann M, Schrappe M, et al. Acute leukaemias of ambiguous lineage in children: characterization, prognosis and therapy recommendations. Br J Haematol 2010;149(1):84–92.
6. Harris MB, Shuster JJ, Carroll A, et al. Trisomy of leukemic cell chromosomes 4 and 10 identifies children with B-progenitor cell acute lymphoblastic leukemia with a very low risk of treatment failure: a Pediatric Oncology Group study. Blood 1992;79(12):3316–24.
7. Seeger K, Stackelberg AV, Taube T, et al. Relapse of TEL-AML1-positive acute lymphoblastic leukemia in childhood: a matched-pair analysis. J Clin Oncol 2001;19(13):3188–93.
8. Pollock BH, DeBaun MR, Camitta BM, et al. Racial differences in the survival of childhood B-precursor acute lymphoblastic leukemia: a Pediatric Oncology Group Study. J Clin Oncol 2000;18(4):813–23.
9. Rubnitz JE, Wichlan D, Devidas M, et al, Children's Oncology Group. Prospective analysis of TEL gene rearrangements in childhood acute lymphoblastic leukemia: a Children's Oncology Group study. J Clin Oncol 2008;26(13):2186–91.
10. Heerema NA, Carroll AJ, Devidas M, et al. Intrachromosomal amplification of chromosome 21 is associated with inferior outcomes in children with acute

lymphoblastic leukemia treated in contemporary standard-risk children's oncology group studies: a report from the children's oncology group. J Clin Oncol 2013;31(27):3397–402.

11. Schrappe M, Hunger SP, Pui CH, et al. Outcomes after induction failure in childhood acute lymphoblastic leukemia. N Engl J Med 2012;366(15):1371–81.

12. Borowitz MJ, Devidas M, Hunger SP, et al, Children's Oncology Group. Clinical significance of minimal residual disease in childhood acute lymphoblastic leukemia and its relationship to other prognostic factors: a Children's Oncology Group study. Blood 2008;111(12):5477–85.

13. Conter V, Bartram CR, Valsecchi MG, et al. Molecular response to treatment redefines all prognostic factors in children and adolescents with B-cell precursor acute lymphoblastic leukemia: results in 3184 patients of the AIEOP-BFM ALL 2000 study. Blood 2010;115(16):3206–14.

14. Escherich G, Zimmermann M, Janka-Schaub G, et al. Doxorubicin or daunorubicin given upfront in a therapeutic window are equally effective in children with newly diagnosed acute lymphoblastic leukemia. A randomized comparison in trial CoALL 07-03. Pediatr Blood Cancer 2013;60(2):254–7.

15. Mitchell CD, Richards SM, Kinsey SE, et al. Benefit of dexamethasone compared with prednisolone for childhood acute lymphoblastic leukaemia: results of the UK Medical Research Council ALL97 randomized trial. Br J Haematol 2005;129(6): 734–45.

16. Avramis VI, Sencer S, Periclou AP, et al. A randomized comparison of native *Escherichia coli* asparaginase and polyethylene glycol conjugated asparaginase for treatment of children with newly diagnosed standard-risk acute lymphoblastic leukemia: a Children's Cancer Group study. Blood 2002;99(6):1986–94.

17. Seibel NL, Steinherz PG, Sather HN, et al. Early postinduction intensification therapy improves survival for children and adolescents with high-risk acute lymphoblastic leukemia: a report from the Children's Oncology Group. Blood 2008;111(5):2548.

18. Bhatia S, Landier W, Shangguan M, et al. Nonadherence to oral mercaptopurine and risk of relapse in Hispanic and non-Hispanic white children with acute lymphoblastic leukemia: a report from the children's oncology group. J Clin Oncol 2012;30(17):2094–101.

19. Brackett J, Schafer ES, Leung DH, et al. Use of allopurinol in children with acute lymphoblastic leukemia to reduce skewed thiopurine metabolism. Pediatr Blood Cancer 2014;61(6):1114–7.

20. Schmiegelow K, Schröder H, Gustafsson G, et al. Risk of relapse in childhood acute lymphoblastic leukemia is related to RBC methotrexate and mercaptopurine metabolites during maintenance chemotherapy. Nordic Society for Pediatric Hematology and Oncology. J Clin Oncol 1995;13(2):345–51.

21. Schmiegelow K, Heyman M, Gustafsson G, et al. The degree of myelosuppression during maintenance therapy of adolescents with B-lineage intermediate risk acute lymphoblastic leukemia predicts risk of relapse. Leukemia 2010; 24(4):715–20.

22. Eden TO, Pieters R, Richards S, et al. Systematic review of the addition of vincristine plus steroid pulses in maintenance treatment for childhood acute lymphoblastic leukaemia—an individual patient data meta-analysis involving 5,659 children. Br J Haematol 2010;149(5):722–33.

23. Evans AE, Gilbert ES, Zandstra R. The increasing incidence of central nervous system leukemia in children. (Children's Cancer Study Group A). Cancer 1970; 26:404.

24. Matloub Y, Lindemulder S, Gaynon PS, et al. Intrathecal triple therapy decreases central nervous system relapse but fails to improve event-free survival when compared with intrathecal methotrexate: results of the Children's Cancer Group (CCG) 1952 study for standard-risk acute lymphoblastic leukemia, reported by the Children's Oncology Group. Blood 2006;108(4):1165–73.

25. Pui CH, Campana D, Pei D, et al. Treating childhood acute lymphoblastic leukemia without cranial irradiation. N Engl J Med 2009;360(26):2730–41.

26. Sirvent N, Suciu S, Rialland X, et al. Prognostic significance of the initial cerebrospinal fluid (CSF) involvement of children with acute lymphoblastic leukaemia (ALL) treated without cranial irradiation: results of European Organization for Research and Treatment of Cancer (EORTC) Children Leukemia Group study 58881. Eur J Cancer 2011;47(2):239–47.

27. Hochberg J, Khaled S, Forman SJ, et al. Criteria for and outcomes of allogeneic haematopoietic stem cell transplant in children, adolescents and young adults with acute lymphoblastic leukaemia in first complete remission. Br J Haematol 2013;161(1):27–42.

28. Hilden JM, Dinndorf PA, Meerbaum SO, et al. Analysis of prognostic factors of acute lymphoblastic leukemia in infants: report on CCG 1953 from the Children's Oncology Group. Blood 2006;108(2):441–51.

29. Pieters R, Schrappe M, De Lorenzo P, et al. A treatment protocol for infants younger than 1 year with acute lymphoblastic leukaemia (Interfant-99): an observational study and a multicentre randomised trial. Lancet 2007;370(9583): 240–50.

30. Pichler H, Reismüller B, Steiner M, et al. The inferior prognosis of adolescents with acute lymphoblastic leukaemia (ALL) is caused by a higher rate of treatment-related mortality and not an increased relapse rate–a population-based analysis of 25 years of the Austrian ALL-BFM (Berlin-Frankfurt-Münster) Study Group. Br J Haematol 2013;161(4):556–65.

31. O'Brien SH, Klima J, Termuhlen AM, et al. Venous thromboembolism and adolescent and young adult oncology inpatients in US children's hospitals, 2001 to 2008. J Pediatr 2011;159(1):133–7.

32. Ram R, Wolach O, Vidal L, et al. Adolescents and young adults with acute lymphoblastic leukemia have a better outcome when treated with pediatric-inspired regimens: systematic review and meta-analysis. Am J Hematol 2012; 87(5):472–8.

33. Berg SL, Blaney SM, Devidas M, et al. Phase II study of nelarabine (compound 506U78) in children and young adults with refractory T-cell malignancies: A report from the Children's Oncology Group. J Clin Oncol 2005;15:3376–82.

34. Rubnitz JE, Onciu M, Pounds S, et al. Acute mixed lineage leukemia in children: the experience of St Jude Children's Research Hospital. Blood 2009;113(21): 5083–9.

35. Whitlock JA. Down syndrome and acute lymphoblastic leukaemia. Br J Haematol 2006;135(5):595–602.

36. Schultz KR, Bowman WP, Aledo A, et al. Improved early event-free survival with imatinib in Philadelphia chromosome-positive acute lymphoblastic leukemia: a children's oncology group study. J Clin Oncol 2009;27(31): 5175–81.

37. Locatelli F, Schrappe M, Bernardo ME, et al. How I treat relapsed childhood acute lymphoblastic leukemia. Blood 2012;120(14):2807–16.

38. Chessells JM. Relapsed lymphoblastic leukaemia in children: a continuing challenge. Br J Haematol 1998;102(2):423–38.

39. Nguyen K, Devidas M, Cheng SC, et al. Factors influencing survival after relapse from acute lymphoblastic leukemia: a Children's Oncology Group study. Leukemia 2008;22(12):2142–50.
40. Coustan-Smith E, Gajjar A, Hijiya N, et al. Clinical significance of minimal residual disease in childhood acute lymphoblastic leukemia after first relapse. Leukemia 2004;18(3):499–504.
41. Eckert C, von Stackelberg A, Seeger K, et al. Minimal residual disease after induction is the strongest predictor of prognosis in intermediate risk relapsed acute lymphoblastic leukaemia - long-term results of trial ALL-REZ BFM P95/96. Eur J Cancer 2013;49(6):1346–55.
42. Gandemer V, Chevret S, Petit A, et al. Excellent prognosis of late relapses of ETV6/RUNX1-positive childhood acute lymphoblastic leukemia: lessons from the FRALLE 93 protocol. Haematologica 2012;97(11):1743–50.
43. Hof J, Krentz S, van Schewick C, et al. Mutations and deletions of the TP53 gene predict nonresponse to treatment and poor outcome in first relapse of childhood acute lymphoblastic leukemia. J Clin Oncol 2011;29(23):3185–93.
44. Parker C, Waters R, Leighton C, et al. Effect of mitoxantrone on outcome of children with first relapse of acute lymphoblastic leukaemia (ALL R3): an open-label randomised trial. Lancet 2010;376(9757):2009–17.
45. Rivera GK, Hudson MM, Liu Q, et al. Effectiveness of intensified rotational combination chemotherapy for late hematologic relapse of childhood acute lymphoblastic leukemia. Blood 1996;88(3):831–7.
46. Wofford MM, Smith SD, Shuster JJ, et al. Treatment of occult or late overt testicular relapse in children with acute lymphoblastic leukemia: a Pediatric Oncology Group study. J Clin Oncol 1992;10(4):624–30.
47. Levine JE, Barrett AJ, Zhang MJ, et al. Donor leukocyte infusions to treat hematologic malignancy relapse following allo-SCT in a pediatric population. Bone Marrow Transplant 2008;42(3):201–5.
48. Brentjens RJ, Curran KJ. Novel cellular therapies for leukemia: CAR-modified T cells targeted to the CD19antigen. Hematology Am Soc Hematol Educ Program 2012;2012:143–51.
49. Hoffman LM, Gore L. Blinatumomab, a Bi-Specific Anti-CD19/CD3 BiTE(®) antibody for the treatment of acute lymphoblastic leukemia: perspectives and current pediatric applications. Front Oncol 2014;4:63.
50. Kreitman RJ, Pastan I. Antibody fusion proteins: anti-CD22 recombinant immunotoxin moxetumomab pasudotox. Clin Cancer Res 2011;17(20):6398–405.
51. Burke MJ, Bhatla T. Epigenetic modifications in pediatric acute lymphoblastic leukemia. Front Pediatr 2014;2:42.
52. Pui CH, Jeha S. New therapeutic strategies for the treatment of acute lymphoblastic leukaemia. Nat Rev Drug Discov 2007;6:149–65.

Pediatric Acute Myeloid Leukemia

Biology and Therapeutic Implications of Genomic Variants

Katherine Tarlock, MD, Soheil Meshinchi, MD, PhD*

KEYWORDS

- Acute myeloid leukemia • Pediatrics • Epigenetic • Genomic • Therapy

KEY POINTS

- Pediatric acute myeloid leukemia (AML) has a genomic and epigenetic profile distinct from that of adult AML.
- Somatic mutations and epigenetic alterations contribute to myeloid leukemogenesis, and can evolve from diagnosis to relapse.
- Next-generation sequencing technologies are providing novel insights into the biology of AML and are highlighting potential targets for therapeutic intervention.
- Cytogenetic alterations, somatic mutations, and response to induction therapy contribute to current risk stratification and appropriate therapy allocation.

INTRODUCTION

Acute myeloid leukemia (AML) is a hematopoietic malignancy that is the culmination of genetic and epigenetic alterations in the hematopoietic stem/progenitor cells, leading to dysregulation of critical signal transduction pathways and resulting in the expansion of undifferentiated myeloid cells. AML can be broadly divided into 2 categories, de novo AML and secondary AML. Secondary AML refers to evolution of AML subsequent to prior exposure to cytotoxic therapy or antecedent hematopoietic insufficiency (eg, myelodysplastic syndrome [MDS], marrow failure), leading to evolution of distinct karyotypic and molecular alterations including *MLL* translocations following exposure to topoisomerase inhibitors. In contrast to secondary AML, AML that evolves without a prior cytotoxic exposure is referred to as de novo AML.

Clinical Research Division, Fred Hutchinson Cancer Research Center, 1100 Fairview Avenue North, Seattle, WA 98109, USA
* Corresponding author. 1100 Fairview Avenue North, D5-380, PO Box 19024, Seattle, WA 98109-1024.
E-mail address: smeshinc@fhcrc.org

Pediatr Clin N Am 62 (2015) 75–93
http://dx.doi.org/10.1016/j.pcl.2014.09.007
0031-3955/15/$ – see front matter
pediatric.theclinics.com

Numerous somatic, karyotypic and molecular alterations have been identified in de novo AML; however, despite association of many of these alterations with clinical phenotype, most have no prognostic value, nor do they identify a specific target or a distinct pathway that can be readily exploited for therapeutic intervention. The observed age-associated evolution of molecular alterations reveals a profile for younger children with AML distinct from that of older children and adolescents with AML. Furthermore, the landscape of genetic alterations differs markedly from AML in adults and the paucity of potential therapeutic targets is more notable in childhood AML.

EPIDEMIOLOGY OF ACUTE MYELOID LEUKEMIA

AML is diagnosed in very young children and comprises nearly 25% of pediatric leukemias; however, it is far more prevalent in adults, and is generally considered a disease of older adults whereby the median age at diagnosis is nearly 70 years. Incidence of AML can be better appreciated by close evaluation of the most recent SEER (Surveillance, Epidemiology, and End Results) data. Initial evaluation demonstrates low incidence of AML in children and young adults, with a significant increase in older adults (**Fig. 1A**).[1] However, closer examination of the data demonstrates highest incidence of AML in younger patients (<40 years) to be in infancy with an incidence of 1.6 cases per 100,000, similar to that in the fourth decade of life. After infancy, there is a declining incidence of approximately 0.12 cases per 100,000 per year in the first decade of life (see **Fig. 1B**) to an incidence of 0.4 per 100,000 by age 10. In the following 3 decades, there is a steady increase in AML incidence of approximately 0.02 cases per 100,000 per year to 1.3 cases per 100,000 per year by age 45 years, nearly equivalent to that seen in infants. A substantial increase in the rate of AML diagnosis occurs in the fifth decade to nearly 10 times the observed rate in the previous 3 decades, to an incidence of 6.2 per 100,000 by age 65. After age 65, AML diagnosis increases again substantially, more than 30-fold higher than that seen in younger patients (age 10–40), likely attributable in part to its evolution from an underlying MDS. This epidemiologic observation parallels the underlying known and emerging karyotypic and genomic makeup of AML, and provides insight into the contribution of genomic alterations to the evolution of AML.

Inherited Susceptibility of Acute Myeloid Leukemia

Although AML is a rare event in childhood, there are a wide range of inherited chromosomal and gene defects and marrow failure syndromes that predispose to the development of AML. Some of the more common AML predisposition syndromes include trisomy 21 (Down syndrome [DS]), Fanconi anemia, dyskeratosis congenita (DC), Shwachman-Diamond syndrome (SDS), and Kostmann syndrome (severe congenital neutropenia or SCN). Down syndrome is associated with 10- to 20-fold increased risk of leukemia, as well as high incidence of development of transient myeloproliferative disorder (TMD) in the first 3 months of life that resembles AML, but in most cases the disease undergoes spontaneous resolution.[2] Fanconi anemia is an autosomal recessive disorder caused by mutations in DNA repair genes, and has been estimated to show a cumulative incidence of AML/MDS of approximately 50% by age 40 years.[3] DC is an X-linked disorder caused by mutations in the dyskerin gene, *DKC1*, which is a key subunit of ribosomal RNA processing and the telomerase complex. Autosomal recessive forms of DC exist and are due to mutations in *TERC*, the RNA component of telomerase, or *TERT*, the enzymatic component of telomerase.[4] SDS is an autosomal recessive disorder caused by mutations in the *SBDS*

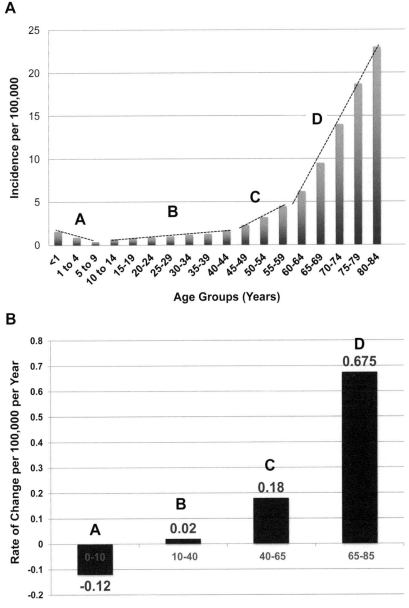

Fig. 1. Incidence of acute myeloid leukemia (AML) by age (A)[1] and rate of change in AML incidence (per 100,000 per year; B) in age groups calculated from **Fig. 1A.**

gene, which functions in ribosome processing and function and is characterized by neutropenia and pancreatic insufficiency.[5] Kostmann syndrome is progressive neutropenia caused by defects in neutrophil elastase (*ELA2*), and is associated with evolution into AML.[6]

GENOMIC LANDSCAPE OF CHILDHOOD ACUTE MYELOID LEUKEMIA

Until recently, most genomic events defined in children were derived from adult studies, thus demonstrating a lower prevalence or lack of such AML-associated genomic lesions in childhood AML.[7] More recently, focused characterization on the somatic genomic changes in childhood AML have provided new insights into the biology of pediatric AML, affording an opportunity to begin to correlate these changes with clinical and biological phenotypes. To date, disease-associated genomic alterations, including translocations, numerical structural alterations (eg, monosomies, trisomies), or sequence variations (mutations, indels), have been used as powerful tools for prediction of response to therapy and outcome in a subset of patients.

Karyotypic Alterations

Cytogenetic alterations have been a cornerstone in the diagnosis of AML, and an invaluable tool for consideration of stratification for treatment based on risk categorization. Although a large number of chromosomal alterations can be identified in AML, most pediatric AML cases separate into distinct cytogenetic categories based on specific chromosomal events: 25% have t(8;21) or Inv(16)/t(16;16), which are collectively referred to as core binding factor AML (CBF AML); 12% have t(15;17); 20% have rearrangements involving the *MLL* gene; and 20% do not have a discernible karyotypic abnormality (normal karyotype). Such cytogenetic alterations have significant age-associated variations (**Fig. 2**), with some highly prevalent in younger patients (eg, *MLL*) and others more prevalent in teenagers (CBF). In addition to karyotypic alterations, disease-associated mutations have been identified in AML; greater than 90% of pediatric AML cases have at least 1 genomic alteration that can be detected by current methods, with the highest fraction occurring in those with a normal karyotype.

Subkaryotypic (cryptic) chromosomal abnormalities

Cytogenetic abnormalities involving large chromosomal regions can be detected by conventional cytogenetics. However, karyotypic analysis in AML is limited by the ability to culture leukemic cells in vitro before analysis in addition to the size of the region involved. Cryptic translocations, those not amenable to identification by conventional karyotyping, may require more specialized techniques such as polymerase chain reaction or fluorescence in situ hybridization studies (FISH) for identification. Several cryptic translocations, including *NUP98/NSD1*, *CBFA2T3/GLIS2*, and *NUP98/KDM5A*, have been discovered recently and shown to be prevalent in children with AML, and may provide significant insight into the pathogenesis of childhood AML.[8–10] Segmental or whole chromosome deletions and their associated

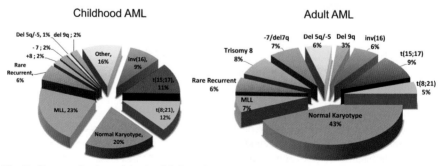

Fig. 2. Karyotypic alterations in childhood versus adult AML.

loss of heterozygosity (LOH) lead to haploinsufficiency of involved genes, and may contribute to malignant transformation. More recent sequencing and array technologies have identified regions of LOH without associated deletions (copy-neutral LOH [CN-LOH]), also referred to as acquired uniparental disomy,[11,12] a homologous recombination-mediated process whereby a homozygous state is achieved after an initial acquisition of a heterozygous mutation. With the use of array and sequencing technologies, regions of CN-LOH have been shown to be prevalent in AML, but their contribution to malignant transformation or progression remains unclear.[13,14]

Somatic Mutations in Childhood Acute Myeloid Leukemia

Somatic mutations in genes known to regulate hematopoiesis have been identified in a significant proportion of AML, and the presence of these mutations has been shown to be associated with clinical outcome. At present, numerous mutations have been implicated in AML pathogenesis, with the number rising with new discovery phase initiatives.[15,16] At present, mutations in 3 genes (*FLT3*, *NPM1*, and *CEBPA*) have been shown to have clinical implications in childhood AML and have been incorporated in clinical trials as prognostic markers, therapeutic targets, or both.

FLT3 mutations

The most commonly mutated gene in childhood AML is FMS-like tyrosine kinase 3 (*FLT3*), which results in constitutive activation of the receptor kinase activity, and can be due to the internal tandem duplication (*FLT3*/ITD) of the juxtamembrane domain coding sequence, or a missense mutation in the activation loop domain (*FLT3*/ALM).[17,18] *FLT3*/ITD is detected in 15% of all children with AML, and has been shown to be highly associated with poor response to induction chemotherapy and high relapse rate.[19,20] Despite biological similarity to *FLT3*/ITD, those with *FLT3*/ALM do not have increased rates of treatment failure.[19] Several studies have shown that patients with *FLT3*/ITD who receive allogeneic stem cell transplantation in complete remission have an improved outcome, thus providing a rationale for therapy allocation in this high-risk cohort of patients.[19,21,22] Furthermore, tyrosine kinase inhibitors (TKI) targeting FLT3 have shown efficacy in inducing high rates of remission in patients with *FLT3*/ITD, although the long-term benefits of such interventions are yet to be determined.[23] In contrast to *FLT3*/ITD, *FLT3*/ALM has not been shown to be similarly amenable to TKI-mediated FLT3 inhibition, which may be in part due to FLT3 conformational changes resulting from the distinct mutations and TKI-binding affinity.[24–26]

Nucleophosmin (NPM1) mutations

NPM1 encodes a ubiquitously expressed molecular chaperone that shuttles rapidly between the nucleus and cytoplasm. Mutations in *NPM1* are common in AML, with a prevalence of 30% in adult and 8% to 10% in pediatric AML.[27–30] *NPM1* mutations appear to be more prevalent in AML with normal karyotype, with a prevalence of nearly 40% to 50% in adults and 20% in pediatric AML. Disease-associated mutations, characterized by 4 base insertions in exon 12 of the *NPM* gene, lead to impaired nuclear localization of the nucleophosmin protein. Presence of *NPM1* mutations portends a favorable outcome with reduced relapse risk and improved survival, similar to the favorable outcome achieved in patients with CBF AML. In pediatric AML, the presence of *NPM1* mutations appears to overlap in a subset of patients with *FLT3*/ITD, and its coexpression seems to partially ameliorate the poor prognosis conferred by *FLT3*/ITD alone.[29]

CEBPA mutations

The *CEBPA* gene encodes CCAAT/enhancer binding protein alpha (C/EBPa), which functions as a transcription factor that regulates granulocytic proliferation and terminal differentiation. Mutations in the *CEBPA* occur in approximately 5% of childhood AML, and most cases with this mutation occur in a biallelic manner whereby two distinct mutations occur, one in the N-terminal domain (NTD) and the second in the opposite allele affecting the bZip domain.[31] Such a biallelic mutation results in the expression of a truncated protein, which has been shown to be sufficient for the development of AML.[32] *CEBPA* mutations tend to occur in patients with normal cytogenetics, and are associated with decreased relapse risk and improved survival.[31]

EPIGENETIC ALTERATIONS

Some of the differences observed in gene and protein expression are regulated by alterations that are not encoded in the genome. Alterations in DNA methylation can lead to silencing of genes, similar to that of a functional mutation. Silencing of the *CEBPA* gene by promoter methylation appears to have a functional consequence similar to that seen with mutations in the *CEBPA* gene[33] and, on a genome-wide scale, altered CpG methylation profiles have been associated with distinct subsets of adult AML.[34] Aberrant methylation can be caused by genomic alterations (mutations, deletions, or translocations) in genes regulating methylation, including a large number of methyltransferase genes (eg, *MLL1*, *DNMT3A*, *TET2*). The strategy of targeting aberrant methylation for therapeutic benefit with demethylating agents is currently under investigation.

AGE-ASSOCIATED GENOMIC VARIATION IN ACUTE MYELOID LEUKEMIA

There is a significant age-associated variation in the incidence of AML, with infants and older adults having an elevated incidence. There is a close association between the biology of AML and its age-based incidence, as evidenced by the significant variability of genomic alterations in AML from infancy to adulthood.

The age-based variation in the prevalence of structural and sequence variations is notable in childhood AML (**Figs. 3** and **4**). Examination of the karyotypic alterations demonstrates significant age-based variation, with *MLL* translocations being highly prevalent in infants whereby those younger than 1 year harbor *MLL* alterations in nearly 60% of cases. This rapid evolution of disease, within weeks to months of birth, signifies the impact and high penetrance of *MLL* translocations in causing leukemia. The *MLL* prevalence declines over the following decade of life to less than 10%, similar to what is observed in younger adults (see **Fig. 3**A). In addition, CBF AML is relatively rare in infants, but increases in prevalence to that seen in adults by the second decade of life. It is notable that CBF AML, which is associated with favorable outcome, decreases in prevalence in older adults. Similarly, patients with normal karyotype are rare in younger patients (likely owing to the high prevalence of *MLL* translocations), and their prevalence increases to nearly adult prevalence of nearly 50% in older pediatric patients.

The aforementioned alterations are present in nearly 70% of all childhood AML; however, less common structural alterations are described with variable biology and prognostic significance. Notable examples are monosomy 7 (-7), monosomy 5, and deletion 5q (-5/del5q), which cumulatively account for 2% to 4% of cases of childhood AML and greater than 10% of adult AML. Although specific genes in these chromosomal regions that contribute to disease pathogenesis have not been identified, the

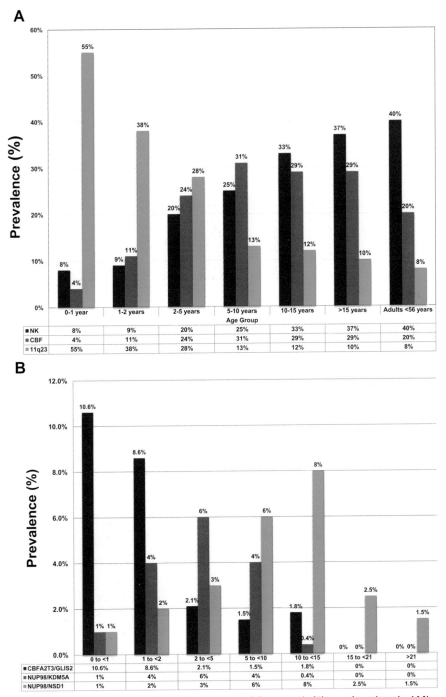

A

Age Group	0-1 year	1-2 years	2-5 years	5-10 years	10-15 years	>15 years	Adults <56 years
NK	8%	9%	20%	25%	33%	37%	40%
CBF	4%	11%	24%	31%	29%	29%	20%
11q23	55%	38%	28%	13%	12%	10%	8%

B

	0 to <1	1 to <2	2 to <5	5 to <10	10 to <15	15 to <21	>21
CBFA2T3/GLIS2	10.6%	8.6%	2.1%	1.5%	1.8%	0%	0%
NUP98/KDM5A	1%	4%	6%	4%	0.4%	0%	0%
NUP98/NSD1	1%	2%	3%	6%	8%	2.5%	1.5%

Fig. 3. Age-based prevalence of specific karyotypic (*A*) or cryptic (*B*) translocations in AML.

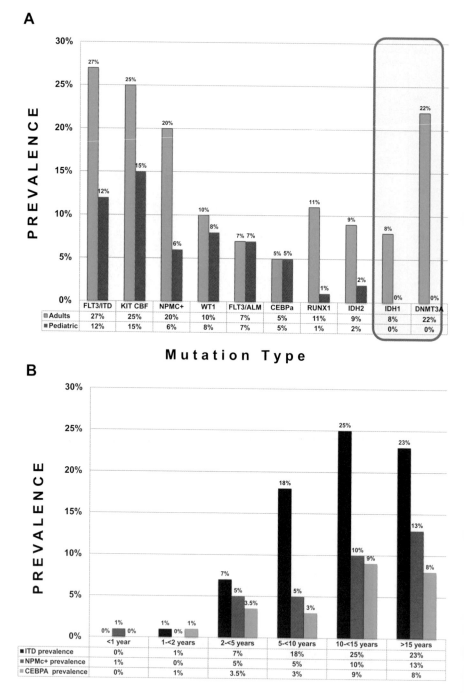

A

Mutation Type

	FLT3/ITD	KIT CBF	NPMC+	WT1	FLT3/ALM	CEBPa	RUNX1	IDH2	IDH1	DNMT3A
Adults	27%	25%	20%	10%	7%	5%	11%	9%	8%	22%
Pediatric	12%	15%	6%	8%	7%	5%	1%	2%	0%	0%

B

Age Group

	<1 year	1-<2 years	2-<5 years	5-<10 years	10-<15 years	>15 years
ITD prevalence	0%	1%	7%	18%	25%	23%
NPMc+ prevalence	1%	0%	5%	5%	10%	13%
CEBPA prevalence	0%	1%	3.5%	3%	9%	8%

Fig. 4. (*A*) Prevalence of AML-associated mutations in pediatric versus adult AML, demonstrating lower incidence of mutations in pediatric AML. Bordered panel shows 2 newly discovered mutations in adults that are absent in pediatric AML. (*B*) Age-based prevalence of common AML-associated mutations.

presence of these alterations is associated with resistance to chemotherapy and extremely poor survival.[35]

Acute promyelocytic leukemia (APL), whereby normal hematopoiesis is replaced by immature granulocytes (promyelocytes), is the consequence of chromosomal translocation between chromosomes 15 and 17 (t(15;17)), involving the PML gene on chromosome 15 and the retinoic acid receptor alpha (*RARα* or *RARA*) gene on chromosome 17 (t(15;17)). The t(15;17) translocation juxtaposes the *PML* and *RARA* gene and leads to the expression of a novel fusion product, which is a potent recruiter of transcriptional repressors, resulting in the arrest of leukemic cells in the immature, promyelocyte stage.[36–38]

Cryptic translocations that previously have gone undetected are emerging as significant contributors to childhood AML, with a relatively high prevalence in younger children and significant decline in adults (see **Fig. 3**B). These cryptic structural events include translocations involving methyltransferase genes (*NSD1* and *KDM5A*), which were not previously implicated in AML pathogenesis. Most notable is the fact that somatic mutations affecting the methylation pathway (*DNMT3A*, *IDH*, *TET2*) are highly prevalent in adults but rare or absent in children (see **Fig. 4**A), whereas structural alterations in methyltransferase genes are prevalent in young children but are rare or absent in adults (see **Fig. 3**B). These data highlight the significant contribution of epigenetic derangements to myeloid leukemogenesis that is achieved by different mechanisms in children in comparison with adults.

Similar to the cytogenetic alterations, sequence variations also vary by age, and, as most of these mutations were identified in adults, these AML-associated genes are rare in pediatric AML. However, assessment of prevalence of these mutations has demonstrated paucity of these mutations at a younger age, with rapid evolution of these lesions to adult prevalence by the second decade of life. For example, mutations in *FLT3*, *NPM*, and *CEBPA* are the most prevalent and clinically relevant mutations in childhood AML but are not usually detected in the first year of life, with increasing age-related prevalence to a level commensurate to what is observed in adults by the second decade of life (see **Fig. 4**B).

In the past decade, advances in next-generation sequencing (NGS) technologies have revolutionized the ability to interrogate cancer genomes, culminating in whole-genome sequencing (WGS), whole-exome sequencing (WES), and transcriptome sequencing (RNA Seq). These approaches provide comprehensive coverage of most of the genome at a single base resolution of the genome, exome, or transcriptome, respectively. WGS, in addition to identifying sequence variations (SNVs and indels), provides additional layers of information, including structural alterations such as deletions, duplications, and inter- and intrachromosomal junctions. Transcriptome sequencing provides sequence and fusion data, in addition to mRNA expression levels that are not available by WGS. NGS technologies have rapidly transformed the genomic landscape in cancer by providing high-throughput, comprehensive genomic profiles in a large number of patients.[39] Ley and colleagues[40] identified *IDH1* and *DNMT3A* to be 2 highly prevalent, clinically significant somatic alterations in adult AML.[15] Despite confirmation of the prevalence and clinical utility of these mutations in adult AML, they appear to be rare or absent in childhood AML (see **Fig. 2**),[41,42] highlighting the significant differences between AML in older and younger patients. More recent data from The Cancer Genome Atlas Research Network (TCGA) AML study demonstrated that 23 genes were significantly mutated in this adult cohort. Of the 23 genes, 14 are well-known mutations in AML that have also been well studied in childhood AML and, with the exception of a few (*FLT3*, *NPM*, *WT1*), have been shown to be rare events in childhood AML.

Based on the significant age-associated differences in somatic alterations in AML, a concerted effort has been devoted to the characterization of genomic and epigenomic profiles for the spectrum of childhood AML. Two such projects, the Children's Oncology Group (COG)/National Cancer Institute (NCI) Therapeutically Applicable Research to Generate Effective Treatments (TARGET) AML initiative, and the St Jude/Washington University Pediatric Cancer Genome Project (PCGP), have initiated comprehensive evaluations of the genomic landscape of childhood AML using currently available NGS approaches.[16,43] Early data emerging from these studies has provided new biological insights, and will only further the investigation of the molecular basis of childhood AML.

Already new insights have emerged from these projects. For instance, based on an analysis of RNA Seq, the St Jude PCGP project evaluated the transcriptome profile of a subset of patients with megakaryocytic leukemia (FAB M7), known to be associated with a poor outcome in children. This study identified a cryptic translocation between CBFA2T3 and GLIS2 genes in nearly 30% of children with FAB M7 AML, and further demonstrated that the CBFA2T3/GLIS2 fusion provides enhanced self-renewal capacity in colony-forming assay and that its presence is associated with adverse outcomes in FAB M7 AML.[9] Subsequent studies have demonstrated the presence of this translocation in other AML subsets and its association with adverse outcome.[44,45]

The COG/NCI-sponsored TARGET AML initiative is using WGS and RNA Seq to establish the genomic profile of childhood AML in a large cohort of children with AML and to establish the nature of genomic evolution of childhood AML from diagnosis to relapse. The pilot phase of the TARGET AML initiative used WES to evaluate diagnostic and relapse specimens from 20 patients who lacked karyotypic high-risk features to identify somatic alterations that contribute to AML pathogenesis, and to study genomic evolution from diagnosis to relapse.[16] In this study, of the 195 distinct nonsynonymous mutations present in 180 genes, mutations in 6 genes were detected in more than 1 patient, including ETV6, KIT, KRAS, and NRAS in 2 patients and TET2 or WT1 in 3 patients, suggesting that, in contrast to adult AML, there may not be a set of highly recurrent mutations in childhood AML. Although most of the identified mutations had been previously described as somatic alterations in pediatric AML, subsequent frequency validation of somatic mutations in ETV6 showed the mutations to be present in 6% of childhood AML and in less than 1% of adult AML. In this study the presence of ETV6 mutations, which were primarily observed in those without previously known risk factors, were highly associated with a significantly higher risk of relapse and worse survival.[46] In addition to identification of the somatic mutations in AML at diagnosis, this study surveyed the genomic landscape at relapse compared with that seen at diagnosis, demonstrating significant clonal evolution from diagnosis to relapse, whereby nearly one-third of total mutations identified at diagnosis persisted at relapse with acquisition of a myriad of new mutations at relapse, indicating significant genomic evolution of diagnostic clone en route to relapse. Furthermore, a large number of diagnostic events, primarily minor and subclonal events, resolved from diagnosis to relapse.[16] These findings were in line with observations in 8 matched diagnostic/relapse pairs previously reported by Ding and colleagues[47] in adult AML using WGS, whereby they identified "founding" clones in the primary tumor that gained novel mutations evolving into the relapse clone. This observation signifies that in addition to the genomic alterations that may lead to disease evolution, additional events, whether genomic or epigenomic, may arise or be selected for, and may mediate resistance to therapy and the emergence of new leukemic clones with a genomic profile distinct from that of the diagnostic one.

THERAPEUTIC APPROACHES IN ACUTE MYELOID LEUKEMIA

Survival in childhood AML has improved from less than 10% to nearly 60% over the last several decades.[48] In the process, several unique genomic subsets of patients have been identified to receive specific therapies based on their unique susceptibilities as a result of their genomic makeup. In particular, the therapeutic approach for AML in patients with DS-AML and those with APL have been tailored to meet the unique susceptibilities to conventional therapy (DS AML) or response to molecularly directed therapy (APL).[2,49]

In APL, identification of its underlying genomic etiology led the discovery that pharmacologic doses of retinoic acid overcome the transcription repression induced by the *PML/RARA* fusion product, allowing for forced differentiation of the leukemic cells along the granulocytic pathway. As a result, APL became the first disease to be treated by a molecularly targeted therapy. With the incorporation of all-*trans* retinoic acid (ATRA) into the conventional therapeutic regimen, survival for APL dramatically improved to 75% to 85%, leading to treatment of APL differently from those having other types of AML.[36] More recently, arsenic trioxide (ATO) was shown to have significant efficacy in the management of APL.[37] Lo-Coco and colleagues[38] demonstrated that in combining ATO with ATRA, all other cytotoxic agents can be safely eliminated from APL therapeutic regimens, maintaining the outstanding survival in APL while sparing the patient the short-term and long-term toxicities of cytotoxic therapies. Understanding the biological basis and genomic alterations of APL allowed for the development of a rational, targeted therapy for this subtype of AML. The resultant fusion transcript can also be used for monitoring response to therapy and predicting relapse as emergence of the fusion transcript can be detected in advance of morphologic relapse, allowing for initiation of treatment at the time of submorphologic disease, thus permitting intervention and improved survival for those with impending relapse.

In those with de novo AML, therapeutic modalities have been based on demonstrated efficacy of anthracycline and the nucleoside analogue class of chemotherapies, whereby combination of daunorubicin and cytarabine remains the mainstay of induction therapy in AML. The current approach to remission induction at diagnosis includes treatment with daunorubicin and cytarabine with or without etoposide at varying doses and schedules. Although this therapy leads to an 80% or higher remission rate, it is also associated with significant cytopenias, leading to toxicities and life-threatening events that may lead to treatment-related mortality (TRM) in 3% to 6% of patients. Use of the 3 + 7 combination of daunorubicin and cytarabine for induction of remission, and postinduction therapy with multiagent drug combinations and high-dose cytarabine, improved the results, however cure rates remained at less than 40% in the early 1980s.[50,51]

Emerging data about the resistance of "dormant" leukemia stem cells (LSC) to chemotherapy (not in cell cycle during exposure) led to attempts at targeting the dormant LSC. Trials led by Woods and colleagues[52] demonstrated that intensifying the induction chemotherapy (time sequential induction), though leading to elevated induction TRM, significantly improved survival by decreasing the postinduction relapse rate. A similar strategy at targeting the LSC using prolonged exposure to cytarabine was conducted by investigators in the United Kingdom,[53] demonstrating overall survival rates similar to those achieved by Woods and colleagues.[54] These studies also demonstrated the efficacy of allogeneic hematopoietic cell transplantation (allo HCT) as a postinduction consolidation strategy in AML, in which those who received postinduction consolidation with allo HCT had a significantly improved survival in comparison with those who received conventional chemotherapy. As a result, postinduction consolidation with allo HCT became the standard of care in those with a matched sibling donors in the United States. Although initial trials limited allo HCT to those with matched sibling donors, evolving improvements in molecular human leukocyte antigen typing, graft-versus-host disease management, and supportive care has led to similar survival in allo HCT from matched unrelated donors and has expanded the population who may benefit from allo HCT. The routine use of autologous stem cell transplantation as a means of consolidation, however, did not show improvement in results over intensified chemotherapy.[55] Current postinduction consolidation uses relapse risk as a determining factor for allocation to the high-risk consolidation arm of the therapy, whereby those deemed to be at a high risk of relapse receive more intensive postinduction chemotherapy followed by allo HCT from the most suitable related or unrelated donor. The clinical trials that led to the current general strategy of therapy for childhood AML were recently reviewed.[56–59] Thus a standard protocol includes cytarabine (10 days), daunorubicin (3 days), and etoposide (3 days), followed by 3 to 4 courses of intensive drug combinations consisting of high-dose cytarabine by itself or with other agents. Unlike in childhood acute lymphoblastic leukemia, central nervous system relapse is uncommon and is well controlled with a single dose of intrathecal cytarabine with each of the drug courses. Prolonged neutropenia is common with standard AML therapy, and requires intensive supportive care to minimize morbidity from bacterial and fungal infections. Because of the unique gram-positive infections from the central lines and cytarabine, special precautions are needed, and some investigators have used antibiotic prophylaxis with some success.[60] With the current improved overall results and better understanding of the risk factors (see the following discussion), allo HCT in first remission is now recommended only to patients at high risk for relapse.[61,62] Therapeutic innovations used for improving the results in high-risk patients include use during induction of high-dose cytarabine ($1–3$ g/m^2/dose $\times$ 6 doses), and use of idarubicin or targeted therapy with gemtuzamab (anti-CD33 antibody) conjugated with ozogamicin.[63–66] Postremission strategies used for modulation of multidrug-resistance gene (MDR1) include cyclosporine and the use of the FLT3 inhibitor, lestaurtinib.[63] These strategies have yielded mixed results. Most promising of these was the unexpected finding that gemtuzamab ozogamicin may improve outcome further in the CBF leukemias.[65]

RISK-BASED THERAPY IN CHILDHOOD ACUTE MYELOID LEUKEMIA

Until recently, cytogenetic alterations were the only means of risk identification in AML, whereby those with CBF AML were understood to have a lower risk of relapse, whereas those with -7 or 5/del5q were at high risk of treatment failure. However, most children with AML lack clinically informative karyotypes and were not amenable to risk-based therapy allocation based solely on cytogenetic subgroups. More recently, somatic mutations in FLT3, NPM1, and CEBPA have been shown to correlate with outcome,[19,30,33] and were incorporated into clinical practice for treatment allocation. Cumulatively, clinically significant cytogenetic alterations and somatic mutations account for nearly 35% of AML in children; however, most children with AML still lack a prognostic biomarker. Although other clinically significant mutations have been demonstrated in adult AML, such mutations are either not seen in childhood AML (eg, IDH1, DNMT3A mutations)[41,42] or are not independently prognostic (WT1 mutations).[67] In patients without an informative genomic biomarker, response to therapy as defined by the presence or absence of minimal residual disease (MRD) based on

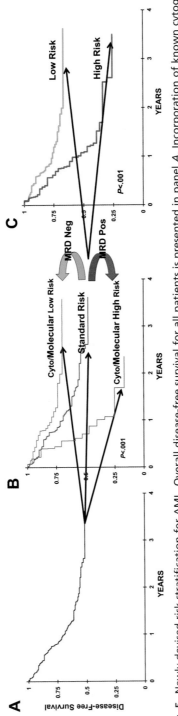
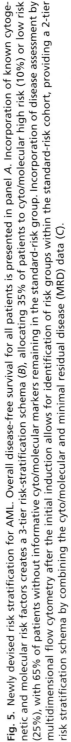

Fig. 5. Newly devised risk stratification for AML. Overall disease-free survival for all patients is presented in panel A. Incorporation of known cytogenetic and molecular risk factors creates a 3-tier risk-stratification schema (B), allocating 35% of patients to cyto/molecular high risk (10%) or low risk (25%), with 65% of patients without informative cyto/molecular markers remaining in the standard-risk group. Incorporation of disease assessment by multidimensional flow cytometry after the initial induction allows for identification of risk groups within the standard-risk cohort, providing a 2-tier risk stratification schema by combining the cyto/molecular and minimal residual disease (MRD) data (C).

detection by multidimensional flow cytometry (MDF) has been used to inform relapse risk.[67,68]

In the ongoing COG de novo AML trial, the combination of diagnostic molecular risk factors with the postinduction response assessment by MRD detection has allowed risk assessment in all patients with AML. This strategy allows for patients with informative molecular markers to be assigned to the appropriate risk class and those lacking any prognostic biomarkers to be risk stratified based on the presence or absence of MRD at the end of induction therapy. Such an approach allows appropriate risk-based therapy allocation for nearly all patients by creating a 2-tier risk allocation system whereby patients are assigned to either a high-risk (cyto/molecular high risk or standard risk with MRD) or low-risk (cyto/molecular low risk or standard risk without MRD) arm based on the most comprehensive set of prognostic data available (**Fig. 5**). This trial is also allocating patients with high-risk *FLT3*/ITD to receive targeted therapy with the addition of sorafenib, a second-generation TKI with FLT3 inhibitory activity, to conventional chemotherapy. Emergence of novel biomarkers will further enhance the existing risk-based therapy schema, whereby those with either high risk of relapse or those with appropriate targets for directed therapy can be allocated to an alternative therapy to optimize outcome and minimize undue toxicity.

SUMMARY

AML is an enormously complex disease characterized by a myriad of genomic and epigenomic alterations that interact to create a wide variety of distinct subtypes with significantly different outcomes. This level of heterogeneity has precluded uniform outcome, given the uniform approach to AML therapy for all patients. Genomic alterations, whether karyotypic abnormalities or specific disease-associated mutations, have been essential in informing clinical decision making. Until recently, genomic profiling only provided clinical prognostic information based on intensity-modulated therapy and, with the exception of *PML-RARA*, there has been a paucity of potential therapeutic targets. More recently, *FLT3*/ITD has emerged as another lesion to potentially benefit from therapeutic targeting. Comprehensive genomic profiling will not only enhance the ability of physicians to provide more individualized prognosis and treatment information to patients with AML, but has the potential to identify lesions that could be targeted for more personalized and directed therapy, negating the need for highly intensive, cytotoxic therapies with their short-term and long-term side effects. New discovery phase initiatives including the NCI-sponsored TARGET AML initiative are aimed at discovering novel biomarkers to be used for more precise risk identification and identify potential therapeutic targets. With the increase in the number of tools for interrogation of the AML genome and epigenome, the ability to allocate patients to individualized therapy directed by the underlying biology of their disease is anticipated. Researchers are emerging from one the most exciting eras in cancer biology in which NGS has provided the tools for comprehensive interrogation of the cancer genome, whose data will be mined for years to come in identifying new biomarkers for risk and target identification, leading to more appropriate risk-based and target-based therapeutic interventions that can make personalized medicine a reality in the near future.

REFERENCES

1. Altekruse S, Kosary C, Krapcho M, et al. SEER cancer statistics review, 1975-2007. Bethesda (MD): National Cancer Institute; 2010. based on November

2009 SEER data submission, posted to the SEER website, 2010. Available at: http://seercancergov/csr/1975_2007/.

2. Ravindranath Y, Abella E, Krischer JP, et al. Acute myeloid leukemia (AML) in Down's syndrome is highly responsive to chemotherapy: experience on Pediatric Oncology Group AML Study 8498. Blood 1992;80(9):2210–4.

3. Alter BP. Cancer in Fanconi anemia, 1927-2001. Cancer 2003;97(2):425–40. http://dx.doi.org/10.1002/cncr.11046.

4. Marrone A, Dokal I. Dyskeratosis congenita: molecular insights into telomerase function, ageing and cancer. Expert Rev Mol Med 2004;6(26):1–23. http://dx. doi.org/10.1017/S1462399404008671.

5. Shimamura A. Shwachman-diamond syndrome. Semin Hematol 2006;43(3): 178–88. http://dx.doi.org/10.1053/j.seminhematol.2006.04.006.

6. Dale DC, Person RE, Bolyard AA, et al. Mutations in the gene encoding neutrophil elastase in congenital and cyclic neutropenia. Blood 2000;96(7): 2317–22.

7. Appelbaum FR, Gundacker H, Head DR, et al. Age and acute myeloid leukemia. Blood 2006;107(9):3481–5. http://dx.doi.org/10.1182/blood-2005-09-3724.

8. Ostronoff F, Othus M, Gerbing RB, et al. Co-expression of NUP98/NSD1 and FLT3/ITD is more prevalent in younger AML patients and leads to high-risk of induction failure: a COG and SWOG report. Blood 2014. http://dx.doi.org/10. 1182/blood-2014-04-570929.

9. Gruber TA, Larson Gedman A, Zhang J, et al. An Inv(16)(p13.3q24.3)-encoded CBFA2T3-GLIS2 fusion protein defines an aggressive subtype of pediatric acute megakaryoblastic leukemia. Cancer Cell 2012;22(5):683–97. http://dx.doi.org/10. 1016/j.ccr.2012.10.007.

10. de Rooij JD, Hollink IH, Arentsen-Peters ST, et al. NUP98/JARID1A is a novel recurrent abnormality in pediatric acute megakaryoblastic leukemia with a distinct HOX gene expression pattern. Leukemia 2013;27(12):2280–8. http://dx. doi.org/10.1038/leu.2013.87.

11. Raghavan M, Smith LL, Lillington DM, et al. Segmental uniparental disomy is a commonly acquired genetic event in relapsed acute myeloid leukemia. Blood 2008;112(3):814–21.

12. Gupta M, Raghavan M, Gale RE, et al. Novel regions of acquired uniparental disomy discovered in acute myeloid leukemia. Genes Chromosomes Cancer 2008;47(9):729–39.

13. Radtke I, Mullighan CG, Ishii M, et al. Genomic analysis reveals few genetic alterations in pediatric acute myeloid leukemia. Proc Natl Acad Sci U S A 2009; 106(31):12944–9. http://dx.doi.org/10.1073/pnas.0903142106. pii:0903142106.

14. Walter MJ, Payton JE, Ries RE, et al. Acquired copy number alterations in adult acute myeloid leukemia genomes. Proc Natl Acad Sci U S A 2009;106(31): 12950–5. http://dx.doi.org/10.1073/pnas.0903091106. pii:0903091106.

15. Mardis ER, Ding L, Dooling DJ, et al. Recurring mutations found by sequencing an acute myeloid leukemia genome. N Engl J Med 2009;361(11):1058–66. http:// dx.doi.org/10.1056/NEJMoa0903840.

16. Meshinchi S, Ries RE, Trevino LR, et al. Identification of novel somatic mutations, regions of recurrent loss of heterozygosity (LOH) and significant clonal evolution from diagnosis to relapse in childhood AML determined by exome capture sequencing - an NCI/COG Target AML Study. ASH Annual Meeting Abstracts 2012;120(21):123.

17. Nakao M, Yokota S, Iwai T, et al. Internal tandem duplication of the flt3 gene found in acute myeloid leukemia. Leukemia 1996;10(12):1911–8.

18. Yamamoto Y, Kiyoi H, Nakano Y, et al. Activating mutation of D835 within the activation loop of FLT3 in human hematologic malignancies. Blood 2001;97(8): 2434–9.

19. Meshinchi S, Alonzo TA, Stirewalt DL, et al. Clinical implications of FLT3 mutations in pediatric AML. Blood 2006;108(12):3654–61.

20. Meshinchi S, Woods WG, Stirewalt DL, et al. Prevalence and prognostic significance of Flt3 internal tandem duplication in pediatric acute myeloid leukemia. Blood 2001;97(1):89–94.

21. Meshinchi S, Arceci RJ, Sanders JE, et al. Role of allogeneic stem cell transplantation in FLT3/ITD-positive AML. Blood 2006;108(1):400 [author reply: 400–1].

22. Bornhauser M, Illmer T, Schaich M, et al. Improved outcome after stem-cell transplantation in FLT3/ITD-positive AML. Blood 2007;109(5):2264–5 [author reply: 2265].

23. Ravandi F, Cortes JE, Jones D, et al. Phase I/II study of combination therapy with sorafenib, idarubicin, and cytarabine in younger patients with acute myeloid leukemia. J Clin Oncol 2010;28(11):1856–62. http://dx.doi.org/10.1200/JCO.2009.25.4888.

24. Kelly LM, Yu JC, Boulton CL, et al. CT53518, a novel selective FLT3 antagonist for the treatment of acute myelogenous leukemia (AML). Cancer Cell 2002;1(5): 421–32.

25. Weisberg E, Boulton C, Kelly LM, et al. Inhibition of mutant FLT3 receptors in leukemia cells by the small molecule tyrosine kinase inhibitor PKC412. Cancer Cell 2002;1(5):433–43.

26. Spiekermann K, Dirschinger RJ, Schwab R, et al. The protein tyrosine kinase inhibitor SU5614 inhibits FLT3 and induces growth arrest and apoptosis in AML-derived cell lines expressing a constitutively activated FLT3. Blood 2003; 101(4):1494–504.

27. Dohner K, Schlenk RF, Habdank M, et al. Mutant nucleophosmin (NPM1) predicts favorable prognosis in younger adults with acute myeloid leukemia and normal cytogenetics: interaction with other gene mutations. Blood 2005;106(12): 3740–6. http://dx.doi.org/10.1182/blood-2005-05-2164. pii:2005-05-2164.

28. Gale RE, Green C, Allen C, et al. The impact of FLT3 internal tandem duplication mutant level, number, size and interaction with NPM1 mutations in a large cohort of young adult patients with acute myeloid leukemia. Blood 2008;111: 2776–84.

29. Hollink IH, Zwaan CM, van den Heuvel-Eibrink MM, et al. Nucleophosmin gene mutations identify a favorable risk group in childhood acute myeloid leukemia with a normal karyotype. ASH Annual Meeting Abstracts 2007;110(11):366.

30. Brown P, McIntyre E, Rau R, et al. The incidence and clinical significance of nucleophosmin mutations in childhood AML. Blood 2007;110(3):979–85. http://dx.doi.org/10.1182/blood-2007-02-076604.

31. Ho PA, Alonzo TA, Gerbing RB, et al. Prevalence and prognostic implications of CEBPA mutations in pediatric acute myeloid leukemia (AML): a report from the Children's Oncology Group. Blood 2009;113(26):6558–66. http://dx.doi.org/10.1182/blood-2008-10-184747.

32. Kirstetter P, Schuster MB, Bereshchenko O, et al. Modeling of C/EBPalpha mutant acute myeloid leukemia reveals a common expression signature of committed myeloid leukemia-initiating cells. Cancer Cell 2008;13(4):299–310. http://dx.doi.org/10.1016/j.ccr.2008.02.008.

33. Wouters BJ, Jorda MA, Keeshan K, et al. Distinct gene expression profiles of acute myeloid/T-lymphoid leukemia with silenced CEBPA and mutations in NOTCH1. Blood 2007;110(10):3706–14.

34. Chen J, Odenike O, Rowley JD. Leukaemogenesis: more than mutant genes. Nat Rev Cancer 2010;10(1):23–36. http://dx.doi.org/10.1038/nrc2765. pii:nrc2765.
35. Hasle H, Alonzo TA, Auvrignon A, et al. Monosomy 7 and deletion 7q in children and adolescents with acute myeloid leukemia: an international retrospective study. Blood 2007;109(11):4641–7. http://dx.doi.org/10.1182/blood-2006-10-051342.
36. Tallman MS, Andersen JW, Schiffer CA, et al. All-trans-retinoic acid in acute promyelocytic leukemia. N Engl J Med 1997;337(15):1021–8.
37. Douer D, Tallman MS. Arsenic trioxide: new clinical experience with an old medication in hematologic malignancies. J Clin Oncol 2005;23(10):2396–410. http://dx.doi.org/10.1200/JCO.2005.10.217.
38. Lo-Coco F, Avvisati G, Vignetti M, et al. Gruppo Italiano Malattie Ematologiche dell'Adulto, German-Austrian Acute Myeloid Leukemia Study Group, Study Alliance Leukemia. Retinoic acid and arsenic trioxide for acute promyelocytic leukemia. N Engl J Med 2013;369(2):111–21. http://dx.doi.org/10.1056/NEJMoa1300874.
39. Ley TJ, Mardis ER, Ding L, et al. DNA sequencing of a cytogenetically normal acute myeloid leukaemia genome. Nature 2008;456(7218):66–72. http://dx.doi.org/10.1038/nature07485. pii:nature07485.
40. Ley TJ, Ding L, Walter MJ, et al. DNMT3A mutations in acute myeloid leukemia. N Engl J Med 2010;363(25):2424–33. http://dx.doi.org/10.1056/NEJMoa1005143.
41. Ho PA, Alonzo TA, Kopecky KJ, et al. Molecular alterations of the IDH1 gene in AML: a Children's Oncology Group and Southwest Oncology Group study. Leukemia 2010;24(5):909–13. http://dx.doi.org/10.1038/leu.2010.56.
42. Ho PA, Kutny MA, Alonzo TA, et al. Leukemic mutations in the methylation-associated genes DNMT3A and IDH2 are rare events in pediatric AML: a report from the Children's Oncology Group. Pediatr Blood Cancer 2011;57(2):204–9. http://dx.doi.org/10.1002/pbc.23179.
43. Downing JR, Wilson RK, Zhang J, et al. The pediatric cancer genome project. Nat Genet 2012;44(6):619–22. http://dx.doi.org/10.1038/ng.2287.
44. Schuback HL, Alonzo T, Gerbing R, et al. CBFA2T3-GLIS2 fusion is prevalent in younger patients with acute myeloid leukemia and associated with high risk of relapse and poor outcome: A Children's Oncology Group Report. ASH Annual Meeting Abstracts 2014.
45. Masetti R, Pigazzi M, Togni M, et al. CBFA2T3-GLIS2 fusion transcript is a novel common feature in pediatric, cytogenetically normal AML, not restricted to FAB M7 subtype. Blood 2013;121(17):3469–72. http://dx.doi.org/10.1182/blood-2012-11-469825.
46. Helton HL, Ries RE, Alonzo TA, et al. Clinically significant mutations, deletions and translocations involving ETV6 identified by whole genome and whole exome sequencing; report from NCI/COG target AML initiative. ASH Annual Meeting Abstracts 2012;120(21):125.
47. Ding L, Ley TJ, Larson DE, et al. Clonal evolution in relapsed acute myeloid leukaemia revealed by whole-genome sequencing. Nature 2012;481(7382):506–10. http://dx.doi.org/10.1038/nature10738.
48. Gamis AS, Alonzo TA, Perentesis JP, et al. Children's Oncology Group's 2013 blueprint for research: acute myeloid leukemia. Pediatr Blood Cancer 2012. http://dx.doi.org/10.1002/pbc.24432.
49. Degos L, Dombret H, Chomienne C, et al. All-trans-retinoic acid as a differentiating agent in the treatment of acute promyelocytic leukemia. Blood 1995;85(10):2643–53.

50. Weinstein HJ, Mayer RJ, Rosenthal DS, et al. Chemotherapy for acute myelogenous leukemia in children and adults: VAPA update. Blood 1983;62(2):315–9.
51. Ravindranath Y, Steuber CP, Krischer J, et al. High-dose cytarabine for intensification of early therapy of childhood acute myeloid leukemia: a Pediatric Oncology Group study. J Clin Oncol 1991;9(4):572–80.
52. Woods WG, Kobrinsky N, Buckley JD, et al. Timed-sequential induction therapy improves postremission outcome in acute myeloid leukemia: a report from the Children's Cancer Group. Blood 1996;87(12):4979–89.
53. Stevens RF, Hann IM, Wheatley K, et al. Marked improvements in outcome with chemotherapy alone in paediatric acute myeloid leukaemia: results of the United Kingdom Medical Research Council's 10th AML trial. MRC Childhood Leukaemia Working Party. Br J Haematol 1998;101(1):130–40.
54. Woods WG, Neudorf S, Gold S, et al. A comparison of allogeneic bone marrow transplantation, autologous bone marrow transplantation, and aggressive chemotherapy in children with acute myeloid leukemia in remission. Blood 2001;97(1):56–62.
55. Ravindranath Y, Yeager AM, Chang MN, et al. Autologous bone marrow transplantation versus intensive consolidation chemotherapy for acute myeloid leukemia in childhood. Pediatric Oncology Group. N Engl J Med 1996;334(22):1428–34. http://dx.doi.org/10.1056/NEJM199605303342203.
56. Ravindranath Y, Chang M, Steuber CP, et al, Pediatric Oncology Group. Pediatric Oncology Group (POG) studies of acute myeloid leukemia (AML): a review of four consecutive childhood AML trials conducted between 1981 and 2000. Leukemia 2005;19(12):2101–16. http://dx.doi.org/10.1038/sj.leu.2403927.
57. Creutzig U, Zimmermann M, Ritter J, et al. Treatment strategies and long-term results in paediatric patients treated in four consecutive AML-BFM trials. Leukemia 2005;19(12):2030–42. http://dx.doi.org/10.1038/sj.leu.2403920.
58. Gibson BE, Wheatley K, Hann IM, et al. Treatment strategy and long-term results in paediatric patients treated in consecutive UK AML trials. Leukemia 2005;19(12):2130–8. http://dx.doi.org/10.1038/sj.leu.2403924.
59. Smith FO, Alonzo TA, Gerbing RB, et al. Long-term results of children with acute myeloid leukemia: a report of three consecutive Phase III trials by the Children's Cancer Group: CCG 251, CCG 213 and CCG 2891. Leukemia 2005;19(12):2054–62. http://dx.doi.org/10.1038/sj.leu.2403925.
60. Kurt B, Flynn P, Shenep JL, et al. Prophylactic antibiotics reduce morbidity due to septicemia during intensive treatment for pediatric acute myeloid leukemia. Cancer 2008;113(2):376–82. http://dx.doi.org/10.1002/cncr.23563.
61. Oliansky DM, Rizzo JD, Aplan PD, et al. The role of cytotoxic therapy with hematopoietic stem cell transplantation in the therapy of acute myeloid leukemia in children: an evidence-based review. Biol Blood Marrow Transplant 2007;13(1):1–25. http://dx.doi.org/10.1016/j.bbmt.2006.10.024.
62. Horan JT, Alonzo TA, Lyman GH, et al. Impact of disease risk on efficacy of matched related bone marrow transplantation for pediatric acute myeloid leukemia: the Children's Oncology Group. J Clin Oncol 2008;26(35):5797–801. http://dx.doi.org/10.1200/JCO.2007.13.5244.
63. Becton D, Dahl GV, Ravindranath Y, et al. Randomized use of cyclosporin A (CsA) to modulate P-glycoprotein in children with AML in remission: Pediatric Oncology Group Study 9421. Blood 2006;107(4):1315–24. http://dx.doi.org/10.1182/blood-2004-08-3218.
64. Creutzig U, Ritter J, Zimmermann M, et al. Improved treatment results in high-risk pediatric acute myeloid leukemia patients after intensification with high-dose

cytarabine and mitoxantrone: results of Study Acute Myeloid Leukemia-Berlin-Frankfurt-Munster 93. J Clin Oncol 2001;19(10):2705–13.

65. Gamis AS, Alonzo TA, Meshinchi S, et al. Gemtuzumab ozogamicin in children and adolescents with de novo acute myeloid leukemia improves event-free survival by reducing relapse risk: results from the randomized phase III Children's Oncology Group Trial AAML0531. J Clin Oncol 2014. http://dx.doi.org/10.1200/JCO.2014.55.3628.

66. Ho PA, Zeng R, Alonzo TA, et al. Prevalence and prognostic implications of WT1 mutations in pediatric acute myeloid leukemia (AML): a report from the Children's Oncology Group. Blood 2010;116(5):702–10. http://dx.doi.org/10.1182/blood-2010-02-268953.

67. Loken MR, Alonzo TA, Pardo L, et al. Residual disease detected by multidimensional flow cytometry signifies high relapse risk in patients with de novo acute myeloid leukemia: a report from Children's Oncology Group. Blood 2012; 120(8):1581–8. http://dx.doi.org/10.1182/blood-2012-02-408336.

68. San Miguel JF, Vidriales MB, Lopez-Berges C, et al. Early immunophenotypical evaluation of minimal residual disease in acute myeloid leukemia identifies different patient risk groups and may contribute to postinduction treatment stratification. Blood 2001;98(6):1746–51.

Juvenile Myelomonocytic Leukemia

CrossMark

Prakash Satwani, MD[a],*, Justine Kahn, MD[b], Christopher C. Dvorak, MD[c]

KEYWORDS

- RAS pathways • PTPN11mutation • Allogeneic hematopoietic cell transplantation
- Children • Leukemia

KEY POINTS

- Juvenile myelomonocytic leukemia (JMML) is a rare myeloid malignancy that occurs only in young children and has a variable clinical course.
- The pathogenesis of JMML involves hyperactivation of the RAS pathways.
- Significant progress has been made in understanding aspects of the molecular basis of JMML. It is now known that 85% to 90% of patients can be firmly diagnosed with the help of molecular studies.
- Allogeneic hematopoietic stem cell transplant is the only curative option for children with JMML, and unfortunately it is an option fraught with frequent relapse and significant toxicity.

INTRODUCTION

Juvenile myelomonocytic leukemia (JMML) is a rare myeloid malignancy that occurs in young children. Similar to other myeloid neoplasms, such as chronic myeloid leukemia (CML) and some cases of acute myeloid leukemia (AML), or to premalignant disorders, such as myelodysplastic syndrome (MDS), JMML is a disorder of myeloid progenitors, or stem cells.

Because of its rarity and because of its varied clinical presentations, JMML is often difficult for general pediatricians, pediatric oncologists, and even for hematopathologists to diagnose. Clinically, a child with JMML may exhibit symptoms that suggest a

Financial Disclosure Statement: None.
[a] Division of Pediatric Hematology/Oncology and Stem Cell Transplantation, Columbia University Medical Center Morgan Stanley Children's Hospital of New York-Presbyterian, 3959 Broadway, CHN-1002, New York, NY 10032, USA; [b] Division of Pediatric Hematology/Oncology and Stem Cell Transplantation, Columbia University Medical Center Morgan Stanley Children's Hospital of New York-Presbyterian, 3959 Broadway, CHN-1002, New York, NY 10032, USA; [c] Division of Pediatric Allergy, Immunology, and Bone Marrow Transplant, Benioff Children's Hospital, University of California San Francisco, 505 Parnassus Ave., M-659, San Francisco, CA, 94143-1278, USA
* Corresponding author.
E-mail address: ps2087@columbia.edu

common viral syndrome. Blood counts and hematologic features may mimic AML. Over the last decade, however, significant progress has been made toward understanding the unique molecular mechanisms and features that render JMML distinct from similar conditions.

EPIDEMIOLOGY, NOMENCLATURE, CLINICAL PRESENTATION, AND DIFFERENTIAL DIAGNOSIS

Epidemiology

JMML is a rare pediatric disease with an annual incidence of approximately 1.2–1.8 cases per million in the United States.[1,2] More recent data suggest that this is an underestimate, because JMML is frequently misclassified and misdiagnosed. Chan and colleagues[3] suggest that based on recently established clinical, cytogenetic, and molecular characteristics, the incidence of JMML in the coming years will increase because of improved diagnostics. Certain genetic syndromes are associated with a propensity to develop JMML or JMML-like disease. The incidence of true JMML is increased 200- to 500-fold in neurofibromatosis (NF)-1.[4] Conversely, some children with Noonan syndrome (NS) display a hematologic phenotype, including a self-resolving myeloproliferative disorder in infancy, which resembles JMML and may last for 1 to 2 years.[5,6]

Clinical Presentation

JMML most often occurs in children younger than 2 years old, and almost always before puberty. Children affected with JMML usually present with fever, respiratory symptoms, skin rash, and hepatosplenomegaly. In children with high burden of disease, hepatosplenomegaly may be significant and respiratory symptoms may be severe. JMML can be associated with NF-1 and in these patients the classic café-au-lait spots may take on a slightly unusual form. Laboratory tests are significant for elevated white blood cell counts with an atypical monocytosis and associated thrombocytopenia. Immature granulocytic precursors and nucleated red cells are evident in most cases, and the peripheral blood blast cell percentage averages 2% and rarely exceeds 20%.[7] The diagnosis of JMML is supported when, in the setting of the previously mentioned symptoms, a patient has an absolute monocyte count exceeding 1×10^9/L in the peripheral blood. However, other possible causes, such as CML, must be excluded.

Bone marrow aspirate is not always required to make the diagnosis of JMML; however, it can be suggestive of the diagnosis in the right clinical setting. Unlike in AML, the bone marrow in patients with JMML demonstrates no blockage of differentiation of myeloid elements (**Fig. 1**). Rather, as is seen in CML, the bone marrow in JMML exhibits myeloid hyperplasia with granulocytic cells at varying stages of maturation. The marrow blast count may be slightly elevated but in classic JMML it does not reach the counts seen in AML. Rare cases of JMML have been described with a predominance of erythroid precursors in the marrow and mimicking acute erythroblastic leukemia. Megakaryocytes are reduced in number and this is mirrored by evidence of thrombocytopenia in the peripheral blood. Of interest, monocytosis seen in the bone marrow is less pronounced than it is in the peripheral blood.[7]

Differential Diagnosis

At initial presentation JMML is difficult to distinguish from other more common illnesses. Young infants with viral infections, such as human herpes virus-6, parvovirus, or cytomegalovirus, can present with clinical and hematologic features similar to those of JMML. Occasionally, patients with JMML may present with these viral infections in addition to their underlying hematologic malignancy. Very young boys with Wiskott-Aldrich syndrome can occasionally present with clinical features mimicking JMML.[8]

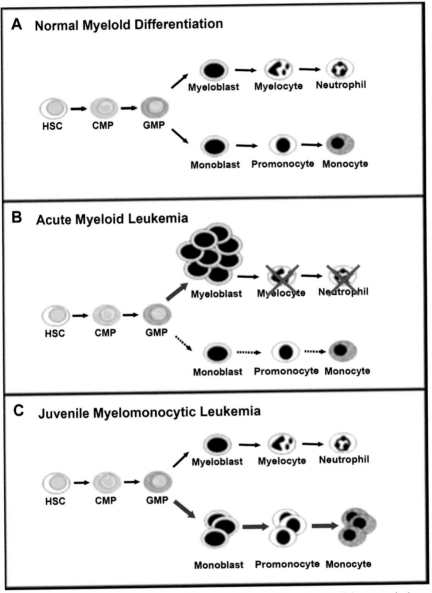

Fig. 1. Schematic diagram of (A) normal hematopoietic differentiation; (B) accumulation of undifferentiated myeloblasts representing acute myeloid leukemia; and (C) increased production of monocytic cells along the full spectrum of differentiation, including blast forms, promonocytes, monocytes, and macrophages, as observed in juvenile myelomonocytic leukemia. CMP, common myeloid progenitor; GMP, granulocyte monocyte progenitor; HSC, hematopoietic stem cell. (*From* Chan RJ, Cooper T, Kratz CP, et al. Juvenile myelomonocytic leukemia: a report from the 2nd International JMML Symposium. Leuk Res 2009;33(3):356; with permission.)

CML, although rare in children, can present with clinical and laboratory features, such as splenomegaly and high white blood cell count with monocytosis, which can render it difficult to distinguish from JMML in the absence of formal testing for the Philadelphia chromosome. AML may also present this way and thus a bone marrow aspirate and biopsy may be required to differentiate the two diseases, because this has prognostic implications. That said, approximately 85% to 90% of patients with JMML have associated cytogenetic and/or molecular abnormalities that are extremely helpful in distinguishing it from viral infections or other leukemias.[9]

Once the diagnosis of JMML is made its clinical course can be variable.[10] Although one-third of patients have a rapidly progressive disease, another third of the patients may have a relatively indolent course.[11] In patients not receiving allogeneic hematopoietic cell transplantation (AlloHCT), the median survival after diagnosis is less than 12 months and the probability of survival at 10 years is only 6%.[12]

Approximately 15% of patients with a diagnosis of JMML eventually progress to AML in a phenomenon referred to as "blast crisis."[13] Rare patients who have certain NRAS or KRAS mutations (glycine to serine substitution) can have spontaneous resolution of the disease,[14] as can some patients with mutations in Casitas B-cell lymphoma (CBL).[15]

CELLULAR BASIS OF JUVENILE MYELOMONOCYTIC LEUKEMIA

JMML is considered a clonal disease originating in pluripotent stem cells of the hematopoietic system. The disease is characterized by clonal proliferation of myeloid, erythroid, and occasionally lymphoid progenitor cells.[16,17]

Using clonality assays based on the differential DNA methylation of X chromosomes and on the detection of a transcriptional polymorphism of the active X chromosome, Busque and colleagues[16] demonstrated the monoclonal origin of JMML (CD34[+]/CD38) cells granulocytes, monocytes, erythroid progenitors, and megakaryocytes. The pathogenesis of JMML involves disruption of signal transduction through the RAS pathway, with resultant selective hypersensitivity of JMML cells to granulocyte-macrophage colony–stimulating factor (GM-CSF).[9]

MOLECULAR ABERRATIONS IN JUVENILE MYELOMONOCYTIC LEUKEMIA

In vitro hypersensitivity to GM-CSF is one of the criteria for the diagnosis of JMML.[4] However, specific molecular aberrations in GM-CSF receptors have never been clearly implicated in the pathogenesis of the disease. RAS proteins are signaling molecules that regulate cellular proliferation and differentiation by switching between an active guanosine triphosphate (GTP)–bound RAS and inactive guanosine diphosphate RAS form. Proteins encoded by the genes of the RAS family play a role in the transduction of extracellular signals to the nucleus and control proliferation and differentiation of many cell types (**Fig. 2**). GM-CSF hypersensitivity results from continuous activation of the GM-CSF receptor–RAS-RAF-MEK-ERK signal transduction pathway.[18] The active GTP RAS activates the RAF kinase, resulting in a downstream proliferative effect (see **Fig. 2**). In JMML, somatic mutations in this pathway are frequent and result in continuous activation and cell proliferation.[18]

Mutations in RAS genes are found in 20% to 30% of all human malignancies.[18] The RAS subfamily includes three members: HRAS, KRAS, and NRAS. In one study, 25% of patients with JMML were found to have a somatic NRAS or KRAS point mutation.[19] In one-quarter of all JMML cases, activating point mutations are found in codon 12, 13, and 61 of NRAS and KRAS resulting in a continuous activation of the RAS pathway. Somatic mutations in HRAS have not been associated with JMML.

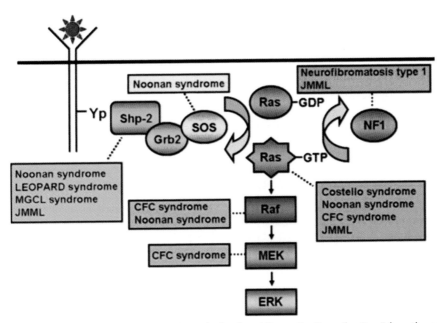

Fig. 2. Schematic diagram showing ligand-stimulated Ras activation, the Ras-Erk pathway, and the gene mutations found to date contributing to the neurocardio-facio-cutaneous congenital disorders and JMML. CFC, cardia-facio-cutaneous; NL/MGCL, Noonan-like/multiple giant cell lesion. (*From* Chan RJ, Cooper T, Kratz CP, et al. Juvenile myelomonocytic leukemia: a report from the 2nd International JMML Symposium. Leuk Res 2009;33(3): 357; with permission.)

GENETIC SYNDROMES AND JUVENILE MYELOMONOCYTIC LEUKEMIA

NF-1 and NS have been instrumental in elucidating key components of the molecular pathogenesis of JMML.[5,20] These genetic syndromes have germline aberrations of the RAS pathway and analysis of their pathophysiology has allowed for improved understanding of JMML pathogenesis and has enabled molecular diagnosis in 85% to 90% of cases.[7]

In 1978 Bader and Miller[21] noted that children affected by NF-1 were particularly prone to developing a CML or AML in the first decade of life. The NF-1 gene acts as a tumor suppressor gene and encodes neurofibromin protein. Absence of normal neurofibromin results in a relative increase in Ras-GTP and elevated levels of Ras-GTP may lead to myeloproliferative neoplasm.[22]

Approximately 50% of children with NS have a missense germline mutation in PTPN11 gene at chromosome 12q24.[23] Approximately 35% of patients with JMML have somatic PTPN11 mutations.[24] In JMML, gain-of-function PTPN11 mutations affect SHP2 protein, which leads to constitutive activation of RAS pathways.[25]

A comparison of the PTPN11 mutations in de novo and syndromic JMML (NS) reveals that many of the same codons in exons 3, 4, and 13 are affected.[26] The precise codon substitutions, however, are distinct. The most common PTPN11 mutation in de novo JMML is the c. 226G>A, which results in E76K, an alteration that has never been documented as a germline lesion in NS. This difference in spectrum and distribution of PTPN11 mutations between de novo JMML and NS may be partly responsible for the different clinical course of myeloproliferation observed in these two groups of patients.[26]

CASITAS B-CELL LYMPHOMA MUTATION

Mutations in CBL were recently described in 17% of patients with JMML who were negative for NF-1, PTPN11, and RAS mutations.[27] Mutations in c-CBL have been shown to result in continuous activation of RAS. The clinical course of JMML with associated c-CBL mutation is of particular interest. In patients with JMML and homozygous CBL mutations, high rates of spontaneous disease resolution have been reported.[28,29] These patients, however, are at increased risk for the development of vasculopathies in the second decade of life unless they undergo AlloHCT. The most frequently observed vasculopathies are optic atrophy, hypertension, cardiomyopathy, and arteritis.[26]

CHROMOSOMAL ABERRATIONS IN JUVENILE MYELOMONOCYTIC LEUKEMIA

Two-thirds of patients with JMML have a completely normal karyotype. Of those who do not have a normal karyotype, the most common chromosomal abnormalities are monosomy 7 or deletion 7q (-/del[7q]).[11] Other rare chromosomal abnormalities observed in patients with JMML are deletion 5q, t(1;5) and 46,XX,der(12)t(3;12).[11] Specific genes associated with these chromosome breakpoints have yet to be identified, and thus their clinical significance remains to be determined.

ESTABLISHING THE DIAGNOSIS OF JUVENILE MYELOMONOCYTIC LEUKEMIA

An understanding of the clinical features and molecular aberrations in JMML is essential in making the diagnosis. In December 2007 the Second International JMML Symposium was held in Atlanta, Georgia. At this meeting, leading experts in JMML established a new set of guidelines for diagnosis of JMML (**Table 1**).[3]

PROGNOSTIC FACTORS IN JUVENILE MYELOMONOCYTIC LEUKEMIA

Unlike in CML, significant advances in understanding the molecular basis of JMML have yet to translate into significant improvement in survival. Because of the disease's rarity, only a small number of patients have been studied in a few retrospective studies and thus clear prognostic factors have not been established. There are a series of

Table 1		
Juvenile myelomonocytic leukemia diagnostic criteria		
Category 1	**Category 2**	**Category 3**
All of the following	At least one of the following	At least two of the following
Splenomegaly[a]	Somatic mutation in *RAS* or	circulating myeloid precursors
Absolute monocyte	*PTPN11*	White blood cells >10,000/μL
count >1000/μL	Clinical diagnosis of NF-1 or	Increased fetal hemoglobin
Blasts in peripheral blood/	*NF1* gene mutation	for age
bone marrow <20%	Homozygous mutation in *CBL*	Clonal cytogenetic
Absence of the t(9;22) *BCR/*	Monosomy 7	abnormality excluding
ABL fusion gene		monosomy 7
		GM-CSF hypersensitivity

The diagnosis of JMML can be made if a patient meets all of the Category 1 criteria and one of the Category 2 criteria. If there are no Category 2 criteria met, then the Category 3 criteria must be met.
  [a] For the 7% to 10% of patients without splenomegaly, the diagnostic criteria must include all other features in Category 1 plus either one of the parameters in Category 2 or two features in Category 3.
  (*Modified from* Chan RJ, Cooper T, Kratz CP, et al. Juvenile myelomonocytic leukemia: a report from the 2nd International JMML Symposium. Leuk Res 2009;33(3):358; with permission.)

clinical and molecular characteristics that have been identified as contributing factors to the prognosis of a patient with JMML. It is well documented that patients who present in JMML blast crisis have a dismal prognosis. Older patients (>4 years at the time of diagnosis) also tend to have a poorer prognosis; however, age cutoff as a prognostic risk factor varies between 1.4 and 4 years depending on the study.[30,31] One Japanese study demonstrated that PTPN11 was associated with poor prognosis.[32] However, in the larger European Working Group of MDS and JMML in Childhood (EWOG-MDS) and Eurocord studies, PTPN11 mutation was not associated with poor prognosis.[28,29] Low platelet count (<40 × 10⁹/L) and fetal hemoglobin greater than 40% at the diagnosis may also be associated with poor prognosis.[1,28] Evidence for monosomy 7 as a risk factor for poor prognosis is conflicting.[28–30]

In a recent study published by Bresolin and colleagues[33] 44 cases of JMML were classified as AML-like and non–AML-like based on specific gene expression criteria. In this group of patients, those who had genetic aberrations rendering their disease AML-like (ie, monosomy 7) had significantly poorer outcomes than their non–AML-like counterparts (10-year overall survival, 7% vs 74%; $P = .0005$). Outcomes after AlloHCT were similarly dismal in the AML-like cohort with 81% of patients experiencing relapse. Bresolin thus suggests that identifying specific gene expressions in JMML cases may be used to classify the disease into risk categories and thus to guide treatment decisions based on these prognostic indicators.

MANAGEMENT OF JUVENILE MYELOMONOCYTIC LEUKEMIA PREALLOGENEIC HEMATOPOIETIC STEM CELL TRANSPLANTATION

To date AlloHCT is the only curative therapy available for most patients diagnosed with JMML. From the time of initial disease presentation it takes approximately 1 to 3 months until the initiation of conditioning for AlloHCT. Because JMML has a variable clinical course, the rapidity with which one proceeds to transplant depends first on the patient's clinical status.

Children who are clinically stable can be observed or receive 6-mercaptopurine either alone or in combination with other drugs. The common treatment approach for stable patients with confirmed JMML is the administration of 6-mercaptopurine (50 mg/m²/day) with or without cis-retinoic acid or low-dose intravenous cytarabine.[15,34] Patients who do not respond to 6-mercaptopurine or who present with more severe symptomatology are administered high-dose cytarabine (2 g/m²/day × 5 days) plus fludarabine (FLU; 30 mg/m²/day × 5 days) to temporize the clinical course. After receiving chemotherapy patients should be closely monitored for pulmonary rebound.

THE IMPACT OF RECEIVING CHEMOTHERAPY PREALLOGENEIC HEMATOPOIETIC STEM CELL TRANSPLANTATION

Theoretically, as is the case with other hematologic malignancies, chemotherapy administered for JMML before AlloHCT should decrease disease burden and by extension, should decrease relapse rates. Only a handful of studies with relatively small numbers have analyzed the relationship between pre-AlloHCT chemotherapy and AlloHCT outcome and thus there is no conclusive evidence regarding the survival benefit of receiving chemotherapy pretransplant.[28,30] In the previously mentioned studies the pretransplant treatment regimens were not identical (low- vs high-dose chemotherapy). Additionally, patients with JMML in blast crisis do poorly regardless of pre-HCT chemotherapy and the inclusion of these patients may have skewed the results.

The current prospective clinical trial for JMML run by the Children's Oncology Group (COG) Study ASCT-1221(NCT01824693) is measuring allelic disease burden (copy numbers of mutated genes) before AlloHCT.[35] The hope is that information gathered from this prospective study will aid in understanding the clinical impact of either receiving or not receiving pretransplant chemotherapy.

TARGETED THERAPY PREALLOGENEIC HEMATOPOIETIC STEM CELL TRANSPLANTATION

In CML, an understanding of the molecular mechanisms implicated in the disease process has revolutionized the treatment of this cancer by enabling the use of targeted therapy. However, targeted treatment of JMML continues to lag behind CML in this regard. Despite significant advances in deciphering molecular pathways involved in JMML, targeted therapy has not shown promising results. Because RAS/MAPK pathways are most critical in pathogenesis of JMML, inhibition of RAS/MAPK pathways would be the most logical target. Tipifarnib (Zarnestra) is a farnesyl transferase inhibitor. In a 2001 COG study (AAML0122 trial), patients with JMML received tipifarnib before AlloHCT but this was not associated with improved disease-free survival compared with patients who did not receive this drug (Stieglitz E, 2014, unpublished data).

Studies in NF1 and KRAS mutant mice have demonstrated promising results with MEK inhibitors.[36,37] Aberrant DNA methylation has also been associated with increased risk of relapse in patients with JMML and azacitidine, a DNA hypomethylating agent, proved effective in one patient with monosomy 7 and an associated KRAS mutation.[38]

ADDITIONALLY MANAGEMENT QUERIES: SPLENECTOMY IN JUVENILE MYELOMONOCYTIC LEUKEMIA

Splenectomy is associated with an increased risk of infections with encapsulated organisms. Splenectomy in patients with JMML is sometimes used to decrease disease burden and improve transplant outcomes. However, the role of splenectomy in the management of JMML is controversial. In the setting of AlloHCT, enlarged spleens may potentially interfere with engraftment because of sequestration of infused stem cells. Two large studies addressed the impact of splenectomy on the outcomes of patients with JMML. The first, EWOG-MDS study, looked at spleen size (<5 cm vs >5 cm) and demonstrated that splenectomy did not have an impact on the relapse incidence or transplant-related mortality (TRM).[30] In the Eurocord study, there was a trend toward an improved event-free survival in patients who underwent splenectomy compared with patients who did not (56% vs 36%; $P = .098$).[31] One potential explanation for this finding is that patients receiving umbilical cord blood had relatively smaller cell doses infused and this, in the presence of an enlarged spleen, could have resulted in slow or no engraftment. Ultimately, this could have led to an increase in TRM secondary to slow (or no) donor immune reconstitution and thus may have contributed to increased incidence of relapse. Patients receiving umbilical cord blood transplant may potentially benefit from splenectomy or from splenic shrinkage with radiation. This subject matter needs further evaluation.

ALLOGENEIC HEMATOPOIETIC CELL TRANSPLANTATION IN PATIENTS WITH JUVENILE MYELOMONOCYTIC LEUKEMIA

At present, AlloHCT is the only curative therapy available for most patients with JMML. However, even with transplant, the cure rates of JMML remain suboptimal. The largest study of JMML and transplant looked at 100 patients and was published by EWOG-MDS.[30] This study demonstrated a 5-year event-free survival of only 52%.

There are two major obstacles impeding the success of AlloHCT for JMML: relapse and TRM. Because most patients have significant disease burden before AlloHCT, one might speculate that myeloablative conditioning regimens could be of benefit and result in fewer relapses. However, myeloablative conditioning regimens in infants and young children are associated with significant transplant-related morbidity and mortality.

The EWOG-MD trial used a conditioning regimen consisting of busulfan (BU) at myeloablative doses (16–20 mg/kg orally over 4 days), cyclophosphamide (CY; 120 mg/kg over 2 days), and melphalan (MEL; 140 mg/m^2).[30] The COG AAML0122 trial used a conditioning regimen consisting of CY (120 mg/kg over 2 days) and 1200-cGy total body irradiation but compliance was poor with the intended total body irradiation regimen, particularly after the BU-based EWOG-MDS trial was published. Given that the average age of children with JMML is 2 years old, the young age at AlloHCT renders it preferable to avoid total body irradiation–based regimens so as to avoid long-term endocrine and neurocognitive damage.

Despite the intense conditioning regimen used in EWOG-MDS, the 5-year cumulative incidence of TRM and JMML recurrence were 13% and 35%, respectively.[30] Further intensifying conditioning regimen may not decrease relapses but may potentially increase morbidity and mortality after AlloHCT and thus the risks of either choice must be weighed accordingly.

Bartelink and colleagues[39] compared a reduced toxicity but myeloablative regimen consisting of BU-FLU to myeloablative BU-CY-MEL in a mixed group of pediatric patients, and found decreased toxicity with equivalent survival. In conjunction with the knowledge that no amount of chemotherapy is curative for the standard patient with JMML, these findings call into question the strategy of maximally intensifying pretransplant conditioning for patients with JMML. An alternative hypothesis is that the sole purpose of the conditioning regimen is to reliably and safely establish donor cell engraftment and to provide a platform for the donor's immune system to perform the actual disease control. Another aspect of treatment worth considering is the potential benefit of the graft-versus-leukemia effect, which could be the best option to improve JMML-free survival.[40] This hypothesis is being prospectively tested in the ongoing COG trial, ASCT1221: A Randomized Phase II Study Comparing Two Different Conditioning Regimens Prior to Allogeneic HCT for Children with JMML (NCT01824693), in which BU-FLU is being studied against BU-CY-MEL.

Patients with early signs of relapse (dropping donor chimerism or detection of gene mutation) might benefit from rapid withdrawal of immunosuppression and/or infusion of donor lymphocytes.[41–43] In patients who suffer relapse, a second AlloHCT is a viable option that salvages a reasonable percentage of patients.[44–46]

SUMMARY

Over the last decade significant progress has been made in understanding aspects of the molecular basis of JMML. It is now known that 85% to 90% of patients can be firmly diagnosed with the help of molecular studies. What remains to be elucidated, however, is how these molecular mechanisms may lead to targeted therapeutics and to improved outcomes. AlloHCT transplant is the only curative option for most children with JMML and, unfortunately, it is an option fraught with frequent relapse and significant toxicity. Further improvements will be achieved with the development of multinational studies that seek to discover and optimize the diagnosis, treatment, and survival of children with JMML.

REFERENCES

1. Hasle H, Arico M, Basso G, et al. A population-based study of childhood myelo-dysplastic syndrome in British Columbia, Canada. Br J Haematol 1999;106(4): 1027–32.
2. Passmore SJ, Chessells JM, Kempski H, et al. Paediatric myelodysplastic syndromes and juvenile myelomonocytic leukaemia in the UK: a population-based study of incidence and survival. Br J Haematol 2003;121(5):758–67.
3. Chan RJ, Cooper T, Kratz C, et al. Juvenile myelomonocytic leukemia: a report from the 2nd International JMML Symposium. Leuk Res 2009;33(3):355–62.
4. Side LE, Emanuel PD, Taylor B, et al. Mutations of the NF1 gene in children with juvenile myelomonocytic leukemia without clinical evidence of neurofibromatosis, type 1. Blood 1998;92(1):267–72.
5. Side LE, Shannon KM. Myeloid disorders in infants with Noonan syndrome and a resident's "rule" recalled. J Pediatr 1997;130(6):857–9.
6. Bader-Meunier B, Tchernia G, Mielot F, et al. Occurrence of myeloproliferative disorder in patients with Noonan syndrome. J Pediatr 1997;130(6):885–9.
7. Niemeyer CM, Kratz CP. Paediatric myelodysplastic syndromes and juvenile myelomonocytic leukaemia: molecular classification and treatment options. Br J Haematol 2008;140(6):610–24.
8. Yoshimi A, Kamachi Y, Imai K, et al. Wiskott-Aldrich syndrome presenting with a clinical picture mimicking juvenile myelomonocytic leukaemia. Pediatr Blood Cancer 2013;60(5):836–41.
9. Dvorak CC, Loh ML. Juvenile myelomonocytic leukaemia: molecular pathogenesis informs current approaches to therapy and hematopoietic cell transplantation. Front Pediatr 2014;2:25, 1–9.
10. Koike K, Matsuda K. Recent advances in the pathogenesis and management of juvenile myelomonocytic leukaemia. Br J Haematol 2008;141(5):567–75.
11. Arico M, Biondi A, Pui CH. Juvenile myelomonocytic leukaemia. Blood 1997;90(2): 479–88.
12. Niemeyer CM, Arico M, Basso G, et al. Chronic myelomonocytic leukemia in childhood: a retrospective analysis of 110 cases. European Working Group on Myelodysplastic Syndromes in Childhood (EWOG-MDS). Blood 1997;89(10):3534–43.
13. Luna-Fineman S, Shannon KM, Atwater SK, et al. Myelodysplastic and myeloproliferative disorders of childhood: a study of 167 patients. Blood 1999;93(2): 459–66.
14. Matsuda K, Shimada A, Yoshida N, et al. Spontaneous improvement of hematologic abnormalities in patients having juvenile myelomonocytic leukaemia with specific RAS mutations. Blood 2007;109(12):5477–80.
15. Bergstraesser E, Hassle H, Rogge T, et al. Non-hematopoietic stem cell transplantation treatment of juvenile myelomonocytic leukemia: a retrospective analysis and definition of response criteria. Pediatr Blood Cancer 2007;49(5):629–33.
16. Busque L, Gilliland DG, Prchal JT, et al. Clonality in juvenile chronic myelogenous leukemia. Blood 1995;85(1):21–30.
17. Inoue S, Shibata T, Ravindranath Y, et al. Clonal origin of erythroid cells in juvenile chronic myelogenous leukemia. Blood 1987;69(3):975–6.
18. de Vries AC, Zwaan CM, van den Heuvel-Eibrink MM. Molecular basis of juvenile myelomonocytic leukemia. Haematologica 2010;95(2):179–82.
19. Flotho C, Valcamonica S, Mach-Pascual S, et al. RAS mutations and clonality analysis in children with juvenile myelomonocytic leukemia (JMML). Leukemia 1999;13(1):32–7.

20. Shannon KM, O'Connell P, Martin GA, et al. Loss of the normal NF1 allele from the bone marrow of children with type 1 neurofibromatosis and malignant myeloid disorders. N Engl J Med 1994;330(9):597–601.
21. Bader JL, Miller RW. Neurofibromatosis and childhood leukemia. J Pediatr 1978; 92(6):925–9.
22. Bollag G, Clap DW, Shih S, et al. Loss of NF1 results in activation of the Ras signaling pathway and leads to aberrant growth in haematopoietic cells. Nat Genet 1996;12(2):144–8.
23. Tartaglia M, Mehler EL, Goldberg R, et al. Mutations in PTPN11, encoding the protein tyrosine phosphatase SHP-2, cause Noonan syndrome. Nat Genet 2001;29(4):465–8.
24. Loh ML, et al. Mutations in PTPN11 implicate the SHP-2 phosphatase in leukemogenesis. Blood 2004;103(6):2325–31.
25. Loh ML, Reynolds MG, Vattikutti S, et al. PTPN11 mutations in pediatric patients with acute myeloid leukemia: results from the Children's Cancer Group. Leukemia 2004;18(11):1831–4.
26. Kratz CP, Niemeyer CM, Castleberry RP, et al. The mutational spectrum of PTPN11 in juvenile myelomonocytic leukemia and Noonan syndrome/myeloproliferative disease. Blood 2005;106(6):2183–5.
27. Loh ML, Sakai DS, Flotho C, et al. Mutations in CBL occur frequently in juvenile myelomonocytic leukemia. Blood 2009;114(9):1859–63.
28. Niemeyer CM, Kang MW, Shin DH, et al. Germline CBL mutations cause developmental abnormalities and predispose to juvenile myelomonocytic leukemia. Nat Genet 2010;42(9):794–800.
29. Perez B, Mechinaud F, Galamburn C, et al. Germline mutations of the CBL gene define a new genetic syndrome with predisposition to juvenile myelomonocytic leukaemia. J Med Genet 2010;47(10):686–91.
30. Locatelli F, et al. Hematopoietic stem cell transplantation (HSCT) in children with juvenile myelomonocytic leukemia (JMML): results of the EWOG-MDS/EBMT trial. Blood 2005;105(1):410–9.
31. Locatelli F, Nolke P, Zecca M, et al. Analysis of risk factors influencing outcomes after cord blood transplantation in children with juvenile myelomonocytic leukemia: a EUROCORD, EBMT, EWOG-MDS, CIBMTR study. Blood 2013;122(12): 2135–41.
32. Yoshida N, Yagasaki H, Xu Y, et al. Correlation of clinical features with the mutational status of GM-CSF signaling pathway-related genes in juvenile myelomonocytic leukemia. Pediatr Res 2009;65(3):334–40.
33. Bresolin S, Zecca M, Flotho C, et al. Gene expression-based classification as an independent predictor of clinical outcome in juvenile myelomonocytic leukemia. J Clin Oncol 2010;28(11):1919–27.
34. Castleberry RP, Emanuel PD, Zuckerman KS, et al. A pilot study of isotretinoin in the treatment of juvenile chronic myelogenous leukemia. N Engl J Med 1994; 331(25):1680–4.
35. Archambeault S, Flores NJ, Yoshimi A, et al. Development of an allele-specific minimal residual disease assay for patients with juvenile myelomonocytic leukemia. Blood 2008;111(3):1124–7.
36. Chang T, Krisman K, Theobald EH, et al. Sustained MEK inhibition abrogates myeloproliferative disease in Nf1 mutant mice. J Clin Invest 2013;123(1): 335–9.
37. Lyubynska N, Gorman MF, Lauchle JO, et al. A MEK inhibitor abrogates myeloproliferative disease in Kras mutant mice. Sci Transl Med 2011;3(76):76ra27.

38. Furlan I, Batz C, Flotho C, et al. Intriguing response to azacitidine in a patient with juvenile myelomonocytic leukemia and monosomy 7. Blood 2009;113(12): 2867–8.

39. Bartelink IH, Van Reji EM, Gerhardt CE, et al. Fludarabine and exposure-targeted busulfan compares favorably with busulfan/cyclophosphamide-based regimens in pediatric hematopoietic cell transplantation: maintaining efficacy with less toxicity. Biol Blood Marrow Transplant 2014;20(3):345–53.

40. Orchard PJ, Miller JS, McGlennen R, et al. Graft-versus-leukemia is sufficient to induce remission in juvenile myelomonocytic leukemia. Bone Marrow Transplant 1998;22(2):201–3.

41. Yoshimi A, Niemeyer CM, Bohmer V, et al. Chimaerism analyses and subsequent immunological intervention after stem cell transplantation in patients with juvenile myelomonocytic leukaemia. Br J Haematol 2005;129(4):542–9.

42. Yoshimi A, Bader P, Matthes-Martin S, et al. Donor leukocyte infusion after hematopoietic stem cell transplantation in patients with juvenile myelomonocytic leukemia. Leukemia 2005;19(6):971–7.

43. Worth A, Rao K, Webb D, et al. Successful treatment of juvenile myelomonocytic leukemia relapsing after stem cell transplantation using donor lymphocyte infusion. Blood 2003;101(5):1713–4.

44. Chang YH, Jou ST, Lin DT, et al. Second allogeneic hematopoietic stem cell transplantation for juvenile myelomonocytic leukemia: case report and literature review. J Pediatr Hematol Oncol 2004;26(3):190–3.

45. Faraci M, Micalizzi C, Lanino E, et al. Three consecutive related bone marrow transplants for juvenile myelomonocytic leukaemia. Pediatr Transplant 2005; 9(6):797–800.

46. Eapen M, Giralt SA, Horowitz MM, et al. Second transplant for acute and chronic leukemia relapsing after first HLA-identical sibling transplant. Bone Marrow Transplant 2004;34(8):721–7.

Chronic Myeloid Leukemia in Children

⊛ CrossMark

Clinical Findings, Management, and Unanswered Questions

Nobuko Hijiya, MD[a,b,*], Frederic Millot, MD[c], Meinolf Suttorp, MD[d]

KEYWORDS

- Chronic myeloid leukemia • Tyrosine kinase inhibitor
- Hematopoietic stem cell transplant • BCR-ABL1

KEY POINTS

- There are few data showing biological differences between adult and pediatric chronic myelogenous leukemia (CML), but the clinical presentations are distinct and the host factors are different in adults and growing children, which raises issues specific to the care of pediatric patients with CML.
- Children have longer life expectancies than adults; therefore, the goal of CML treatment in children should be cure rather than disease suppression.
- Because of the possibility of decades-long tyrosine kinase inhibitor (TKI) treatment, which also occurs during periods of active growth, morbidity related to TKI therapy for CML is different in children than in adults. Careful monitoring of bone growth and other possible long-term morbidity is crucial.
- The role of hematopoietic stem cell transplant in the first chronic phase should be defined for pediatric patients with CML.

INTRODUCTION

Chronic myelogenous leukemia (CML) is diagnosed in approximately 6000 patients every year in the United States according to the Surveillance Epidemiology and End Results (SEER) Program.[1–3] CML in children is usually considered to be rare, but it

[a] Division of Hematology, Oncology, and Stem Cell Transplantation, Ann & Robert H. Lurie Children's Hospital of Chicago, 225 East Chicago Avenue, Box #30, Chicago, IL 60611, USA; [b] Department of Pediatrics, Northwestern University Feinberg School of Medicine, Chicago, IL, USA; [c] Centre d'Investigation Clinique 1402, Institut National de la Santé et de la Recherche Médicale (INSERM), University Hospital of Poitiers, 2 rue de la Milétrie, 86000 Poitiers, France; [d] Department of Pediatrics, University Hospital "Carl Gustav Carus", Fetscherstrasse 74, D-01307 Dresden, Germany
* Corresponding author. Division of Hematology, Oncology, Stem Cell Transplantation, Ann & Robert H. Lurie Children's Hospital of Chicago, 225 East Chicago Avenue, Box #30, Chicago, IL 60611.
E-mail address: nhijiya@luriechildrens.org

Pediatr Clin N Am 62 (2015) 107–119
http://dx.doi.org/10.1016/j.pcl.2014.09.008
0031-3955/15/$ – see front matter © 2015 Elsevier Inc. All rights reserved.

accounts for 10% to 15% of myeloid leukemia and is more common than acute promyelocytic leukemia, which accounts for 5% to 10% of cases. At one time, hematopoietic stem cell transplant (HSCT) was the only curative treatment of CML in children as well as in adults; however, the treatment landscape has changed drastically over the last 15 years since the introduction of the tyrosine kinase inhibitor (TKI) imatinib.[4–6] Continuing TKI treatment indefinitely has become standard practice for adult patients in chronic phase (CP), and the feasibility of discontinuing TKI therapy in patients in deep molecular remission has been studied.[7] However, because of a lack of data from large clinical studies, standardized treatment and interventions have not been established in the pediatric CML population. This article discusses some controversial issues and unanswered questions (**Table 1**), as well as current recommendations, in the management of pediatric CML (**Boxes 1** and **2, Fig. 1**).

Table 1
Unanswered questions and issues specific to pediatric CML

Issues and Questions	Notes
Children have longer life expectancy than adults	• No studies have proved the efficacy of TKIs to suppress disease beyond 15 y • There may be unexpected morbidities after decades of TKI treatment
Morbidities from TKIs in children are different from those in adults	• Children require multiple decades of TKI treatment • TKIs cause growth disturbances • There is no human study showing the effect of TKIs on the future fertility of young children • Immune dysfunction, thyroid, cardiac, vascular, and liver toxicities have been reported in adults, but there are no long-term data in children
Treatment should be designed for cure, rather than suppression, of the disease	• New agents that target leukemic stem cells or overcome TKI resistance may be particularly helpful in pediatric patients
HSCT may still play a role in children in first CP	• The outcome of HSCT is better in children in general • HSCT may provide sustained remission or cure by eradicating leukemic stem cells • Recent techniques such as reduced-intensity conditioning may be effective • There are very few large studies on long-term outcomes and morbidity of HSCT for CML • Very late relapse is possible
Efficacy of newer TKIs has not been validated	• There are ongoing phase 2 studies of 2G TKIs
Pediatric-specific treatment guidelines are lacking	• Modification of ELN and NCCN guidelines may be needed • Recommendations from the I-BFM study group based on adult data have been published • International harmonization is needed
CML scoring system has not been validated in children	• Sokal, Hasford, and EUTOS scores are not reliable in children • Prognostic value of early response and kinetics of *BCR-ABL1* transcript ratio need to be validated in children

Abbreviations: 2G, second generation; ELN, European Leukemia Net; iBFM, international Berlin-Frankfurt-Münster study group; NCCN, National Comprehensive Cancer Network.

Box 1
Recommended tests to monitor disease status

At diagnosis:

1. Bone marrow (cytogenetics, FISH)

2. Qualitative PCR for *BCR-ABL1*

3. Consider HLA typing of the patient and siblings

During TKI treatment:

1. Bone marrow every 3 months until complete cytogenetic remission (no Philadelphia chromosome is identified)

2. RQ-PCR by peripheral blood every 3 months

3. *BCR-ABL1* mutation analysis if response is not optimal

Abbreviations: FISH, fluorescence in situ hybridization; HLA, human leukocyte antigen; RQ-PCR, real-time quantitative polymerase chain reaction.

DIFFERENCES IN CHRONIC MYELOGENOUS LEUKEMIA CLINICAL PRESENTATION IN CHILDREN AND ADULTS

There are some differences in the clinical presentation of CML at diagnosis in children and adults, which suggests different underlying biology. The median baseline white blood cell count (WBC) in adult patients with CML ranges from 80×10^9/L to 150×10^9/L,[8–10] but is higher in children with CML; WBC was reported to be approximately 250×10^9/L in an international registry of 200 children with CML (median age, 11.6 years; range, 8 months to 18 years).[11] Compared with older adults, adolescents and young adults (16–29 years) also present with higher WBC as well as other aggressive disease features (larger spleen, higher peripheral blast counts, and lower hemoglobin levels), although one study showed similar outcomes.[12] Another study showed less favorable cytogenetic and molecular response rates and a trend for shorter event-free survival in a similar age group (15–29 years) of patients with CML compared with older adults, although overall survival rates were not different.[13] The median size of the spleen is 8 cm below the costal margin (range, 0–25 cm)[11] in children, which is not very different from adults.[14] However, the age-based normal size of the spleen in children is smaller than in adults; therefore,

---

Box 2
Recommended monitoring of morbidities and supportive care

- Height, weight and Tanner staging on every visit. If there are abnormal patterns, consult endocrinology and consider bone age and DEXA scan.

- Thyroid function after 4 to 6 weeks of TKI and repeat thereafter periodically.

- Echocardiogram and ECG annually.

- Inactivated vaccines may be given anytime during TKI treatment, although efficacy is not confirmed.

- Live vaccines are not recommended during TKI therapy. May be given after discontinuing TKI for several weeks when the patient is in deep molecular response.

Abbreviations: ECG, electrocardiogram; DEXA, dual-energy X-ray absorptiometry.

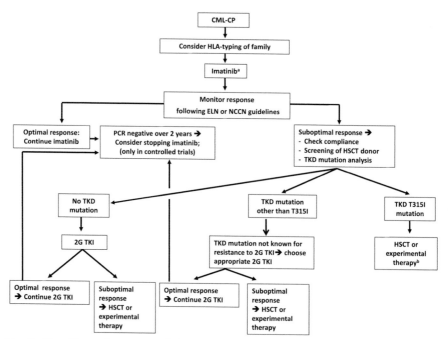

Fig. 1. Algorithm of recommended treatment of pediatric CML in first CP. [a] Second-generation (2G) TKI, if a study is available. [b] Ponatinib, if available for children. ELN, European Leukemia Net; HLA, human leukocyte antigen; NCCN, National Comprehensive Cancer Network; PCR, polymerase chain reaction; TKD, BCR-ABL1 tyrosine kinase domain.

children have proportionally larger spleens. Advanced phases of CML (accelerated phase [AP] or blast crisis [BC]) seem to be diagnosed more frequently in children than in adults.[11,15–17] Given the differences in clinical presentation and the wide gap in the prevalence of CML in children and adults, it is possible that different mechanisms account for the pathogenesis in each age group; however, to date there are few data to support this idea.[18]

ISSUES IN PEDIATRIC CHRONIC MYELOGENOUS LEUKEMIA
Lack of Standard Guidelines and Prognostic Scores in Children

There are no standard guidelines in pediatric CML such as those produced by the National Comprehensive Cancer Network (NCCN)[19] and European Leukemia Net (ELN)[20] for adults; thus, many pediatric oncologists follow guidelines that are designed for adult patients. However, there are several issues unique to children with CML that need to be carefully considered.

Various prognostic scores (eg, Sokal,[21] Hasford,[8] and Eutos[22] scores) based on clinical and biological features at diagnosis predict the outcomes of adult patients with CML treated with chemotherapy,[21] interferon,[8] or imatinib,[22] but the validity of these scores has not been established in the pediatric population. For instance, the Sokal score[21] uses age, spleen size, platelet counts, and blast count. Using this score, a 10-year-old with CML would have a lower risk of mortality than a 70-year-old patient if they had the same spleen size and blood cell counts, but in practice this is not always true. Suttorp and colleagues[23] evaluated the 3 scores and a Sokal young score[24] in 90 children with CML (median age, 11.6 years; range, 1–18 years) who were treated with imatinib, and prognostic scores were inconsistent in children and did not predict poor response at 3 months.

More recently, cytogenetic and molecular responses to TKI therapy have been used as prognostic markers. NCCN[19] and ELN[20] guidelines use TKI responses at 3, 6, and 12 months to define treatment failure or to recommend change of treatment. The prognostic value of early TKI response and kinetics of *BCR-ABL1* have been also described[25,26] but they need to be evaluated in pediatric patients with CML.

Cure or Suppression of Disease?

Whether or not CML in children is different from adult disease is debatable, but the host factors are different in these two patient populations and may inform treatment goals. Cure of disease is ideal for any age group, but an acceptable goal of treatment in adults, especially in older patients, may be to maintain CP for a few decades with TKI.[27,28] If older patients remain *BCR-ABL1*–positive by real-time quantitative reverse transcription polymerase chain reaction, but are in CP with TKI, they can expect a good quality of life for many years. In contrast, children have a much longer life expectancy, and there are no data on the long-term efficacy of TKI beyond 15 years. If children with CML continue TKI treatment and remain in CP, they may still develop resistance and progress to AP/BC after decades. Noncompliance with TKI is also more prevalent in adolescents and young adults compared with older adults or younger children,[29,30] which makes decades-long use of TKI a less attractive option in these patients. Continuing TKI indefinitely can also cause long-term morbidities in children and, over decades, the cost of TKI becomes significant[28] and may also preclude adherence as reported in adults.[31] When pediatric patients with CML enter young adulthood, they face impaired quality-of-life issues related to TKI therapy, which are reported to be significantly worse in the young adult population compared with the older adult population.[32]

One potential solution is to stop TKIs after a period of undetectable *BCR-ABL1*.[7,28,33–35] The prospective Stop Imatinib (STIM) study evaluated the feasibility of discontinuing imatinib in patients 18 years of age or older who remained in complete molecular response (CMR) for at least 2 years while on imatinib.[7] Sixty-nine of 100 patients enrolled had median follow-up of 24 months (range, 13–30 months) and 42 of 69 patients (61%) experienced relapse; however, all patients who had molecular relapse responded to reintroduction of imatinib. Despite these studies, there is limited information on the longer-term (beyond 5 years) outcomes of patients with CML in CMR after cessation of imatinib.[7,34,35] Although *BCR-ABL1* can be persistent without progression of disease for several years,[36] it is also possible that children in CMR may experience molecular relapse after a longer period of time following TKI discontinuation. However, reintroduction of TKI may bring them back to molecular remission.[7,34] The concept of intermittent TKI dosing[37] to reduce the long-term side effects of TKI and financial burden is intriguing in this regard.[38]

There are several potential therapeutic targets and agents under development that potentially overcome TKI resistance or eradicate CML stem cells, which may achieve cure. These targets and agents include interferon-alfa[39] and components of the JAK/STAT,[40,41] Hedgehog,[41] and Wnt/β-catenin signaling pathways[41]; early-phase studies are ongoing. Immunologic approaches[27] like tumor cell–derived peptide vaccination[42,43] may represent other reasonable strategies to cure CML in the future. New treatment options, particularly those intended to cure, are potentially more beneficial for children than for adults; therefore, it is critical that pediatric studies are pursued as part of the clinical development process.

Hematopoietic Stem Cell Transplant for Children with Chronic Myelogenous Leukemia in First Chronic Phase

HSCT is currently not a first-line treatment of CML in adults; however, whether children with CML should continue on TKI or receive HSCT in the first CP is still a valid question. HSCT is the most established treatment to eliminate leukemic stem cells, although late relapse after HSCT has been reported.[27] HSCT, especially with a myeloablative conditioning regimen, causes significant morbidity, including loss of fertility, but in general, children tolerate HSCT better than adults. The best way to determine the benefit of HSCT for children in first CP is to conduct a prospective randomized trial comparing HSCT and TKI therapy; however, such a trial is not realistic given the small number of pediatric patients with CML.

Data are scarce for the use of HSCT in children with CML in first CP. There are only 3 studies that have reported outcomes of HSCT in this population, including data on more than 100 children (**Table 2**).[44–46] Goldman and colleagues[47] reported relapse and late mortality in 2444 patients with CML who received myeloablative HSCT in first CP between 1978 and 1998 and survived in continuous complete remission for 5 years or longer after HSCT. Although the pediatric population was not specifically analyzed in this study, multivariate analysis of a reference group of patients younger than 20 years of age indicated higher disease-free survival than in older patients; relative risk was 1.96 (95% confidence interval [CI], 1.08–3.54); 2.12 (95% CI, 1.2–3.75); 2.92 (95% CI, 1.65–5.15); and 3.93 (95% CI, 2.06–7.51) for patients aged 20 to 29 years ($P = .03$); 30 to 39 years ($P = .009$); 40 to 49 years ($P<.001$); and 50 years or older ($P<.001$), respectively.[47]

In the TKI era, there is reluctance to perform HSCT in children in first CP because of concerns regarding short-term and long-term morbidities. However, supportive care for HSCT has advanced in the last decade and reduced-intensity conditioning regimens with lower morbidities are now available.[48] Although more studies are needed to establish an indication for HSCT in children with CML in first CP, this option may be considered in certain cases, as described later.

Long-term Side Effects of Tyrosine Kinase Inhibitors in Children and Adolescents

TKIs inhibit not only *BCR-ABL1* but also many other targets.[49] Imatinib is known to cause dysregulation of bone remodeling by affecting osteoblasts and osteoclasts through off-target inhibition.[50] Continuing TKIs indefinitely can cause specific long-term complications in growing children. In the last few years, there has been an

Table 2
Published results of HSCT for children with CML in first CP

Author, Year	No. of Patients	Disease Phase at HSCT	Donor Source	Overall Survival
Muramatsu et al,[44] 2010	125	CP1, n = 88 Other, n = 37	Unrelated	59.3% at 5 y
Suttorp et al,[45] 2009	176	CP1, n = 158 Other, n = 18	MRD MUD	87% ± 11% (MSD, n = 41); 52% ± 9% (MUD, n = 71); 45% ± 16% (MMD, n = 55); at 5 y
Cwynarski et al,[46] 2003	314	CP1, n = 253 Other, n = 61	MSD VUD	75% (CP1, MSD, n = 156); 65% (CP1, VUD, n = 97)

Only studies with data for greater than 100 patients are listed.
Abbreviations: CP1, first chronic phase; MMD, mismatched donor; MRD, matched-related donor; MSD, matched-sibling donor; MUD, matched-unrelated donor; VUD, volunteer-unrelated donor.

increasing number of reports of growth abnormalities related to TKIs.[51–59] It seems that prepubertal children are affected more significantly.[16] In addition, reports of growth hormone deficiency[52,59,60] in patients receiving TKIs indicate additional mechanisms by which these agents may potentially affect the eventual height of pediatric patients.

TKIs may also have an adverse effect on pregnancy outcomes,[61,62] and female patients of childbearing age are advised to avoid pregnancy during TKI treatment because of the risk of serious fetal malformations.[19] The offspring of male patients who are receiving imatinib at the time of conception seem to be healthy.[63] The more relevant issue for children with CML is the effect of TKIs on their future fertility, but there are few data in humans on this issue and the results of animal studies vary with regard to the effect of imatinib.[60,63,64] Nevertheless, there are a few case reports in humans that indicate decreased fertility in a teenage boy[65] and a young adult female patient receiving imatinib.[66] Larger studies with longer follow-up are necessary to evaluate the influence of TKI therapy on the future fertility of children.

To date, there are no published data in children on the incidence of other morbidities associated with TKI that have been reported in adults, including thyroid,[67,68] cardiovascular,[69,70] and liver toxicities.[71] Because all side effects may become more significant with longer periods of TKI treatment, careful monitoring for comorbidities is strongly recommended in pediatric patients with CML receiving long-term TKI therapy.

Role of Newer Tyrosine Kinase Inhibitors for Pediatric Chronic Myelogenous Leukemia

Imatinib has been successfully studied in pediatric phase 1, 2, and 4 studies,[5,6,72] and was approved as first-line treatment of children with CML in 2003 by the US Food and Drug Administration (FDA) and the European Medical Agency (EMA). The second-generation (2G) TKIs dasatinib[73,74] and nilotinib[75] have been shown to produce a more rapid and deeper response in adults, and are now included as first-line treatments for adults with CML in CP in the most recent guidelines from ELN[20] and NCCN.[19] Dasatinib[76,77] and nilotinib (clinicaltrials.gov, NCT01077544) have been tested in phase 1 trials in the pediatric patient population and there are ongoing phase 2 trials (NCT00777036). A phase 2 study of nilotinib (NCT01844765) is currently being conducted in the Children's Oncology Group and Innovative Therapies for Children with Cancer. Another 2G TKI (bosutinib),[78] a third-generation TKI (ponatinib) that has been shown to be active against T315I mutation,[79] and a protein translation inhibitor (omacetaxine mepesuccinate)[80] are all approved for resistant or intolerant CML in adults, but have not yet been investigated in children.

CURRENT RECOMMENDATIONS FOR MANAGEMENT

The International Berlin-Frankfurt-Münster (BFM) Study Group CML Committee recently published their recommendations for the management of CML in children and adolescents, taking into account the existing guidelines for adult patients.[71] We recommend management and monitoring of disease status in newly diagnosed children as summarized in **Boxes 1** and **2** and **Fig. 1**. Imatinib is the only TKI that is currently approved as a first-line treatment in pediatric CML but, when pediatric studies of 2G TKI as first-line therapy are opened, clinicians are encouraged to enroll their patients, because these agents have been shown in adults to elicit a more rapid and deeper response with less chance to progress to AP/BC compared with imatinib.[73,81,82] If the response to first-line treatment is not optimal, especially in teenagers, adherence should be thoroughly evaluated, and then *BCR-ABL1* tyrosine kinase domain (TKD) mutation analysis should be performed. Depending on the TKD mutation and the sensitivity,[20] the patient should receive an alternative TKI,[19,83] if available to children. At the same time, an HSCT donor search is recommended. HSCT should also be considered in certain circumstances such as noncompliance, serious side effects with TKIs, availability of a donor, and patient choice following appropriate counseling on the balance of risk and benefit of cure.

There is no standard for monitoring of morbidities in pediatric CML and more data are needed. The currently suggested monitoring schedule is shown in **Box 2**. Lack of knowledge about immune dysfunction with TKI[84] is hindering routine vaccination for children with CML. A study showed that adult patients treated with TKI had an impaired immunoglobulin M (IgM) humoral response to pneumococcal vaccine compared with healthy controls and reduction of IgM-memory B cells through off-target inhibition of kinases.[84] It is safe to give inactivated vaccines to children on TKI therapy, although there may be an insufficient response as in any immunocompromised patient. However, one report indicated a higher seroconversion rate to H1N1 influenza vaccine in adult patients with CML compared with patients with B-cell malignancies or HSCT recipients.[85] The study evaluated 32 adult patients with CML receiving imatinib (n = 23) or dasatinib (n = 9). Protective antibody titers were observed in 85% (P = .086) and 95% (P = .5) of the patients with CML after the first and second doses, respectively, compared with controls (100% after the first dose).[85] Giving live vaccines during TKI treatment is not recommended in general, although one study suggests that varicella vaccine can be given to some immunocompromised children.[86] As an alternative, when a deep molecular response is achieved after a few years of TKI treatment, the TKI treatment may be interrupted for several weeks to provide a window for administering live vaccines. In the United States, all live vaccines are completed by the age of 4 to 6 years (http://www.cdc.gov/vaccines/). Because CML is rarely seen in children before this age, few patients face this issue.

SUMMARY

There are few data showing differences in the biology of CML in children and adults, but host factors in growing children are distinct from those of adults, which raises issues specific to the care of pediatric patients with CML. The goal of treatment in pediatric CML should be cure rather than disease suppression, which can be the goal in many adult patients. Morbidity associated with TKI therapy is different in growing children than in adults. The possible indication of HSCT in first CP should be defined for the pediatric patient population. Large studies are urgently needed to improve understanding of the unique biology and long-term morbidities in children with CML, thus preparing for the creation of pediatric-specific guidelines for treatment and follow-up.

ACKNOWLEDGMENTS

The authors thank Stacey Tobin, PhD, and Michael Miller, MD, for assistance in preparation of this article, and Briana Patterson, MD, for valuable discussion.

REFERENCES

1. Surveillance Research Program NCI. Fast Stats: An interactive tool for access to SEER cancer statistics. 2013. Available at: http://seer.cancer.gov/faststats/. Accessed November 1, 2013.

2. Cancer incidence and survival among children and adolescents: United States SEER Program 1975–1995. Bethesda, MD: National Cancer Institute, SEER Program; 1999. NIH Pub. No. 99–4649.

3. Childhood acute myeloid leukemia/other myeloid malignancies treatment (PDQ®). 2014. Available at: http://www.cancer.gov/cancertopics/pdq/treatment/childAML/HealthProfessional/page1#Reference1.3. Accessed June 22, 2014.

4. Druker BJ, Sawyers CL, Kantarjian H, et al. Activity of a specific inhibitor of the BCR-ABL tyrosine kinase in the blast crisis of chronic myeloid leukemia and acute lymphoblastic leukemia with the Philadelphia chromosome. N Engl J Med 2001; 344(14):1038–42.

5. Champagne MA, Fu CH, Chang M, et al. Higher dose imatinib for children with de novo chronic phase chronic myelogenous leukemia: a report from the Children's Oncology Group. Pediatr Blood Cancer 2011;57(1):56–62.

6. Millot F, Baruchel A, Guilhot J, et al. Imatinib is effective in children with previously untreated chronic myelogenous leukemia in early chronic phase: results of the French national phase IV trial. J Clin Oncol 2011;29(20):2827–32.

7. Mahon FX, Rea D, Guilhot J, et al. Discontinuation of imatinib in patients with chronic myeloid leukaemia who have maintained complete molecular remission for at least 2 years: the prospective, multicentre Stop Imatinib (STIM) trial. Lancet Oncol 2010;11(11):1029–35.

8. Hasford J, Pfirrmann M, Hehlmann R, et al. A new prognostic score for survival of patients with chronic myeloid leukemia treated with interferon alfa. Writing Committee for the Collaborative CML Prognostic Factors Project Group. J Natl Cancer Inst 1998;90(11):850–8.

9. Bonifazi F, de Vivo A, Rosti G, et al. Chronic myeloid leukemia and interferon-alpha: a study of complete cytogenetic responders. Blood 2001;98(10): 3074–81.

10. Lindoerfer D, Hoffmann V, Rosti G, et al. The EUTOS population-based registry; evaluation of baseline characteristics and first treatment choices of 2983 newly diagnosed chronic myeloid leukemia (CML) patients from 20 European countries. Haematologica 2014;99(s1):238.

11. Millot F, Suttorp M, Guilhot J, et al. The International Registry for Chronic Myeloid Leukemia (CML) in Children and Adolescents (I-CML-Ped-Study): Objectives and preliminary results. Blood 2012;120:3741.

12. Kalmanti L, Saussele S, Lauseker M, et al. Younger patients with chronic myeloid leukemia do well in spite of poor prognostic indicators: results from the randomized CML study IV. Ann Hematol 2013;93(1):71–80.

13. Pemmaraju N, Kantarjian H, Shan J, et al. Analysis of outcomes in adolescents and young adults with chronic myelogenous leukemia treated with upfront tyrosine kinase inhibitor therapy. Haematologica 2012;97(7):1029–35.

14. Savage DG, Szydlo RM, Goldman JM. Clinical features at diagnosis in 430 patients with chronic myeloid leukaemia seen at a referral centre over a 16-year period. Br J Haematol 1997;96(1):111–6.

15. Millot F, Traore P, Guilhot J, et al. Clinical and biological features at diagnosis in 40 children with chronic myeloid leukemia. Pediatrics 2005;116(1):140–3.

16. Suttorp M, Millot F. Treatment of pediatric chronic myeloid leukemia in the year 2010: use of tyrosine kinase inhibitors and stem-cell transplantation. Hematology Am Soc Hematol Educ Program 2010;2010:368–76.

17. Mitra D, Trask PC, Iyer S, et al. Patient characteristics and treatment patterns in chronic myeloid leukemia: evidence from a multi-country retrospective medical record chart review study. Int J Hematol 2012;95(3):263–73.

18. Krumbholz M, Karl M, Tauer JT, et al. Genomic BCR-ABL1 breakpoints in pediatric chronic myeloid leukemia. Genes Chromosomes Cancer 2012; 51(11):1045–53.
19. Network NCC. NCCN Clinical practice guidelines in oncology; chronic myelogenous leukemia. Version 1.2015. Available at: http://www.nccn.org/professionals/physician_gls/f_guidelines.asp#cml. 2013. Accessed October 19, 2014.
20. Baccarani M, Deininger MW, Rosti G, et al. European LeukemiaNet recommendations for the management of chronic myeloid leukemia. Blood 2013;122(6): 872–84.
21. Sokal JE, Cox EB, Baccarani M, et al. Prognostic discrimination in "good-risk" chronic granulocytic leukemia. Blood 1984;63(4):789–99.
22. Hasford J, Baccarani M, Hoffmann V, et al. Predicting complete cytogenetic response and subsequent progression-free survival in 2060 patients with CML on imatinib treatment: the EUTOS score. Blood 2011;118(3):686–92.
23. Suttorp MG, Salas DG, Tauer JT, et al. Scoring systems for predicting outcome of chronic myeloid leukemia in adults are poorly informative in pediatric patients treated with imatinib. Blood 2013;122(21):2725.
24. Sokal JE, Baccarani M, Tura S, et al. Prognostic discrimination among younger patients with chronic granulocytic leukemia: relevance to bone marrow transplantation. Blood 1985;66(6):1352–7.
25. Branford S, Yeung DT, Parker WT, et al. Prognosis for patients with CML and >10% BCR-ABL1 after 3 months of imatinib depends on the rate of BCR-ABL1 decline. Blood 2014;124(4):511–8.
26. Marin D, Ibrahim AR, Lucas C, et al. Assessment of BCR-ABL1 transcript levels at 3 months is the only requirement for predicting outcome for patients with chronic myeloid leukemia treated with tyrosine kinase inhibitors. J Clin Oncol 2012;30(3): 232–8.
27. Goldman J, Gordon M. Why do chronic myelogenous leukemia stem cells survive allogeneic stem cell transplantation or imatinib: does it really matter? Leuk Lymphoma 2006;47(1):1–7.
28. Ross DM, Hughes TP. How I determine if and when to recommend stopping tyrosine kinase inhibitor treatment for chronic myeloid leukaemia. Br J Haematol 2014;166(1):3–11.
29. Reaman GH, Bonfiglio J, Krailo M, et al. Cancer in adolescents and young adults. Cancer 1993;71(Suppl 10):3206–9.
30. Millot F, Claviez A, Leverger G, et al. Imatinib cessation in children and adolescents with chronic myeloid leukemia in chronic phase. Pediatr Blood Cancer 2014;61(2):355–7.
31. Dusetzina SB, Winn AN, Abel GA, et al. Cost sharing and adherence to tyrosine kinase inhibitors for patients with chronic myeloid leukemia. J Clin Oncol 2014; 32(4):306–11.
32. Efficace F, Baccarani M, Breccia M, et al. Health-related quality of life in chronic myeloid leukemia patients receiving long-term therapy with imatinib compared with the general population. Blood 2011;118(17):4554–60.
33. Ross DM, Branford S, Seymour JF, et al. Safety and efficacy of imatinib cessation for CML patients with stable undetectable minimal residual disease: results from the TWISTER study. Blood 2013;122(4):515–22.
34. Rea D, Rousselot P, Guilhot F. Discontinuation of second generation (2G) tyrosine kinase inhibitors (TKI) in chronic phase (CP)-chronic myeloid leukemia (CML) patients with stable undetectable BCR-ABL transcripts. Blood 2012;120:916.

35. Moser O, Krumbholz M, Thiede C, et al. Sustained complete molecular remission after imatinib discontinuation in children with chronic myeloid leukemia. Pediatr Blood Cancer 2014;61(11):2080–2.
36. Ross DM, Branford S, Seymour JF, et al. Patients with chronic myeloid leukemia who maintain a complete molecular response after stopping imatinib treatment have evidence of persistent leukemia by DNA PCR. Leukemia 2010;24(10): 1719–24.
37. La Rosee P, Martiat P, Leitner A, et al. Improved tolerability by a modified intermittent treatment schedule of dasatinib for patients with chronic myeloid leukemia resistant or intolerant to imatinib. Ann Hematol 2013;92(10):1345–50.
38. Russo D, Martinelli G, Malagola M, et al. Effects and outcome of a policy of intermittent imatinib treatment in elderly patients with chronic myeloid leukemia. Blood 2013;121(26):5138–44.
39. Talpaz M, Hehlmann R, Quintas-Cardama A, et al. Re-emergence of interferon-alpha in the treatment of chronic myeloid leukemia. Leukemia 2013;27(4):803–12.
40. Warsch W, Walz C, Sexl V. JAK of all trades: JAK2-STAT5 as novel therapeutic targets in BCR-ABL1+ chronic myeloid leukemia. Blood 2013;122(13):2167–75.
41. Kinstrie R, Copland M. Targeting chronic myeloid leukemia stem cells. Curr Hematol Malig Rep 2013;8(1):14–21.
42. Bocchia M, Defina M, Aprile L, et al. Complete molecular response in CML after p210 BCR-ABL1-derived peptide vaccination. Nat Rev Clin Oncol 2010;7(10): 600–3.
43. Smahel M. Antigens in chronic myeloid leukemia: implications for vaccine development. Cancer Immunol Immunother 2011;60(12):1655–68.
44. Muramatsu H, Kojima S, Yoshimi A, et al. Outcome of 125 children with chronic myelogenous leukemia who received transplants from unrelated donors: The Japan Marrow Donor Program. Biol Blood Marrow Transplant 2010;16(2):231–8.
45. Suttorp M, Claviez A, Bader P, et al. Allogeneic stem cell transplantation for pediatric and adolescent patients with CML: results from the prospective trial CML-paed I. Klin Padiatr 2009;221(6):351–7.
46. Cwynarski K, Roberts IA, Iacobelli S, et al. Stem cell transplantation for chronic myeloid leukemia in children. Blood 2003;102(4):1224–31.
47. Goldman JM, Majhail NS, Klein JP, et al. Relapse and late mortality in 5-year survivors of myeloablative allogeneic hematopoietic cell transplantation for chronic myeloid leukemia in first chronic phase. J Clin Oncol 2010;28(11): 1888–95.
48. Warlick E, Ahn KW, Pedersen TL, et al. Reduced intensity conditioning is superior to nonmyeloablative conditioning for older chronic myelogenous leukemia patients undergoing hematopoietic cell transplant during the tyrosine kinase inhibitor era. Blood 2012;119(17):4083–90.
49. Shami PJ, Deininger M. Evolving treatment strategies for patients newly diagnosed with chronic myeloid leukemia: the role of second-generation BCR-ABL inhibitors as first-line therapy. Leukemia 2012;26(2):214–24.
50. Vandyke K, Fitter S, Dewar AL, et al. Dysregulation of bone remodeling by imatinib mesylate. Blood 2010;115(4):766–74.
51. Rastogi MV, Stork L, Druker B, et al. Imatinib mesylate causes growth deceleration in pediatric patients with chronic myelogenous leukemia. Pediatr Blood Cancer 2012;59(5):840–5.
52. Hobernicht SL, Schweiger B, Zeitler P, et al. Acquired growth hormone deficiency in a girl with chronic myelogenous leukemia treated with tyrosine kinase inhibitor therapy. Pediatr Blood Cancer 2011;56(4):671–3.

53. Bansal D, Shava U, Varma N, et al. Imatinib has adverse effect on growth in children with chronic myeloid leukemia. Pediatr Blood Cancer 2012;59(3):481–4.

54. Schmid H, Jaeger BA, Lohse J, et al. Longitudinal growth retardation in a prepuberal girl with chronic myeloid leukemia on long-term treatment with imatinib. Haematologica 2009;94(8):1177–9.

55. Mariani S, Giona F, Basciani S, et al. Low bone density and decreased inhibin-B/FSH ratio in a boy treated with imatinib during puberty. Lancet 2008;372(9633): 111–2.

56. Kimoto T, Inoue M, Kawa K. Growth deceleration in a girl treated with imatinib. Int J Hematol 2009;89(2):251–2.

57. Hijiya N, Broglie L, Chaudhury S, et al. Survival after hematopoietic stem cell transplantation (HSCT) or tyrosine kinase inhibitors (TKI) in children with chronic myeloid leukemia (CML) in chronic phase; a single institution experience. May 9–12. Ped Blood Cancer 2012;58(7):1049.

58. Shima H, Tokuyama M, Tanizawa A, et al. Distinct impact of imatinib on growth at prepubertal and pubertal ages of children with chronic myeloid leukemia. J Pediatr 2011;159(4):676–81.

59. Giona F, Mariani S, Gnessi L, et al. Bone metabolism, growth rate and pubertal development in children with chronic myeloid leukemia treated with imatinib during puberty. Haematologica 2013;98(3):e25–7.

60. Ulmer A, Tauer JT, Suttorp M. Impact of treatment with tyrosine kinase inhibitors (TKIs) on blood levels of growth hormone-related parameters, testosterone, and inhibin B in juvenile rats and pediatric patients with chronic myeloid leukemia (CML). Blood 2012;120:3752.

61. Pye SM, Cortes J, Ault P, et al. The effects of imatinib on pregnancy outcome. Blood 2008;111(12):5505–8.

62. Berveiller P, Andreoli A, Mir O, et al. A dramatic fetal outcome following transplacental transfer of dasatinib. Anticancer Drugs 2012;23(7):754–7.

63. Apperley J. CML in pregnancy and childhood. Best Pract Res Clin Haematol 2009;22(3):455–74.

64. Schultheis B, Nijmeijer BA, Yin H, et al. Imatinib mesylate at therapeutic doses has no impact on folliculogenesis or spermatogenesis in a leukaemic mouse model. Leuk Res 2012;36(3):271–4.

65. Seshadri T, Seymour JF, McArthur GA. Oligospermia in a patient receiving imatinib therapy for the hypereosinophilic syndrome. N Engl J Med 2004;351(20): 2134–5.

66. Christopoulos C, Dimakopoulou V, Rotas E. Primary ovarian insufficiency associated with imatinib therapy. N Engl J Med 2008;358(10):1079–80.

67. Kim TD, Schwarz M, Nogai H, et al. Thyroid dysfunction caused by second-generation tyrosine kinase inhibitors in Philadelphia chromosome-positive chronic myeloid leukemia. Thyroid 2010;20(11):1209–14.

68. Fallahi P, Ferrari SM, Vita R, et al. Thyroid dysfunctions induced by tyrosine kinase inhibitors. Expert Opin Drug Saf 2014;13(6):723–33.

69. Atallah E. Nilotinib cardiac toxicity: should we still be concerned? Leuk Res 2011; 35(5):577–8.

70. Giles FJ, Mauro MJ, Hong F, et al. Rates of peripheral arterial occlusive disease in patients with chronic myeloid leukemia in the chronic phase treated with imatinib, nilotinib, or non-tyrosine kinase therapy: a retrospective cohort analysis. Leukemia 2013;27(6):1310–5.

71. de la Fuente J, Baruchel A, Biondi A, et al. Managing children with chronic myeloid leukaemia (CML): recommendations for the management of CML in

children and young people up to the age of 18 years. Br J Haematol 2014;167(1): 33–47.

72. Champagne MA, Capdeville R, Krailo M, et al. Imatinib mesylate (STI571) for treatment of children with Philadelphia chromosome-positive leukemia: results from a Children's Oncology Group phase 1 study. Blood 2004;104(9):2655–60.

73. Kantarjian HM, Shah NP, Cortes JE, et al. Dasatinib or imatinib in newly diagnosed chronic-phase chronic myeloid leukemia: 2-year follow-up from a randomized phase 3 trial (DASISION). Blood 2012;119(5):1123–9.

74. Jabbour E, Kantarjian HM, Saglio G, et al. Early response with dasatinib or imatinib in chronic myeloid leukemia: 3-year follow-up from a randomized phase 3 trial (DASISION). Blood 2014;123(4):494–500.

75. Larson RA, Hochhaus A, Hughes TP, et al. Nilotinib vs imatinib in patients with newly diagnosed Philadelphia chromosome-positive chronic myeloid leukemia in chronic phase: ENESTnd 3-year follow-up. Leukemia 2012;26(10):2197–203.

76. Zwaan CM, Rizzari C, Mechinaud F, et al. Dasatinib in children and adolescents with relapsed or refractory leukemia: results of the CA180-018 phase I dose-escalation study of the Innovative Therapies for Children with Cancer Consortium. J Clin Oncol 2013;31(19):2460–8.

77. Aplenc R, Blaney SM, Strauss LC, et al. Pediatric phase I trial and pharmacokinetic study of dasatinib: a report from the children's oncology group phase I consortium. J Clin Oncol 2011;29(7):839–44.

78. Cortes JE, Kim DW, Kantarjian HM, et al. Bosutinib versus imatinib in newly diagnosed chronic-phase chronic myeloid leukemia: results from the BELA trial. J Clin Oncol 2012;30(28):3486–92.

79. Cortes JE, Kim DW, Pinilla-Ibarz J, et al. A phase 2 trial of ponatinib in Philadelphia chromosome-positive leukemias. N Engl J Med 2013;369(19):1783–96.

80. Cortes J, Digumarti R, Parikh PM, et al. Phase 2 study of subcutaneous omacetaxine mepesuccinate for chronic-phase chronic myeloid leukemia patients resistant to or intolerant of tyrosine kinase inhibitors. Am J Hematol 2013;88(5):350–4.

81. Kantarjian HM, Hochhaus A, Saglio G, et al. Nilotinib versus imatinib for the treatment of patients with newly diagnosed chronic phase, Philadelphia chromosome-positive, chronic myeloid leukaemia: 24-month minimum follow-up of the phase 3 randomised ENESTnd trial. Lancet Oncol 2011;12(9):841–51.

82. Larson RA, Saglio G, Kim DW, et al. Nilotinib versus imatinib in patients (pts) with newly diagnosed chronic myeloid leukemia in chronic phase (CML-CP): ENESTnd 4-year (y) update. Paper presented at: American Society of Clinical Oncology (ASCO) Annual '13 meeting. Chicago, 2013. J Clin Oncol 2013;31 (suppl; abstr 7052).

83. Soverini S, Hochhaus A, Nicolini FE, et al. BCR-ABL kinase domain mutation analysis in chronic myeloid leukemia patients treated with tyrosine kinase inhibitors: recommendations from an expert panel on behalf of European LeukemiaNet. Blood 2011;118(5):1208–15.

84. de Lavallade H, Khoder A, Hart M, et al. Tyrosine kinase inhibitors impair B-cell immune responses in CML through off-target inhibition of kinases important for cell signaling. Blood 2013;122(2):227–38.

85. de Lavallade H, Garland P, Sekine T, et al. Repeated vaccination is required to optimize seroprotection against H1N1 in the immunocompromised host. Haematologica 2011;96(2):307–14.

86. Luthy KE, Tiedeman ME, Beckstrand RL, et al. Safety of live-virus vaccines for children with immune deficiency. J Am Acad Nurse Pract 2006;18(10):494–503.

Down Syndrome Preleukemia and Leukemia

Kelly W. Maloney, MD[a], Jeffrey W. Taub, MD[b],*, Yaddanapudi Ravindranath, MBBS[b], Irene Roberts, MD[c], Paresh Vyas, MD[d]

KEYWORDS

- Down syndrome • Preleukemia • Leukemia
- Myeloid leukemia of Down syndrome • B-ALL • GATA1
- Transient abnormal hematopoiesis/transient myeloproliferative disorder

KEY POINTS

- Children with Down syndrome manifest multiple hematologic manifestations: (1) transient myeloproliferative disorder (TMD)/transient abnormal myelopoiesis (TAM) at birth, (2) acute myeloid leukemia (ML-DS), and (3) acute lymphoblastic leukemia (ALL).
- The underlying primary basis for the varied hematologic manifestations is linked to the gene dosage effect of chromosome 21–encoded genes.
- TMD/TAM and ML-DS are characterized by the presence of truncating mutations in exon 2 of the hematopoietic transcription factor *GATA1*. Spontaneous resolution is common in TMD/TAM, and ML-DS is highly responsive to chemotherapy with resultant high cure rates compared with acute myeloid leukemia in non-DS children.
- DS-ALL is characterized by the presence of mutations in *JAK2* tyrosine kinase and *IKZF1*. In contrast to the high cure rates in ML-DS, the results in DS-ALL are same are inferior to non-DS ALL, in part, because of the lower frequency of good-response ALL subtypes and also the higher systemic toxicity of agents used in children with DS.

INTRODUCTION

For more than 150 years, Down syndrome (DS) has been linked to the English physician John Langdon Down. His essay published in 1866, "Observations on an Ethnic Classification of Idiots," described a group of cognitively impaired individuals with common physical features. DS is now recognized as the most common chromosomal

[a] Center for Cancer & Blood Disorders, Children's Hospital Colorado, 13123 East 16th Avenue, B115, Aurora, CO 80045, USA; [b] Division of Pediatric Hematology/Oncology, Children's Hospital of Michigan, Wayne State University School of Medicine, 3901 Beaubien Boulevard, Detroit, MI 48201, USA; [c] Department of Paediatrics and Molecular Haematology Unit, University of Oxford and Oxford University Hospitals NHS Trust, Oxford, OX3 9DS, UK; [d] MRC Molecular Haematology Unit, Department of Haematology, Weatherall Institute of Molecular Medicine, Oxford University Hospitals NHS Trust, University of Oxford, Oxford OX3 9DS, UK
* Corresponding author.
E-mail address: jtaub@med.wayne.edu

Pediatr Clin N Am 62 (2015) 121–137
http://dx.doi.org/10.1016/j.pcl.2014.09.009
0031-3955/15/$ – see front matter © 2015 Elsevier Inc. All rights reserved.

abnormality, occurring in 1 in every 800 to 1000 live births. Neonates, children, and adults with DS develop multiple medical disorders; hematologic disorders being one of the most well known. It has long been recognized that children with constitutional trisomy 21 (DS) have a markedly increased risk of acute leukemia. The first description of a child with DS who developed acute leukemia was published in 1930. Subsequently, a national survey in the United States provided support to the notion that children with DS had an increased risk of developing leukemia.[1] Remarkably, children with DS are at an increased risk both of acute megakaryocyte-erythroid leukemia (known as myeloid leukemia of DS [ML-DS]) by 150-fold and of acute B-lineage lymphoblastic leukemia by 33-fold compared with children without DS.

In ML-DS, it is now clear that the initial event is perturbation of fetal hemopoiesis by trisomy 21 (T21) itself. This perturbation leads to complex defects in fetal hemopoiesis and newborn hematology. In up to 28% of fetuses/newborns with DS, hemopoietic cells acquire mutations in the gene encoding the key megakaryocyte-erythroid transcription factor GATA1. Acquisition of *GATA1* mutations can either be clinically silent or result in a clinically important preleukemic fetal/neonatal disorder transient abnormal myelopoiesis (TAM). Most cases of TAM resolve without long-term clinical sequelae; but in a proportion of cases with TAM, neonates/young children acquire additional genetic mutations that immortalize the TAM clone and result in frank ML-DS. There are parallel defects in DS fetal B-cell lymphopoiesis caused by T21 that most likely result in acquisition of a series of cooperating and transforming mutations in genes encoding key regulators of B-lymphopoiesis (eg, *JAK2* and *CLRF2*).

Thus, the unique features of DS-associated leukemias arise because of the crucial role played by T21 that then creates the right cellular and molecular environment for the acquisition of additional genetic mutations that together lead to acute leukemia. Thus, DS-associated leukemias represent potentially one of the most tractable human models to understand the biological basis of multistep leukemogenesis and the impact of aneuploidy on cancer. Next, the authors highlight some of the recent clinical and biological advances in these preleukemic and leukemic conditions.

TRISOMY 21 AND HUMAN FETAL HEMATOPOIESIS
Fetal Origin of Trisomy 21–Associated Leukemias

Human T21 itself perturbs second-trimester fetal liver hemopoietic stem/progenitor (HSPC) function.[2–4] T21 increases the frequency of immunophenotypic hemopoietic stem cell (HSC) that has a biased erythroid-megakaryocyte primed gene expression profile compared with disomic HSC. Furthermore, multiple HSPC populations show increased megakaryocyte-erythroid output in colony assays. Coupled with this, there is an expansion of megakaryocyte-erythroid progenitors themselves. Consistent with this increased megakaryocyte output, immunohistochemical studies of T21 fetal liver sections show increased megakaryocyte numbers. However, megakaryocyte differentiation may be compromised, as fetal liver megakaryocytes are morphologically abnormal. Corroborating data from human T21 embryonic stem cells and induced pluripotent stem cells show increased erythroid and possible megakaryocyte production.[5,6] In addition to increased, but likely perturbed megakaryocyte-erythroid differentiation, there is a severe impairment of B-lymphoid development in DS fetal liver; with an approximately 10-fold reduction in pre-pro B cells and B-cell potential of HSC, in tandem with reduced HSC lymphoid gene expression priming.[4]

Abnormalities of Blood Counts in Newborns with Down Syndrome

Fetal liver hemopoietic defects most likely result in multi-lineage blood count changes in newborns with DS. These changes were initially noted in several small retrospective studies[7–9] and, more recently, in a recent large prospective study.[10] Neonates with DS had higher hemoglobin concentrations, increased circulating erythroblasts, and abnormal red cell morphology, including macrocytosis, target cells, and basophilic stippling. Median platelet counts were also lower than normal in neonates with DS. Thrombocytopenia was common; although the median mean platelet volume was similar to neonates without DS, platelet morphology was abnormal (giant platelets, circulating megakaryocytes, and/or megakaryocyte fragments) in greater than 95% of cases. Neonates with DS had higher numbers of granulocytes and monocytes despite the reduction in granulocyte-monocyte progenitors in fetal liver.[4] This finding may reflect a greater reliance on bone marrow hematopoiesis in late gestation and after birth. The total lymphocyte count (and particularly B-lymphocyte count) was reduced in the neonates with DS.

Molecular Basis for Perturbed Fetal/Neonatal Hematology Caused by Trisomy 21

The molecular basis for trisomy 21-mediated abnormal hematopoiesis is still largely unclear. The complex HSPC and peripheral defects suggest multiple genes are likely to be involved at distinct fetal stages of hematopoiesis. These genes could include the approximately 300 protein- and RNA-encoding on chromosome 21 through gene dosage and/or more global impact on disomic gene regulation. At least 2 approaches have been used to identify genes linked to increased leukemia susceptibility. First, studies in rare patients and mouse models have tried to narrow down the anatomic region of chromosome 21 responsible for the hemopoietic phenotype. Occasional patients with partial trisomy suggest that the leukemia risk is confined to an 8.5-Mb region on chromosome 21, although conclusions here are limited by the very small number of cases of leukemia identified in these patients.[11] The study of murine models trisomic for a variable number of human chromosome 21 genes has provided some insight but are somewhat limited, as none fully recapitulates the human hemopoietic phenotype in fetal and neonatal human DS.[12–16] In summary, overexpression of the genes *ERG, DYRK1A, CHAF1B*, and *HLCS* have all been implicated in a late-onset adult myeloproliferative disorder and in facilitating the transformation to acute myeloid leukemia (AML). Second, analysis of gene expression in primary T21 fetal liver samples and hemopoietic cells derived from human T21 embryonic stem cells or induced pluripotent cells suggest that increased expression of several genes may contribute to deregulated hemopoiesis. These genes include *RUNX1, BACH1, ETS2, ERG, DYRK1A, GABPA*, and *SON*. However, careful functional experiments will be central to understanding if altered expression of any gene is causal to the T21 hemopoietic phenotype.

In addition, it is unclear if the T21 phenotype is hemopoietic cell autonomous or is, in part, mediated by cells constituting the hemopoietic microenvironment. Several lines of indirect evidence suggest that fetal liver may provide the specialized microenvironment necessary for instigating and/or maintaining abnormal hematopoiesis in DS. First, as mentioned earlier, the observation that abnormal hemopoiesis occurs in fetal life suggests a yolk sac/fetal microenvironment is important. Second, differential production and responsiveness of fetal tissues, including hematopoietic cells, to insulin-like growth factors is one of the few consistently reported differences between adult and fetal hematopoiesis.[17–19]

TRANSIENT ABNORMAL MYELOPOIESIS: MYELOID PRELEUKEMIA OF DOWN SYNDROME
Clinical Findings

Although TAM is usually seen in newborns with DS, 7% to 16% of TAM cases have mosaic T21. TAM can also present as hydrops fetalis with hepatosplenomegaly. The current definition of TAM is imprecise. It is defined as the presence of circulating blood blasts in a baby with typical clinical features of TAM who may or may not have hematologic abnormalities. Previous studies have used differing clinical and/or hematologic criteria to define TAM.[20] At one end of the spectrum, TAM is detected as an incidental finding on review of a blood smear in an otherwise well baby. Often there will be an associated mild leucocytosis and thrombocytopenia but these findings are also common in neonates with DS who do not have TAM. At the other of the spectrum, babies can be extremely sick with bruising, ascites, jaundice, hepatosplenomegaly, respiratory distress associated with pleural effusions, and a low cardiac output state associated with a pericardial effusion. In one series, 25% of the babies with TAM were referred to an intensive care unit.[21]

Transient Abnormal Myelopoiesis: Laboratory Findings

Laboratory tests (reviewed in[22]) can show leucocytosis (20%–30% of cases with a mean white cell count of 20–40 $\times$ 10^9/L, with occasional cases having a white count of >100 $\times$ 10^9/L), though. There is variable thrombocytopenia in approximately 40% of cases (mean 80–100 $\times$ 10^9/L) but thrombocytopenia is not more common in TAM than in neonates with DS who do not have TAM and occasionally severe anemia (hemoglobin <8 g/dL) is seen. Basophilia and an eosinophilia are often seen. Blasts often, but not invariably, have the appearance of megakaryoblasts (with cytoplasmic blebbing). Flow cytometry of blasts may be helpful, as they often express CD34, CD38, CD117, CD7, CD45, the erythroid antigen CD235, the megakaryocyte antigens CD41, CD42b, and CD61 and CD56 and almost always express CD33. The bone marrow aspirate is not often helpful. The cellularity can be increased, normal, or decreased. There is a deranged coagulation profile in 20% to 25% of cases, with disseminated intravascular coagulation (DIC) in approximately 7% to 10% of cases. Hepatic dysfunction is usually associated with hyperbilirubinemia, ascites, elevated transaminases, and hepatic infiltration with blasts. In more severe cases, there is hepatic fibrosis.

GATA1 Mutation, Definition of Transient Abnormal Myelopoiesis and Silent Transient Abnormal Myelopoiesis, and Identification of Children at Risk of Myeloid Leukemia of Down Syndrome

A diagnostic test in nearly many cases have a normal white cell count babies with TAM is the presence of acquired N-terminal truncating mutations[23–27] and, more rarely internal in frame deletions,[28] within exon 2 and, occasionally, exon 3 in the gene encoding the megakaryocyte-erythroid transcription factor GATA1. GATA1 mutations are required for TAM. The detection of N-terminal truncating GATA1 mutations also extends to cases of TAM in neonates with DS mosaicism. There is a unique association with these types of GATA1 mutation and leukemogenesis in hemopoietic cells with T21. Although rare, families and individuals have been described with N-terminal truncating GATA1 mutations in non-DS individuals; there is no documented increased risk of AML in these cases. Non-DS patients with N-terminal truncating GATA1 mutations present with a variety of hematologic phenotypes, including multiple cytopenias[29] and Diamond-Blackfan anemia phenotype.[30]

The incidence of TAM has been the subject of debate. Retrospective studies suggest TAM affects approximately 10% of neonates with DS; but these studies have used differing clinical and/or hematologic criteria to define TAM, none of which is specific for TAM.[20,21,31] Importantly, no retrospective studies have systematically screened neonates for *GATA1* mutations, a genetic marker specific for TAM and ML-DS. Thus, current definitions of TAM neither specify the percentage of blasts considered abnormal in DS neonates nor the role of *GATA1* mutation analysis in the diagnosis. As a result, asymptomatic TAM may be missed in some neonates, as blood counts and smears are often not performed. However, in others babies, TAM may be overdiagnosed by relying on nonspecific clinical and hematologic features. This possibility is borne out by the only large systematic *GATA1* mutation screen, performed by Sanger sequencing of genomic DNA extracted from dried blood spots, which found a prevalence of *GATA1* mutations in neonates with DS of only 3.8%,[32] in contrast to the 5% to 10% prevalence of TAM diagnosed by clinical and hematologic criteria (see review by[22]).

The perception of the incidence and definition of TAM has been changed by a recent prospective study that systematically documented clinical features, blood counts, blood smears, and *GATA1* mutation in a large population-based cohort of newborns with DS.[10] Surprisingly, 195 out of 200 (97.5%) neonates with DS had circulating blasts (range: 1%–77%). In approximately 8.5% of cases, the blast count was greater than 10%; a *GATA1* mutation was detected by conventional Sanger sequencing and mutation detection techniques (direct high-pressure liquid chromatography [DHPLC]). In a further approximately 20% of babies with blast counts less than 10%, *GATA1* mutations were detected by the more sensitive next-generation sequencing mutation detection.[10] No clinical or hematologic features distinguished these neonates from *GATA1* mutation-negative neonates with DS or cases of TAM. Thus, *GATA1* mutations are common, occur in approximately 28% of all neonates with DS, but are often unsuspected and detectable only with sensitive methods. The authors suggest TAM is defined as blasts greater than 10% and a *GATA1* mutation detected by conventional sequencing and/or DHPLC. The authors suggest the term *silent TAM* for those with a *GATA1* mutation detectable only by more sensitive sequencing techniques. In the authors' series, both TAM and silent TAM can transform to ML-DS. Longer-term follow-up is required to determine rates of transformation. To diagnose silent TAM and TAM, an initial evaluation of blood smears as well as full blood counts, as recommended by the American Academy of Pediatrics,[33] is a useful, immediate screening step to identify neonates with DS with classic TAM who may require early treatment (especially where *GATA1* analysis is unavailable or delayed). If possible, all neonates with DS should also have *GATA1* mutation analysis by Sanger sequencing and DHPLC to quickly identify those with large mutant *GATA1* clones. For neonates with DS without mutations by Sanger sequencing or DHPLC, next-generation resequencing can be used to identify those with small mutant *GATA1* clones. By comprehensively detecting *GATA1* mutations, pediatric hematology follow-up can be limited to those at risk of transformation rather than all babies with blasts (ie, almost all babies with DS).

Outcome and Management of Transient Abnormal Myelopoiesis

In most babies (80%–90%), the condition only requires observation and blood count monitoring, as it resolves spontaneously over a 1- to 3-month period (median time to resolution 47 days[31]). However, a proportion of babies require therapy for clinical symptoms (eg, cardiac failure or DIC). However, it is unclear which infants will benefit from treatment and what the most effective treatment is. Accordingly, treatment policies vary considerably between centers. Both the US Pediatric/Children's Oncology Group (POG/COG) and the German International Berlin-Frankfurt-Munster (BFM) group have developed treatment guidelines for TAM that can be instituted at the physician's discretion.[21,31]

As TAM blasts are highly sensitive to cytarabine, it is the basis of cytoreductive therapy. The response is generally rapid with disappearance of peripheral blasts within 7 days of treatment. However, in babies with severe liver disease associated with fibrosis, the response to chemotherapy is poor. In the POG study 9481, cytosine arabinoside (araC) was given either as 10 mg/m^2 per dose or 1.2 to 1.5 mg/kg per dose subcutaneously or intravenously by slow injection twice a day for 7 days.[20] In the AML-BFM study, 0.5 to 1.5 mg/kg was administered for 3 to 12 days.[21] The higher dose of cytarabine (3.33 mg/kg/24 h given by continuous infusion for 5 days) used in the COG A2971 study is probably not required and was associated with significant toxicity.[31] Despite therapy, 10% to 20% of babies die of TAM within 3 months with hepatic and renal failure and DIC. These babies often present with a higher white count (>100 $\times$ 10^9/L), ascites, effusions, and coagulopathy and develop hepatic fibrosis.

Transformation to Myeloid Leukemia of Down Syndrome

Following the clinical resolution of TAM with normalization of blood counts either spontaneously or after treatment with very low-dose cytarabine, up to 30% of these neonates with clinical TAM will subsequently develop ML-DS.[34] In a baby with a history of TAM, often the same GATA1 mutation is detected when the child presents with ML-DS proving that the two disorders are clonally linked.[24,25,27] In approximately 15% to 25% of cases, multiple GATA1 mutations are detected in both TAM and ML-DS suggesting that multiple GATA1 mutant clones exist.[27]

Clinical Features of Myeloid Leukemia of Down Syndrome

Children with ML-DS with DS represent approximately 15% of the pediatric AML cases.[35] Reports from both the United Kingdom Childhood Cancer Study and the Children's Cancer Group (CCG) identified that the mean age at diagnosis of ML-DS was lower than the age for children without DS (2.2 years versus 6.7 years and 1.8 versus 7.5 years, respectively).[35,36] Overall, 95% of ML-DS cases are diagnosed before 4 years of age.[37] Progression to ML-DS does not occur in children beyond 5 years of age.[37]

Progression to ML-DS occurs at a variable tempo. In some children, progression is heralded by a period of falling blood counts, especially thrombocytopenia and leukopenia. Cytopenia may be short or prolonged over months before a formal diagnosis of ML-DS. It is often associated with dysplastic changes in peripheral blood cells. At presentation of ML-DS, children with DS may not seem acutely ill compared with children without DS. This circumstance is caused, in part, by closer clinical monitoring of these children based on their known increased risk to develop leukemia and early evidence of abnormalities in blood count parameters indicating evidence of potential progression to leukemia in the absence of clinical symptoms. These early signs of myelodysplasia are characterized by progressive anemia and thrombocytopenia in association with dysplastic erythroid cells and megakaryocytes in the bone marrow.[38] This myelodysplastic phase frequently precedes the development of AML, and the spectrum of both myelodysplastic syndrome (MDS) and AML have been known collectively as ML-DS.[38,39] Rarely ML-DS can progress directly from aggressive TAM. In these cases, the diagnosis is problematic, as it is difficult to distinguish between TAM that is not resolving and the development of ML-DS. A bone marrow aspirate and trephine can be helpful to confirm greater than 30% blasts. Often the blast count is lower as the marrow sample on aspirate is hemodilute. In these cases, the trephine shows marrow fibrosis echoing the liver fibrosis seen in some cases of TAM. If the marrow is aspirable or if there are circulating blasts, flow cytometry is valuable, as blasts express the same cell surface markers as TAM blasts.

Laboratory Features of Myeloid Leukemia of Down Syndrome

Several other distinctive differences exist in the biological features of ML-DS compared with AML in children without DS. Among the 8 different French-American-British subtypes of AML, children with DS have a disproportionately high proportion with the acute megakaryocytic/megakaryoblastic (AMKL, M7) phenotype. Zipursky[38] estimated that children with DS have a 500-fold increased risk of developing ML-DS compared with children without DS, with some clinical studies identifying the ML-DS phenotype in more than 90% of ML-DS cases.[38] Besides the morphologic identification of the ML-DS phenotype, megakaryoblasts are identified by their immunophenotype expression of the platelet-associated membrane antigens (glycoprotein IIb/IIIa) using CD41/61 antibodies and frequently the aberrant expression of the T-cell antigen, CD7, and the thrombospondin receptor, CD36.[40,41] High expression of CD36 marker distinguishes ML-DS from most cases of de novo AMKL and may be a surrogate for the developmental stage of the megakaryoblasts identified by molecular studies.[18,19,41]

The proportion of patients with DS who fit the criteria of MDS based on the bone marrow involvement containing less that 30% blasts was approximately 30% for both the COG A2971 and CCG-2891 studies.[35,42] Structural chromosomal abnormalities detected in ML-DS include trisomy 8, trisomy 11, and T21 (besides the constitutional T21), dup (1p), del (6q), del (7p), dup (7q), and del (16q).[43] In contrast, the classic cytogenetic abnormalities seen in AML cases in children without DS, including *AML-ETO* t (8;21), *PML-RARA* t (15;17), *CBFB-MYH11* inv (16), and *MLL* 11q23 rearrangements, are not seen in ML-DS. Furthermore, neonates and children with DS developing ML-DS usually do not acquire the specific non-DS childhood AMKL cytogenetic abnormality *RBM15-MKL1* t (1;22)[44] or the cryptic inversion of chromosome 16 that produces the CBFA2T3-GLIS2 fusion gene.[45,46]

Molecular Abnormalities in Myeloid Leukemia of Down Syndrome

Whole genome/exome sequencing identified that the mean number of somatic mutations in TAM cases (with *GATA1* mutations in all cases) was 1.5, whereas the number of mutations was significantly higher in ML-DS cases than in TAM.[47,48] Acquired mutations were identified in genes encoding components of the cohesin complex (*RAD21, STAG2, NIPBL, SMC3, SMC1A*); chromatin regulators (*EZH2, SUZ12, ASXL1, DNMT3A*), cytokine signaling pathway regulators (*JAK1, JAK3, MPL, KRAS, NRAS, PTPN11, SH2B3*), and other genes that have also been previously shown to be been mutated in leukemia (*TP53, ETV6, SRSF2*). These observations indicate that TAM is caused by a *GATA1* mutation together with T21 and progresses to ML-DS because of the acquisition of additional mutations.[48]

THERAPY FOR MYELOID LEUKEMIA OF DOWN SYNDROME

Although the chemotherapy agents used in the treatment of ML-DS are the same as for children without DS, current treatment strategies differ significantly between the DS and non-DS patient groups and, in particular, balance curative therapy against the risk of treatment-associated morbidity and mortality for children with DS. The POG 8498 trial was the first to identify that ML-DS had very high cure rates when children with DS were treated with equivalent protocols as for children without DS.[49] Previous to this report, less-than-optimal leukemia therapy for children with DS seemed to be a significant factor in their poor survival rates because of a perception that children with DS would not tolerate contemporary AML therapies. Subsequent studies from the CCG, POG, Medical Research Council, Nordic Society of Pediatric/Hematology Oncology, and the BFM cooperative groups confirmed the high cure rates for ML-DS with overall event-free survival (EFS) rates of approximately 80%.[50–54] The utilization of high-dose araC-based therapy for patients with ML-DS seemed to have contributed to the improved survival rates.[55]

The time-intensive strategy for treating pediatric AML (without evidence of full marrow recovery from neutropenia and thrombocytopenia) was found to be too toxic for patients with ML-DS as highlighted by the CCG-2861/2891 studies in which there was a 32% treatment-associated mortality rate for patients treated on the intensive-timed treatment arm.[52] The Mecial Research Council AM 10/12 studies reported that children with DS experienced a 27% treatment-related mortality (TRM) rate and received equivalent drug dosing as for children without DS.[54] Cardiotoxicity was a significant treatment-related complication for children with DS treated on POG 9421 (which used a high total cumulative anthracycline dose); 21% of children developed late-onset congestive heart failure, including several treatment-associated (and non-leukemic) deaths.[56]

The CCG-2891 study found that patients with ML-DS experience similar toxicities compared with non-DS patients when a decreased dose-intensity regimen was administered.[35] This finding has also led to the design of DS-specific AML protocols including COG A2971[42] and AAML 0431.

In order to reduce therapy-associated toxicity, other groups have reported the use of either intermediate-dose or very-low-dose araC. Studies from Japan used an intermediate-dose araC-based regimen (5 cycles of araC 100 $mg/m^2/d \times 7$ days with an 83% EFS rate).[57] Canadian studies have used repetitive courses of very-low-dose araC (10 mg/m^2 per dose), with several nonresponsive patients being able to be salvaged with intensive AML therapies.[58] A study of patients with ML-DS treated in France from 1990 to 2003, however, reported that low-dose chemotherapy regimens including araC were inferior compared with standard-dose chemotherapy regimens.[59]

The current COG AAML 0431 trial is investigating the clinical significance of minimal residual disease (MRD) testing for ML-DS, which may identify patients who could be treated with reduced-intensity therapy.

PROGNOSTIC FACTORS

Several prognostic factors have been reported for patients with ML-DS, which are associated with outcome. The BFM group identified that a prior diagnosis of TAM was associated with superior EFS rates compared with patients without a TMD history,[21] though the results of the COG studies reported equivalent outcomes.[35,42] Patients with ML-DS older than 4 years of age (who compose ~5% of the patient group) have a poor outcome; for the CCG-2891 study, EFS rates were only 33%.[35] This finding may indicate differences in leukemia biology among patients with DS, including a low detection rate of GATA1 mutations in blast cells among the older patients.[37]

An international retrospective analysis of 451 patients with ML-DS had an overall survival (OS) rate of 79% and identified several factors: (1) patients with normal karyotypes had an overall relapse rate of 21% compared with 9% with patients with an aberrant karyotype; (2) patients with a white blood cell count of 20,000/μL or more and aged greater than 3 years were independent predictors for poor EFS. Patients with ML-DS with monosomy 7 had a moderately worse outcome with EFS rates of 69%, though still superior than monosomy 7 AML in children without DS.[60]

Although the ML-DS group overall has an excellent prognosis, a minority of patients with either refractory or relapsed disease have a poor prognosis. Patients with DS with relapsed leukemia treated on the POG 9421 and CCG-2891 AML studies had an OS rate of only 12%.[61] Twenty-six Japanese patients with DS AML (including 22 with ML-DS) with relapsed or refractory disease had an OS rate of only 25.9%.[62] In another study, patients with ML-DS only had a 19% probability of survival following stem cell transplant (SCT). These studies all highlight that patients with DS with refractory/relapsed leukemia have very chemotherapy-resistant disease. A recent Japanese study reported an 80% EFS rate for ML-DS using a lower-intensity conditioning regimen preceding SCT for ML-DS,[63] though the inclusion of patients in first remission who may have already been cured by frontline chemotherapy may have biased the very favorable results.

Several new therapeutic approaches may offer promising treatments for relapsed ML-DS cases: (1) Preventing cell cycle checkpoint activation by inhibiting the upstream kinase wee1 with the inhibitor MK-1775 in combination with araC. MK-1775 was able to synergistically enhance araC cytotoxic effects in ML-DS cell lines and ex vivo patient samples by abrogation of an intra-S phase DNA damage checkpoint and enhancement of araC-induced DNA damage.[64] (2) Inhibition of aurora A kinase with MLN9237 was able to induce polyploidization and differentiation of non-DS ML-DS cells and an ML-DS cell line.[65] (3) Histone deacetylase inhibitors inducing apoptosis by suppressing autophagy.[66]

ACUTE LYMPHOBLASTIC LEUKEMIA IN DOWN SYNDROME
Incidence

Studies suggest a 10- to 20-fold increased risk of leukemia in children with DS, with acute lymphoblastic leukemia (ALL) occurring in 1 in 300 children with DS versus 1 in 3500 children without DS.[67,68] Hasle and colleagues[69] described the incidence of malignancy in 2814 individuals with DS registered in the Danish Cytogenetic Registry from 1968 to 1995 and reported that leukemia made up 60% of the malignant diseases overall, with the majority occurring before 15 years of age. In this registry study of individuals with DS, no cases of leukemia were seen after 29 years of age.

Clinical Features, Therapy, and Outcome in Children with Down Syndrome Acute Lymphoblastic Leukemia

Children with DS and ALL do have a few unique clinical characteristics as compared with those without DS as well as more therapy-related challenges. The age distribution at presentation of the leukemia is similar in children with and without DS, with most children presenting at greater than 1 year of age. ALL is very rarely diagnosed in children with DS who are less than 1 year of age, whereas approximately 2.6% of non-DS ALL cases occur in infants less than 1 year of age.[70–74] Most studies also report no significant difference in initial white blood cell count, racial or ethnic differences in the population, or assignment to National Cancer Institute (NCI) risk groups.[70,71,73–77] Although not uniformly reported, the incidence of a mediastinal mass or the presence of central nervous system disease at diagnosis is similar between DS ALL and non-DS ALL.[70,71,76]

However, there are clear immunophenotypic differences between DS and non-DS ALL. T-cell phenotype (T-ALL) and mature B-cell phenotype are very rare in patients with DS but occur at higher incidences in non-DS leukemia.[73] A recent review of

708 patients with DS ALL found only 5 patients with DS with T-ALL, compared with the expected 10% to 15% in non-DS ALL.[78]

Induction therapy for DS ALL and non-DS ALL is now essentially the same with only minimal differences in DS ALL to enhance safety in most of the treatment protocols. In most modern therapeutic trials, clinical remission (CR) at the end of induction is found to be similar between DS ALL and non-DS ALL.[70,71,77] The rates of CR at the end of induction are reported to range from 96% to 99% and were not statistically significant from the CR rates of non-DS ALL patients in these studies.[73,75,79] However, a large retrospective study evaluated 653 patients with DS ALL and found induction failures to occur in 3% of DS ALL versus 1% of non-DS ALL ($P<.001$).[78] Increased mortality, primarily caused by infection, during remission induction in DS ALL has been well described and contributes to induction failure.[78,80,81]

Additional measures about the depth of remission or rapidity of response to induction therapy are used to augment the risk classification and prognosis. There is limited data that suggests DS ALL responses in small studies are equivalent to those with non-DS ALL. Prednisone response (prednisone response = number of lymphoblasts in blood after a 7-day exposure to prednisone with a good response being $<1000/\mu$ blood blasts) was not different between DS ALL and non-DS ALL in the BFM protocols with prednisone good response in 90.7% and 98.1%, respectively.[71] Levels of bone marrow MRD as measured by flow cytometry (measured from $<0.1\%$ to $>1\%$) did not show a difference between DS-ALL versus non-DS ALL at day 29 of induction in the most recent COG therapeutic trials.[82] In addition, the corresponding marrow response at day 8 and day 15 was similar between DS ALL and non-DS ALL in this study.

Currently, most ALL cooperative group protocols use the same or very similar therapy for DS ALL as for their patients without DS and have in some cases successfully increased the intensity of therapy (L Silverman, personal communication, 2014).[70,71,75,83] Frequently, however, there may be additional modifications or supportive care guidelines for DS ALL versus non-DS ALL. COG and Medical Research Council United Kingdom Childhood Acute Lymphoblastic Leukemia trials now incorporate discontinuous dexamethasone during delayed intensification. Additionally, the COG therapy trials added leucovorin rescue after intrathecal administration of methotrexate.[80,81] Anthracycline exposure in DS ALL is approached differently among the groups. Two groups are decreasing the anthracycline exposure to high-risk patients with DS ALL by only giving induction daunomycin to those patients with a slow response.[84] However, St. Jude Research Hospital's ALL therapies incorporate anthracycline along with steroids in induction with no excess toxicity or mortality in the DS ALL population (M Relling, personal communication). The balance in modern therapy is to continue to improve the survival of this special group of patients while decreasing the severe adverse effects of therapy in DS ALL.

One of the key agents used in ALL therapy is methotrexate (MTX). It is well known that patients with DS ALL are more susceptible to MTX-induced side effects than non-DS ALL patients. Multiple studies have shown that patients with DS ALL suffer significantly higher incidences of gastrointestinal toxicity primarily as well as more hematologic toxicity.[78,85–88] For this reason, infusional MTX is often started at a more modest dose for patients with DS, increasing if tolerated. TRM is higher for patients with DS ALL as compared with non-DS ALL. In the large retrospective study, the TRM for patients with DS was 7.7% as compared with 2.3% in non-DS patients.[78] Most TRM in DS ALL is caused by infection/sepsis. In fact, the infection-related mortality (IRM) can be as high as 18.6% versus 1.9% in non-DS ALL.[80] Additionally, IRM in non-DS ALL occurs primarily during induction; but for DS ALL, this risk is spread throughout all phases of therapy.[78,80,89] When caring for patients with DS ALL, careful observation and adherence to supportive care measures is quite important. However, further studies are needed to assess the value of additional supportive care, such as prophylactic antibiotics and immunoglobulin use.

The prognosis of children with DS ALL is worse than for those with non-DS ALL in general.[74,78,89] The Ponte di Legno study group reported a lower EFS of 64% versus 81% at 8 years for DS ALL versus non-DS ALL and consequently a lower OS of 74% versus 89%, respectively.[78] Similar results have also been show in smaller studies. COG reported an inferior EFS and OS for patients with DS enrolled on the AALL 0232, the most recently completed high risk trial, largely caused by the increased toxic mortality rates as discussed earlier. The EFS for the patients with DS on the NCI standard risk trial, AALL 0331, were similar to non-DS patients; but the OS was significantly lower, 89% versus 96%, respectively.[89]

Despite a high rate of TRM, relapse is still a main cause of treatment failure in this group of patients.[78] However, enrollment on relapse treatment protocols for this group of patients has not been consistent, so there are limited data about the outcome following relapse. Relapses in patients with DS ALL tend to occur later when compared with non-DS ALL.[78,90] The BFM 106529 relapsed trials (ALL REZ BFM) retrospectively found that a significantly higher proportion of children with DS has fatal treatment-related adverse events during induction therapy (22%) and subsequent treatment phases (10%) as compared with children without DS when treated for relapse (3% and 6%, respectively). In addition, hematopoietic SCT was used less frequently in DS ALL after relapse than in non-DS ALL.[90] As the numbers are small, further understanding of the tolerance of therapy and transplant in this population is important for making therapeutic decisions for relapse.

Biological Features of Down Syndrome Acute Lymphoblastic Leukemia

The biological features of DS ALL are distinctly different than ALL in children without DS. Additionally, DS ALL does not have an overriding lesion responsible for the transformation, as does DS AML. The Ponte di Legno study group reported BCR-ABL1 fusion in 0.7% compared with 2.4% non-DS ALL and MLL rearrangements of less than 1.0% in DS ALL versus 1.2% of non-DS ALL.[78] These findings are also consistent with other studies that have confirmed this lower incidence of hypodiploidy, t(9;22), and 11q23 translocations in DS ALL as compared with non-DS ALL.[43,76,82]

Different frequencies of favorable subtypes in DS ALL may also be responsible for some of the inferior survival seen in DS ALL. COG 9900 series, a series of therapeutic trials with a uniform classification strategy, showed that the incidence of the favorable cytogenetic lesions are different between DS ALL and non-DS ALL.[82] The incidence of ETV6-RUNX1 fusion transcripts were found in 2.5% of DS ALL versus 24% of non-DS ALL. Similarly, trisomy of both chromosomes 4 and 10 occurred in 7.7% of DS ALL versus 23.9% of non-DS ALL. The proportion of high hyperdiploidy as measured by a DNA index of greater than 1.16 was significantly different between the 2 groups with 5% in DS ALL versus 24.6% in non-DS ALL.

Additional genetic abnormalities (JAK mutations, cytokine receptorlike factor 2 [CRLF2] expression, and IKZF1 mutations) have been recognized in pediatric ALL. The aberrant expression of CRLF2 is detected in 50% of DS ALL versus 5% in non-DS ALL.[91] Most of the CRLF2 alterations were observed in cases lacking translocations associated with ALL, suggesting that CFLF2 alteration is a potent leukemogenic event in the setting of T21.[91,92] Although the overexpression of CRLF2 is frequently found in DS ALL, it has not been proven to be associated with a therapeutic outcome, which is in contrast to non-DS ALL whereby CFLF2 overexpression has been associated with a poor EFS.[92,93] *JAK2*-activating mutations have recently been described in approximately 20% of DS ALL cases and approximately 10% of high-risk non-DS ALL.[94,95] Patients with DS ALL with *JAK2* mutations have a similar outcome to those without the mutation.[78,96] The identification of *JAK2* mutations in DS ALL leads to the possibility of targeted therapy with a JAK2 inhibitor. Early trials of these drugs are occurring in myeloproliferative disorders and may then lead to additional therapeutic options for DS ALL with potentially less toxicity. Recently, *IKZF1* gene deletions/alterations have been shown to be associated with a very poor outcome in B-cell–progenitor ALL. *IKZF1* deletions have been reported in approximately 30% of patients with DS ALL. Similar to those with non-DS ALL, these mutations are associated with a poor prognosis, EFS 45% with DS ALL, and *IKZF1* mutation versus 95% for DS ALL without the mutation.[97] As we move forward, larger trials will be needed to confirm the prognostic importance of these more newly described genetic alterations in DS ALL.

SUMMARY

Children with DS and ALL have unique biological, cytogenetic, and intrinsic factors that affect their treatment and outcome. As their EFS and OS are poorer than non-DS ALL, it is important to continue to study the biology of their leukemia; enroll them on therapeutic trials, including relapse trials; investigate new agents that could potentially improve their leukemia-free survival without additional toxicity; and strive to maximize the supportive care these patients need.

REFERENCES

1. Krivit W, Good RA. Simultaneous occurrence of mongolism and leukemia; report of a nationwide survey. AMA J Dis Child 1957;94:289–93.
2. Tunstall-Pedoe O, Roy A, Karadimitris A, et al. Abnormalities in the myeloid compartment in Down syndrome fetal liver precede acquisition of GATA1 mutations. Blood 2008;112:4507–11.
3. Chou ST, Opalinska JB, Yao Y, et al. Trisomy 21 enhances human fetal erythro-megakaryocytic development. Blood 2008;112:4503–6.
4. Roy A, Cowan G, Mead AJ, et al. Perturbation of fetal liver hematopoietic stem and progenitor cell development by trisomy 21. Proc Natl Acad Sci U S A 2012;109:17579–84.
5. Chou ST, Byrska-Bishop M, Tober JM, et al. Trisomy 21-associated defects in human primitive hematopoiesis revealed through induced pluripotent stem cells. Proc Natl Acad Sci U S A 2012;109(43):17573–8.
6. Maclean GA, Menne TF, Guo G, et al. Altered hematopoiesis in trisomy 21 as revealed through in vitro differentiation of isogenic human pluripotent cells. Proc Natl Acad Sci U S A 2012;109(43):17567–72.
7. Starc TJ. Erythrocyte macrocytosis in infants and children with Down syndrome. J Pediatr 1992;121:578–81.
8. Kivivuori SM, Rajantie J, Siimes MA. Peripheral blood cell counts in infants with Down's syndrome. Clin Genet 1996;49:15–9.
9. Henry E, Walker D, Wiedmeier SE, et al. Hematological abnormalities during the first week of life among neonates with Down syndrome: data from a multihospital healthcare system. Am J Med Genet A 2007;143:42–50.
10. Roberts I, Alford K, Hall G, et al. GATA1-mutant clones are frequent and often unsuspected in babies with Down syndrome: identification of a population at risk of leukemia. Blood 2013;122:3908–17.

11. Korbel JO, Tirosh-Wagner T, Urban AE, et al. The genetic architecture of Down syndrome phenotypes revealed by high-resolution analysis of human segmental trisomies. Proc Natl Acad Sci U S A 2009;106:12031–6.
12. Alford KA, Slender A, Vanes L, et al. Perturbed hematopoiesis in the Tc1 mouse model of Down syndrome. Blood 2010;115:2928–37.
13. Kirsammer G, Jilani S, Liu H, et al. Highly penetrant myeloproliferative disease in the Ts65Dn mouse model of Down syndrome. Blood 2008;111:767–75.
14. Stankiewicz MJ, Crispino JD. ETS2 and ERG promote megakaryopoiesis and synergize with alterations in GATA-1 to immortalize hematopoietic progenitor cells. Blood 2009;113:3337–47.
15. Salek-Ardakani S, Smooha G, de Boer J, et al. ERG is a megakaryocytic oncogene. Cancer Res 2009;69:4665–73.
16. Malinge S, Bliss-Moreau M, Kirsammer G, et al. Increased dosage of the chromosome 21 ortholog Dyrk1a promotes megakaryoblastic leukemia in a murine model of Down syndrome. J Clin Invest 2012;122:948–62.
17. Chou S, Lodish HF. Fetal liver hepatic progenitors are supportive stromal cells for hematopoietic stem cells. Proc Natl Acad Sci U S A 2010;107:7799–804.
18. Klusmann JH, Godinho FJ, Heitmann K, et al. Developmental stage-specific interplay of GATA1 and IGF signaling in fetal megakaryopoiesis and leukemogenesis. Genes Dev 2010;24:1659–72.
19. Bourquin JP, Subramanian A, Langebrake C, et al. Identification of distinct molecular phenotypes in acute megakaryoblastic leukemia by gene expression profiling. Proc Natl Acad Sci U S A 2006;103:3339–44.
20. Massey GV, Zipursky A, Chang MN, et al. A prospective study of the natural history of transient leukemia (TL) in neonates with Down syndrome (DS): Children's Oncology Group (COG) study POG-9481. Blood 2006;107:4606–13.
21. Klusmann JH, Creutzig U, Zimmermann M, et al. Treatment and prognostic impact of transient leukemia in neonates with Down syndrome. Blood 2008;111:2991–8.
22. Roy A, Roberts I, Vyas P. Biology and management of transient abnormal myelopoiesis (TAM) in children with Down syndrome. Semin Fetal Neonatal Med 2012;17:196–201.
23. Wechsler J, Greene M, McDevitt MA, et al. Acquired mutations in GATA1 in the megakaryoblastic leukemia of Down syndrome. Nat Genet 2002;32:148–52.
24. Rainis L, Bercovich D, Strehl S, et al. Mutations in exon 2 of GATA1 are early events in megakaryocytic malignancies associated with trisomy 21. Blood 2003;102:981–6.
25. Hitzler JK, Cheung J, Li Y, et al. GATA1 mutations in transient leukemia and acute megakaryoblastic leukemia of Down syndrome. Blood 2003;101:4301–4.
26. Xu G, Nagano M, Kanezaki R, et al. Frequent mutations in the GATA-1 gene in the transient myeloproliferative disorder of Down syndrome. Blood 2003;102:2960–8.
27. Ahmed M, Sternberg A, Hall G, et al. Natural history of GATA1 mutations in Down syndrome. Blood 2004;103:2480–9.
28. Toki T, Kanezaki R, Kobayashi E, et al. Naturally occurring oncogenic GATA1 mutants with internal deletions in transient abnormal myelopoiesis in Down syndrome. Blood 2013;121:3181–4.
29. Hollanda LM, Lima CS, Cunha AF, et al. An inherited mutation leading to production of only the short isoform of GATA-1 is associated with impaired erythropoiesis. Nat Genet 2006;38:807–12.
30. Sankaran VG, Ghazvinian R, Do R, et al. Exome sequencing identifies GATA1 mutations resulting in Diamond-Blackfan anemia. J Clin Invest 2012;122:2439–43.

31. Gamis AS, Alonzo TA, Gerbing RB, et al. Natural history of transient myeloprolif-erative disorder clinically diagnosed in Down syndrome neonates: a report from the Children's Oncology Group Study A2971. Blood 2011;118:6752–9 [quiz: 996].
32. Pine SR, Guo Q, Yin C, et al. Incidence and clinical implications of GATA1 muta-tions in newborns with Down syndrome. Blood 2007;110:2128–31.
33. Bull MJ. Health supervision for children with Down syndrome. Pediatrics 2011; 128:393–406.
34. Zipursky A. Transient leukaemia - a benign form of leukaemia in newborn infants with trisomy 21. Br J Haematol 2003;120:930–8.
35. Gamis AS, Woods WG, Alonzo TA, et al. Increased age at diagnosis has a signif-icantly negative effect on outcome in children with Down syndrome and acute myeloid leukemia: a report from the Children's Cancer Group Study 2891. J Clin Oncol 2003;21:3415–22.
36. James R, Lightfoot T, Simpson J, et al. Acute leukemia in children with Down's syndrome: the importance of population based study. Haematologica 2008;93: 1262–3.
37. Hasle H, Abrahamsson J, Arola M, et al. Myeloid leukemia in children 4 years or older with Down syndrome often lacks GATA1 mutation and cytogenetics and risk of relapse are more akin to sporadic AML. Leukemia 2008;22:1428–30.
38. Zipursky A, Thorner P, De Harven E, et al. Myelodysplasia and acute megakaryo-blastic leukemia in Down's syndrome. Leuk Res 1994;18:163–71.
39. Heerema-McKenney A, Arber DA. Acute myeloid leukemia. Hematol Oncol Clin North Am 2009;23:633–54.
40. Langebrake C, Creutzig U, Reinhardt D. Immunophenotype of Down syndrome acute myeloid leukemia and transient myeloproliferative disease differs signifi-cantly from other diseases with morphologically identical or similar blasts. Klin Padiatr 2005;217:126–34.
41. Savasan S, Buck S, Raimondi SC, et al. CD36 (thrombospondin receptor) expres-sion in childhood acute megakaryoblastic leukemia: in vitro drug sensitivity and outcome. Leuk Lymphoma 2006;47:2076–83.
42. Sorrell AD, Alonzo TA, Hilden JM, et al. Favorable survival maintained in children who have myeloid leukemia associated with Down syndrome using reduced-dose chemotherapy on Children's Oncology Group trial A2971: a report from the Children's Oncology Group. Cancer 2012;118:4806–14.
43. Forestier E, Izraeli S, Beverloo B, et al. Cytogenetic features of acute lympho-blastic and myeloid leukemias in pediatric patients with Down syndrome: an iBFM-SG study. Blood 2008;111:1575–83.
44. Mercher T, Coniat MB, Monni R, et al. Involvement of a human gene related to the Drosophila spen gene in the recurrent t(1;22) translocation of acute megakaryo-cytic leukemia. Proc Natl Acad Sci U S A 2001;98:5776–9.
45. Thiollier C, Lopez CK, Gerby B, et al. Characterization of novel genomic alter-ations and therapeutic approaches using acute megakaryoblastic leukemia xenograft models. J Exp Med 2012;209:2017–31.
46. Gruber TA, Larson Gedman A, Zhang J, et al. An Inv(16)(p13.3q24.3)-encoded CBFA2T3-GLIS2 fusion protein defines an aggressive subtype of pediatric acute megakaryoblastic leukemia. Cancer Cell 2012;22:683–97.
47. Yoshida K, Toki T, Okuno Y, et al. The landscape of somatic mutations in Down syndrome-related myeloid disorders. Nat Genet 2013;45:1293–9.
48. Nikolaev SI, Santoni F, Vannier A, et al. Exome sequencing identifies putative drivers of progression of transient myeloproliferative disorder to AMKL in infants with Down syndrome. Blood 2013;122:554–61.

49. Ravindranath Y, Abella E, Krischer JP, et al. Acute myeloid leukemia (AML) in Down's syndrome is highly responsive to chemotherapy: experience on Pediatric Oncology Group AML Study 8498. Blood 1992;80:2210–4.
50. Zeller B, Gustafsson G, Forestier E, et al. Acute leukaemia in children with Down syndrome: a population-based Nordic study. Br J Haematol 2005;128: 797–804.
51. Creutzig U, Reinhardt D, Diekamp S, et al. AML patients with Down syndrome have a high cure rate with AML-BFM therapy with reduced dose intensity. Leukemia 2005;19:1355–60.
52. Lange BJ, Kobrinsky N, Barnard DR, et al. Distinctive demography, biology, and outcome of acute myeloid leukemia and myelodysplastic syndrome in children with Down syndrome: Children's Cancer Group Studies 2861 and 2891. Blood 1998;91:608–15.
53. Ravindranath Y, Yeager AM, Chang MN, et al. Autologous bone marrow transplantation versus intensive consolidation chemotherapy for acute myeloid leukemia in childhood. Pediatric Oncology Group. N Engl J Med 1996;334:1428–34.
54. Rao A, Hills RK, Stiller C, et al. Treatment for myeloid leukaemia of Down syndrome: population-based experience in the UK and results from the Medical Research Council AML 10 and AML 12 trials. Br J Haematol 2006;132:576–83.
55. Ravindranath Y, Taub JW. Down syndrome and acute myeloid leukemia. Lessons learned from experience with high-dose Ara-C containing regimens. Adv Exp Med Biol 1999;457:409–14.
56. O'Brien MM, Taub JW, Chang MN, et al. Cardiomyopathy in children with Down syndrome treated for acute myeloid leukemia: a report from the Children's Oncology Group Study POG 9421. J Clin Oncol 2008;26:414–20.
57. Kudo K, Kojima S, Tabuchi K, et al. Prospective study of a pirarubicin, intermediate-dose cytarabine, and etoposide regimen in children with Down syndrome and acute myeloid leukemia: the Japanese Childhood AML Cooperative Study Group. J Clin Oncol 2007;25:5442–7.
58. Al-Ahmari A, Shah N, Sung L, et al. Long-term results of an ultra low-dose cytarabine-based regimen for the treatment of acute megakaryoblastic leukaemia in children with Down syndrome. Br J Haematol 2006;133:646–8.
59. Tandonnet J, Clavel J, Baruchel A, et al. Myeloid leukaemia in children with Down syndrome: report of the registry-based French experience between 1990 and 2003. Pediatr Blood Cancer 2010;54:927–33.
60. Blink M, Zimmermann M, von Neuhoff C, et al. Normal karyotype is a poor prognostic factor in myeloid leukemia of Down syndrome: a retrospective, international study. Haematologica 2014;99:299–307.
61. Loew TM, Gamis A, Smith FO, et al. Down syndrome patients with relapsed acute myelogenous leukemia. Blood 2004;104 [abstract: 4526].
62. Taga T, Saito AM, Kudo K, et al. Clinical characteristics and outcome of refractory/relapsed myeloid leukemia in children with Down syndrome. Blood 2012; 120:1810–5.
63. Muramatsu H, Sakaguchi H, Taga T, et al. Reduced intensity conditioning in allogeneic stem cell transplantation for AML with Down syndrome. Pediatr Blood Cancer 2014;61:925–7.
64. Caldwell JT, Edwards H, Buck SA, et al. Targeting the wee1 kinase for treatment of pediatric Down syndrome acute myeloid leukemia. Pediatr Blood Cancer 2014; 61(10):1767–73.
65. Wen Q, Goldenson B, Silver SJ, et al. Identification of regulators of polyploidization presents therapeutic targets for treatment of AMKL. Cell 2012;150:575–89.

66. Stankov MV, El Khatib M, Kumar Thakur B, et al. Histone deacetylase inhibitors induce apoptosis in myeloid leukemia by suppressing autophagy. Leukemia 2014;28:577–88.
67. Lange B. The management of neoplastic disorders of haematopoiesis in children with Down's syndrome. Br J Haematol 2000;110:512–24.
68. Robison LL. Down syndrome and leukemia. Leukemia 1992;6(Suppl 1):5–7.
69. Hasle H, Clemmensen IH, Mikkelsen M. Risks of leukaemia and solid tumours in individuals with Down's syndrome. Lancet 2000;355:165–9.
70. Chessells JM, Harrison G, Richards SM, et al. Down's syndrome and acute lymphoblastic leukaemia: clinical features and response to treatment. Arch Dis Child 2001;85:321–5.
71. Dordelmann M, Schrappe M, Reiter A, et al. Down's syndrome in childhood acute lymphoblastic leukemia: clinical characteristics and treatment outcome in four consecutive BFM trials. Berlin-Frankfurt-Munster Group. Leukemia 1998;12:645–51.
72. Kalwinsky DK, Raimondi SC, Bunin NJ, et al. Clinical and biological characteristics of acute lymphocytic leukemia in children with Down syndrome. Am J Med Genet Suppl 1990;7:267–71.
73. Maloney KW. Acute lymphoblastic leukaemia in children with Down syndrome: an updated review. Br J Haematol 2011;155:420–5.
74. Whitlock JA, Sather HN, Gaynon P, et al. Clinical characteristics and outcome of children with Down syndrome and acute lymphoblastic leukemia: a Children's Cancer Group study. Blood 2005;106:4043–9.
75. Bassal M, La MK, Whitlock JA, et al. Lymphoblast biology and outcome among children with Down syndrome and ALL treated on CCG-1952. Pediatr Blood Cancer 2005;44:21–8.
76. Pui CH, Raimondi SC, Borowitz MJ, et al. Immunophenotypes and karyotypes of leukemic cells in children with Down syndrome and acute lymphoblastic leukemia. J Clin Oncol 1993;11:1361–7.
77. Ragab AH, Abdel-Mageed A, Shuster JJ, et al. Clinical characteristics and treatment outcome of children with acute lymphocytic leukemia and Down's syndrome. A Pediatric Oncology Group study. Cancer 1991;67:1057–63.
78. Buitenkamp TD, Izraeli S, Zimmermann M, et al. Acute lymphoblastic leukemia in children with Down syndrome: a retrospective analysis from the Ponte di Legno study group. Blood 2014;123:70–7.
79. Arico M, Ziino O, Valsecchi MG, et al. Acute lymphoblastic leukemia and Down syndrome: presenting features and treatment outcome in the experience of the Italian Association of Pediatric Hematology and Oncology (AIEOP). Cancer 2008;113:515–21.
80. O'Connor D, Bate J, Wade R, et al. Infection-related mortality in children with acute lymphoblastic leukemia: an analysis of infectious deaths on UKALL2003. Blood 2014;124:1056–61.
81. Maloney KW, Larsen E, Mattano LA Jr, et al. Improvement in the Infection-related Mortality for Children with Down Syndrome (DS) in Contemporary Children's Oncology Group (COG) Acute Lymphoblastic Leukemia (ALL) Clinical Trials. Pediatr Blood Cancer 2010;54:787–864.
82. Maloney KW, Carroll WL, Carroll AJ, et al. Down syndrome childhood acute lymphoblastic leukemia has a unique spectrum of sentinel cytogenetic lesions that influences treatment outcome: a report from the Children's Oncology Group. Blood 2010;116:1045–50.
83. Hargrave DR, Hann II, Richards SM, et al. Progressive reduction in treatment-related deaths in Medical Research Council childhood lymphoblastic leukaemia trials from 1980 to 1997 (UKALL VIII, X and XI). Br J Haematol 2001;112:293–9.

84. Izraeli S, Vora A, Zwaan CM, et al. How I treat ALL in Down's syndrome: pathobiology and management. Blood 2014;123:35–40.
85. Garre ML, Relling MV, Kalwinsky D, et al. Pharmacokinetics and toxicity of methotrexate in children with Down syndrome and acute lymphocytic leukemia. J Pediatr 1987;111:606–12.
86. Peeters MA, Rethore MO, Lejeune J. In vivo folic acid supplementation partially corrects in vitro methotrexate toxicity in patients with Down syndrome. Br J Haematol 1995;89:678–80.
87. Taub JW, Ge Y. Down syndrome, drug metabolism and chromosome 21. Pediatr Blood Cancer 2005;44:33–9.
88. Matloub Y, Bostrom BC, Hunger SP, et al. Escalating intravenous methotrexate improves event-free survival in children with standard-risk acute lymphoblastic leukemia: a report from the Children's Oncology Group. Blood 2011;118:243–51.
89. Maloney KW, Larsen E, Devidas M, et al. Event free (EFS) and overall survival (OS) for children with Down syndrome (DS) and B-lymphoblastic leukemia (B-ALL) in Children's Oncology Group (COG) clinical trials AALL0232 and AALL0331. Pediatr Blood Cancer 2014;61:S1–104.
90. Meyr F, Escherich G, Mann G, et al. Outcomes of treatment for relapsed acute lymphoblastic leukaemia in children with Down syndrome. Br J Haematol 2013; 162:98–106.
91. Hertzberg L, Vendramini E, Ganmore I, et al. Down syndrome acute lymphoblastic leukemia, a highly heterogeneous disease in which aberrant expression of CRLF2 is associated with mutated JAK2: a report from the International BFM Study Group. Blood 2010;115:1006–17.
92. Mullighan CG, Collins-Underwood JR, Phillips LA, et al. Rearrangement of CRLF2 in B-progenitor- and Down syndrome-associated acute lymphoblastic leukemia. Nat Genet 2009;41:1243–6.
93. Cario G, Zimmermann M, Romey R, et al. Presence of the P2RY8-CRLF2 rearrangement is associated with a poor prognosis in non-high-risk precursor B-cell acute lymphoblastic leukemia in children treated according to the ALL-BFM 2000 protocol. Blood 2010;115:5393–7.
94. Bercovich D, Ganmore I, Scott LM, et al. Mutations of JAK2 in acute lymphoblastic leukaemias associated with Down's syndrome. Lancet 2008;372:1484–92.
95. Mullighan CG, Zhang J, Harvey RC, et al. JAK mutations in high-risk childhood acute lymphoblastic leukemia. Proc Natl Acad Sci U S A 2009;106:9414–8.
96. Harvey RC, Mullighan CG, Chen IM, et al. Rearrangement of CRLF2 is associated with mutation of JAK kinases, alteration of IKZF1, Hispanic/Latino ethnicity, and a poor outcome in pediatric B-progenitor acute lymphoblastic leukemia. Blood 2010;115:5312–21.
97. Buitenkamp TD, Pieters R, Gallimore NE, et al. Outcome in children with Down's syndrome and acute lymphoblastic leukemia: role of IKZF1 deletions and CRLF2 aberrations. Leukemia 2012;26:2204–11.

Pediatric Lymphomas and Histiocytic Disorders of Childhood

CrossMark

Carl E. Allen, MD, PhD[a], Kara M. Kelly, MD[b],
Catherine M. Bollard, MD[c],*

KEYWORDS

- Burkitt lymphoma (BL) • Diffuse large B-cell lymphoma (DLBCL)
- Posttransplant lymphoproliferative disease (PTLD)
- Anaplastic large cell lymphoma (ALCL) • Hodgkin lymphoma (HL)
- Langerhans cell histiocytosis (LCH) • Juvenile xanthoganuloma (JXG)
- Rosai-Dorfman disease (RDD)

KEY POINTS

- Non_Hodgkin lymphoma accounts for approximately 7% of cancers in patients under 20 years, or approximately 800 cases annually in the USA with cure rates ranging from 65% to over 90%, even for disseminated disease.
- A major challenge that needs to be overcome for the treatment of NHL is to optimize up-front treatment to prevent relapse since prognosis for patients with refractory of relapsed disease remains exceedingly poor.
- Hodgkin Lymphoma (HL) is diagnosed in approximately 1100 children and adolescents under age 20 years in the USA each year, accounting for 6% of overall childhood cancer diagnoses and its rank as the most common malignancy among adolescents 15–19 years.
- HL is one of the most curable forms of childhood cancer, with estimated 5-year survival rates exceeding 98%, yet long-term overall survival declines primarily from delayed effects of therapy necessitating the development of novel targeted therapies.
- Langerhan cell histiocytosis (LCH) occurs with similar frequency as HL and patients with high-risk disseminated disease have approximately 90% long-term survival; patients with low-risk disease have almost 100% survival but current standard of care therapy for LCH fails to cure over 50% of all patients.

Continued

---

[a] Department of Pediatrics, Texas Children's Cancer Center, Baylor College of Medicine, 1102 Bates St, Houston, TX 77030, USA; [b] Herbert Irving Child and Adolescent Oncology Center, Morgan Stanley Children's Hospital, New York-Presbyterian, Columbia University Medical Center, 161 Fort Washington Ave, New York, NY 10032, USA; [c] Program for Cell Enhancement and Technologies for Immunotherapy, BMT Division, Department of Pediatrics, Children's National Health System, The George Washington University, 111 Michigan Avenue, Northwest, Washington, DC 20010, USA
* Corresponding author.
E-mail address: cbollard@cnmc.org

Pediatr Clin N Am 62 (2015) 139–165
http://dx.doi.org/10.1016/j.pcl.2014.09.010
0031-3955/15/$ – see front matter © 2015 Elsevier Inc. All rights reserved.

Continued

- Emerging biological data support reclassification of LCH and other histiocytic disorders including ECD and JXG as myeloid neoplasias. Inclusion of patients with these diseases in cooperative pediatric cancer network trials is essential to optimize diagnostic and therapeutic strategies.

INTRODUCTION

Lymphomas are the third most common malignancy among children and adolescents.[1,2] In children less than 15 years of age, non-Hodgkin Lymphoma (NHL) is more frequent; however, in patients up to 18 years of age, Hodgkin disease is predominant. Unlike in adults where low and intermediate grade lymphoma predominate, NHLs in children are usually diffuse high-grade tumors possibly reflecting maturational changes in the function and composition of the immune system. The different histologies explain in part the differing disease course and treatment approaches in adults versus children. The differences in treatment strategies and disease subtypes are perhaps less striking in adults and children with Hodgkin Lymphoma (HL). However, there are unique challenges in the management of children with HL because of the late effects which are sequelae of therapy including radiation- and chemotherapy-related second malignancies and late cardiac deaths. For both NHL and HL, ongoing and future trials are examining ways to reduce the toxicity of therapy with targeted therapies in order to maintain the excellent without the unacceptable late effects.

Histiocytic disorders include a spectrum of diseases caused by pathologic proliferation, differentiation and/or function of "histiocytes", an archaic umbrella to describe phagocytic and antigen-presenting cells that now includes dendritic cells, macrophages and monocytes. Langerhans cell histiocytosis is the most common histiocytic disease; the more rare conditions include juvenille xanthogranuloma (JXG), Erdheim-Chester disease, malignant histiocytosis, Rosai-Dorfman disease, and hemophagocytic syndromes. Therapies for children with histiocytic disorders remain limited to empiric strategies. New biological insights are refining our understanding of pathogenesis which may lead to improved approaches to diagnosis, risk-stratification and therapy.

NON-HODGKIN LYMPHOMA
Histopathological Categories

Non-Hodgkin lymphoma (NHL) in children is distinct from the low-grade or intermediate-grade lymphomas seen in adults because almost all NHL that occurs in children is high grade.[3] The World Health Organization (WHO) has classified NHL on the basis of phenotype (B vs T vs NK cell lineage) and differentiation (ie, precursor vs mature).[4] Based on disease response to therapy, NHL in pediatric and young adult age groups falls into the following categories:

1. Mature B-cell NHL (predominantly Burkitt lymphoma [BL] and diffuse large B-cell lymphoma [DLBCL]).
2. Lymphoblastic lymphoma (LBL), which is predominantly a precursor T-cell lymphoma with precursor B-cell lymphoma being a rarer entity.
3. Anaplastic large cell lymphoma (ALCL; mature T-cell or null-cell lymphomas).

4. Posttransplant lymphoproliferative diseases (PTLD) usually have a mature B-cell phenotype including DLBCL and BL, although 10% will be mature (peripheral) T-cell lymphomas. Furthermore, PTLD is classified according to WHO nomenclature as (1) early lesions, (2) polymorphic, and (3) monomorphic.[5]

Current therapies for LBL are now based on acute lymphoblastic leukemia protocols and, therefore, the focus of the NHL section of this article is on mature B-cell NHL, ALCL, and PTLD (**Table 1**).

B-cell non-Hodgkin lymphoma–Burkitt lymphoma and diffuse large B-cell lymphoma
BL accounts for about 30% of childhood NHL in the United States and is generally a highly aggressive tumor.[3] It is higher among boys than girls (approximately 4:1).[6] The most common primary sites of disease are the lymph nodes (especially head and neck) and abdomen, although the disease can present at other sites including bone, skin, bone marrow, testes, and the central nervous system (CNS).[6] The malignant cells show a mature B-cell phenotype and are terminal deoxynucleotidyl transferase–negative. The lymphoma cells usually express surface immunoglobulin with either κ or λ light chains. Additional B-cell markers such as CD20 and CD22 are usually present, and almost all express common acute lymphoblastic leukemia antigen (CD10). BL expresses the characteristic chromosomal translocation juxtaposing the c-*myc* oncogene and immunoglobulin locus regulatory elements such as t(8;14) and more rarely t(8;22) or t(2;8).[3] Cytogenetic evidence of c-*myc* rearrangement is the gold standard for the diagnosis of BL. The distinction between BL and Burkitt-like lymphoma/leukemia is, however, controversial and, on pathology, the latter may appear more consistent with DLBCL if there is a lack of cytogenetic evidence for BL. Studies have demonstrated that most Burkitt-like or "atypical Burkitt" lymphomas have a gene expression signature similar to BL.[7] In addition, as many as 30% of pediatric DLBCLs will have a gene signature similar to BL.[7,8] Despite the histologic differences, BL and Burkitt-like lymphoma/leukemia and DLBCL are clinically very aggressive and, unlike in adults, are treated with similar regimens.[9,10]

DLBCL represents 10% to 20% of pediatric NHL and occurs more frequently in the 10- to 20-year age group than in children less than 10 years of age.[3,11,12] The clinical presentation of pediatric DLBCL is similar to BL, although it is more often localized and less often involves the CNS or bone marrow.[11,12] Approximately 20% of pediatric DLBCL presents as primary mediastinal B-cell lymphoma (PMBL) and is more common in older children/young adults. It is associated with distinctive chromosomal aberrations with gains in chromosome 9p and 2p (regions that involve *JAK2* and c-*rel*, respectively),[13] with inactivation of *SOCS1* also seen. PMBL also has a distinctive gene expression profile compared with other DLBCLs, and some suggest there is a closer relationship of this disease with HL.[14] Apart from PMBL, pediatric DLBCL differs biologically from the disease seen in adults because most pediatric DLBCL have a germinal center B-cell phenotype, unlike adult DLBCL, which is more frequently associated with the ABC phenotype.[15]

Posttransplant lymphoproliferative disease
The incidence of lymphoproliferative disease (LPD) or lymphoma is 100-fold higher in immunocompromised children than in the general population. The cause of such immune deficiencies may be a genetically inherited or an acquired defect (eg, HIV infection) or following transplantation (solid organ transplantation [SOT] or allogeneic hematopoietic stem cell transplantation [HSCT]). Epstein-Barr virus (EBV) is associated with most of these tumors, but some cases are not associated with

Table 1
Major histopathological categories of non-Hodgkin lymphoma in children and young adults

Category (WHO Classification/ Updated REAL)	Category (Working Formulation)	Immunophenotype	Clinical Presentation	Chromosome Translocation	Genes Affected
BLs	Malignant lymphoma small noncleaved cell	Mature B cell	Sporadic: head and neck (not jaw), intra-abdominal, bone marrow, CNS Endemic: >50% head and neck (jaw)	t(8;14) (q24;q32), t(2;8) (p11;q24), t(8;22) (q24;q11)	C-MYC, IGH, IGK, IGL
DLBCL	Malignant lymphoma large cell	Mature B cell; occ CD30+	Nodal, abdominal, bone, and mediastinal Primary CNS generally associated with immunodeficiency	No consistent cytogenetic abnormality identified except in PMBL	PMBL: gains in chromosome 9p and 2p in regions that involve JAK2 and c-rel SOCS1 inactivation
ALCL (systemic)	Malignant lymphoma immunoblastic or malignant lymphoma large cell	CD30+ (Ki-1+) T cell or null cell	Variable. systemic symptoms often prominent	t(2;5) (p23;q35); less common variant translocations involving ALK	ALK, NPM

Abbreviations: occ, occasionally; REAL, Revised European-American Lymphoma classification.

any infectious agent. This section focuses on PTLD, the most common setting of pediatric LPD. This disease represents a spectrum of morphologically and clinically heterogeneous lymphoproliferations. EBV is highly associated with PTLD following HSCT but EBV-negative PTLD can be seen following SOT, especially LPDs that present late post-SOT.[16] The WHO has classified PTLD into the following 3 subtypes[5]:

- Early lesions: early lesions show germinal center expansion, but tissue architecture remains normal.
- Polymorphic PTLD: polymorphic PTLD shows disruption of nodal architecture and necrosis with infiltrating T cells.
- Monomorphic PTLD: monomorphic PTLD shows similar histologies to those observed in NHL, with DLBCL being the most common histology, followed by BL and then rarer subtypes.

EBV PTLD may manifest as isolated hepatitis, interstitial pneumonitis, meningoencephalitis, or an infectious mononucleosis-like syndrome. The definition of PTLD is frequently limited to lymphomatous lesions (low stage or high stage), which are often extranodal (frequently in the allograft). Although less common, PTLD may present as a rapidly progressive disease with multiorgan failure that usually results in death despite therapy.[16]

Anaplastic large cell lymphoma

ALCL accounts for approximately 10% of childhood NHL.[12] Although the predominant immunophenotype of ALCL is mature T-cell, null-cell disease (ie, no T-cell, B-cell, or NK-cell surface antigen expression) does occur. The WHO classification system classifies ALCL as a peripheral T-cell lymphoma.[4] All ALCL are CD30+ and most (>90%) pediatric ALCLs have a chromosomal rearrangement involving the *ALK* gene, and their prognosis tends to be superior to adults who generally have an *ALK*-negative disease.[17] Clinically, systemic ALCL has a broad range of presentations, including lymph node as well as extranodal involvement (skin, bone, and, less commonly, lung, pleura, gastrointestinal tract, and muscle). Involvement of the CNS and bone marrow is uncommon. ALCL is often associated with systemic symptoms (eg, fever, weight loss) that can wax and wane, which may delay diagnosis.

Staging for Childhood Non-Hodgkin Lymphoma

The most widely used staging scheme for childhood NHL is that of the Murphy Staging.[18] However, as shown in **Table 2**, patients with mature B-cell NHL (BL and DLBCL) are generally treated based on features of the disease, other than stage.

Stage I: involvement of a single tumor or nodal area excluding abdomen and mediastinum

Stage II: disease limited to a single tumor with regional node involvement, 2 or more tumors or nodal areas involved on one side of the diaphragm, or a primary gastrointestinal tract tumor (completely resected) with or without regional node involvement

Stage III: tumors or involved lymph node areas occurring on both sides of the diaphragm, including any primary intrathoracic (mediastinal, pleural, or thymic) disease, extensive primary intra-abdominal disease, or any paraspinal or epidural tumors

Stage IV: tumors involving bone marrow (>5% malignant cells in otherwise normal BM or <25% malignant cells for LBL) and/or CNS, irrespective of other sites of involvement.

Apart from LBL, the definition of CNS disease in NHL is any malignant cell present in the CSF regardless of cell count.

Table 2 French-American-British/LMB staging schema for B-cell non-Hodgkin lymphoma		
	Stratum	Disease Manifestation
FAB/LMB International Study[30,114,115]	A	Completely resected stage I and abdominal stage II
	B	Multiple extra-abdominal sites
		Nonresected stage I and II, III, IV (marrow <25% blasts, no CNS disease)
	C	Mature B-cell ALL (>25% blasts in marrow) and/or CNS disease

Abbreviations: ALL, acute lymphoblastic leukemia; FAB, French-American-British; LMB, lymphoma malignancy B-cell.

General Treatment Considerations

Management goals
There are 2 potentially life-threatening clinical situations that are often seen in children with NHL: (1) mediastinal masses and (2) tumor lysis syndrome, most often seen in LBL and BL. These emergent situations should be anticipated in children with NHL and addressed immediately.

Mediastinal masses Patients with large mediastinal masses are at risk of cardiac or respiratory arrest during heavy sedation or general anesthesia. Therefore, a careful physiologic and radiographic evaluation should be carried out and the least invasive procedure should be used to establish the diagnosis, including bone marrow biopsy, pleural tap, or CT-guided core needle biopsy, keeping patients out of a supine position.[19,20]

Tumor lysis syndrome Tumor lysis syndrome results from rapid breakdown of malignant cells, resulting in, most notably, hyperuricemia, hyperkalemia, and hyperphosphatemia. Hyperhydration and allopurinol or rasburicase (urate oxidase) are essential treatments in all patients except those with the most limited disease.[21,22] An initial prephase consisting of low-dose cyclophosphamide and vincristine does not obviate allopurinol or rasburicase and hydration. Gastrointestinal bleeding, obstruction, and (rarely) perforation may occur. Hyperuricemia and tumor lysis syndrome, particularly when associated with ureteral obstruction, frequently result in life-threatening complications.

Role of radiographic imaging in childhood non-Hodgkin lymphoma Radiographic imaging is essential in the staging of patients with NHL. CT scan and, more recently, MRI have been used for staging. Radionucleotide bone scans should be considered for patients wherein bone involvement is suspected. The role of functional imaging in pediatric NHL is controversial. Gallium scans have been replaced by fluorodeoxyglucose PET scanning. The value of PET scanning for staging pediatric NHL is, however, still under investigation. Data support that PET identifies more abnormalities than CT scanning, but it is unclear whether this should be used to change therapy.[23] The use of PET to assess rapidity of response to therapy appears to have prognostic value in HL and some types of NHL observed in adult patients, but requires investigation in pediatric NHL. Caution is also required for surveillance scanning because false-positive results are common. There are also data demonstrating that PET scanning can produce false-negative results; therefore, a biopsy to prove residual or recurrent disease is required.[24]

Pharmacologic and novel targeted strategies
Mature B-cell non-Hodgkin lymphoma (Burkitt lymphoma and diffuse large B-cell lymphoma) Patients with low-stage (stage I/II) disease have an outstanding prognosis, regardless of histology with disease-free survival of about 95% **(Table 3)**. Patients with high-stage (stage III/IV) mature B-lineage NHL have an 80% to 95% long-term survival.[25,26] Unlike mature B-lineage NHL seen in adults, there is no difference in outcome based on histology (BL or Burkitt-like lymphoma or DLBCL) with current therapy in pediatric trials **(Table 4)**.[25,26]

Rituximab is a mouse/human chimeric monoclonal antibody targeting the CD20 antigen, which is expressed by DLBCL and BL in children and has been widely used in the treatment of adult lymphomas (eg, R-CHOP [Rituximab, Cycophosphamide, Doxorubicin Hydrochloride (Hydroxydaunomycin), Vincristine Sulfate (Oncovin) and Prednisone] and EPOCH-R [Etoposide, Prednisone, Vincristine, Cyclophosphamide, Doxorubicin and Rituximab]).[27] In children, a single-agent window phase II study of rituximab performed by the Berlin-Frankfurt-Munster group showed activity in BL.[28] A Children's Oncology Group (COG) pilot study (COG-ANHL01P1) added rituximab to baseline chemotherapy with FAB/lymphoma malignancy B-cell-96 therapy in patients with stage III and stage IV B-cell NHL. ANHL01P1 found no serious toxicities associated with the addition of rituximab, although, especially in adult studies, infectious complications with fatal viral infections have been observed. Rituximab pharmacokinetics found similar drug exposures to adult studies and was detected in serum up to 6 months after last dose. The 3-year event-free survival (EFS) rate was 93% (95% confidence interval [CI]; 78%–98%) for group B and 86% (95% CI; 70%–94%) for group C patients.[29] The study provided the key feasibility data for the current intergroup study (COG ANHL1131), which is currently open within European cooperative groups, and the COG, to patients with advanced stage B-cell NHL (stage III disease with LDH >2 times normal and any stage IV disease) or mature B-cell leukemia (>25% blasts in marrow), excluding patients with PMBL.

Primary mediastinal B-cell lymphoma This entity has been associated with an inferior outcome compared with other pediatric DLBCL (see **Table 4**).[10,29,30] However, a

Table 3
Standard treatment options for low-stage non-Hodgkin lymphoma

Disease	Treatment Options	Outcomes
BL or DLBCL (completely resected)	BFM-90/95 (R1): 2 cycles of chemotherapy[10] COG-C5961 (FAB/LMB-96) (group A): 2 cycles of chemotherapy[115]	EFS >95%
BL or DLBCL (nonresected stage I/II)	BFM-95 (R2): Prephase + 4 cycles of chemotherapy (4-h methotrexate infusion)[10]	EFS 95%
	COG-C5961 (FAB/LMB-96) (group B): prephase + 4 cycles of chemotherapy (reduced-intensity arm)[30]	EFS 98%
ALCL	POG-8314/POG-8719: 3 cycles of CHOP[26]	EFS 88% for DLBCL and ALCL (5 y)
	BFM-90: prephase + 3 cycles of chemotherapy (only for completely resected disease)[116]	90% EFS
	ALCL99: prephase + 6 cycles of chemotherapy (for disease not completely resected)[117]	Completely resected patients: 100% EFS Patients without complete resection: EFS 81% (3 y)

Abbreviations: BFM, Berlin-Frankfurt-Munster; FAB, French-American-British.

Table 4
Standard treatment options for high-stage B-cell non-Hodgkin lymphoma

	Disease Stage	Disease Manifestations	Regimen	Outcome
FAB/LMB-96 International Study COG-C5961[30,114]	B	Multiple extra-abdominal sites Nonresected stage I, II, III, IV Marrow <25% blasts No CNS disease	Prephase + 4 cycles of chemotherapy (reduced intensity arm)[30]	90%–94% 4 y EFS (70% PBML)
	C	Mature B-cell ALL (>25% blasts in marrow) and/or CNS disease	Prephase + 8 cycles of chemotherapy (full intensity arm)[114]	70%–90% EFS Best responders if in CR after 3 cycles standard intensity treatment 70% EFS in patients with CNS disease
BFM Group[10,118]	R2	Nonresected stage I/II and stage III with LDH <500 IU/L	Prephase + 4 cycles of chemotherapy (4 h methotrexate infusion)[10]	EFS >95%
	R3	Stage III with LDH 500–999 IU/L Stage IV, B-cell ALL (>25% blasts) and LDH <1000 IU/L No CNS disease	Prephase + 5 cycles of chemotherapy (24 h methotrexate infusion)[10]	Overall EFS 85% for R3 Overall EFS 81% for R4 Reducing MTX from 24 to 4 h → inferior outcome (75 vs 91% EFS)
	R4	Stage III, IV, B-cell ALL with LDH >1000 IU/L Any CNS disease	Prephase + 6 cycles of chemotherapy (24 h methotrexate infusion)[10]	PMBL: 50% EFS (3 y) CNS presentation: 70% EFS (3 y)

Abbreviations: ALL, acute lymphoblastic leukemia; BFM, Berlin-Frankfurt-Munster; LDH, lactate dehydrogenase.

single-arm study in adults showed excellent disease-free survival using the DA-EPOCH-R regimen (dose-adjusted etoposide, doxorubicin, cyclophosphamide, vincristine, prednisone, and rituximab; usually 6 cycles) with filgrastim and no radiation therapy. The 5-year EFS was 93% and overall survival (OS) was 97%.[31,32] At 10 years after the study, there was no evidence of cardiac toxicity; this is currently being tested in pediatric clinical trials including part of COG-ANHL1131.

Anaplastic large cell lymphoma The optimal treatment strategy for ALCL remains to be defined, with survival ranging from 70% to 85%, regardless of treatment.[26,33,34] For low-stage ALCL, the best results have come from using pulsed chemotherapy similar to mature B-cell NHL therapy with 3-year EFS ranging from 80% to 88% and OS greater than 95% (see **Table 3**) Vinblastine appears to have significant activity in relapsed ALCL[35] and has been incorporated as front-line treatment in 2 randomized trials: ALCL (multinational European trial) and APO (doxorubicin, prednisone, and vincristine) (COG trial). The COG study demonstrated no benefit with the addition of vinblastine.[36] In ALCL99, patients receiving vinblastine maintenance for 1 year had a better 1-year EFS than those without vinblastine (91% vs 74%, respectively); however, by 2 years, the EFS decreased to 73% for both groups.[37] In addition, ALCL99 showed that 1 g/m² methotrexate given over a period of 24 hours was similar to 3 g/m² over a period of 3 hours without intrathecal chemotherapy, but the latter had less acute toxicity.[38] The excellent activity of brentuximab vedotin (Bv; tubulin-inhibitor conjugated monoclonal anti-CD30) and crizotinib (oral ALK inhibitor) in relapsed ALCL patients[39,40] has, however, led the COG to pursue testing the efficacy and toxicity of adding these 2 targeted agents with standard chemotherapy in newly diagnosed pediatric patients with ALCL in COG-ANHL12P1.

Posttransplant lymphoproliferative diseases These highly immunogenic tumors express a type III latency of EBV antigen expression wherein they express all latent EBV proteins and therefore are amenable to immune-based therapies. Numerous therapeutic approaches to PTLD have been explored in children but generally there has been a paucity of multicenter studies for this disease. Withdrawal or reduction of immunosuppression is often considered because first-line therapy response depends on whether the patient can recover sufficient T-cell function to eradicate EBV-infected B cells. After SOT, modalities such as radiotherapy or surgical resection for localized PTLD can result in complete remissions. One study evaluated the efficacy of low-dose cyclophosphamide and prednisone for pediatric patients with PTLD after SOT. All patients had progressed despite reduction of immune suppression and received 6 cycles of chemotherapy. The 2-year EFS and OS were 67% and 73%, respectively.[41] Subsequently, the COG evaluated in a phase II study (COG-ANHL0221) the addition of rituximab to this regimen of low-dose cyclophosphamide and prednisone demonstrating an EFS and OS of 71% and 83%, respectively. To build on the success of this first cooperative group trial for PTLD, the COG now propose to administer "off-the-shelf" third-party allogeneic EBV/latent membrane protein-cytotoxic T lymphocytes[42] to determine the safety and efficacy in patients with PTLD post SOT.

HODGKIN LYMPHOMA
Histopathological Categories

In general, HL in children and adolescents is comparable to HL observed in young adults.[43] HL is characterized by the presence of multinucleated giant cells (Hodgkin/Reed-Sternberg cells, H/RS) or large mononuclear cell variants (lymphocytic and histiocytic cells) in a background of inflammatory cells consisting of small lymphocytes, histiocytes, neutrophils, eosinophils, plasma cells, and fibroblasts. Nearly all cases of HL arise from germinal center B cells that cannot synthesize immunoglobulin, yet these cells account for approximately 1% of the cells in the involved areas.[44] Use of fine needle aspirates for determination of diagnosis is discouraged because of the rarity of the H/RS cells and risk for missing the diagnosis. Two broad pathologic classes exist: classical (cHL) and nodular lymphocyte predominant (NLPHL).[45]

Classical Hodgkin lymphoma

cHL accounts for most childhood HL in the United States and the male-to-female ratio (M:F) varies markedly by age. Children less than 5 years of age show a strong male predominance (M:F = 5.3), whereas adolescents 15 to 19 years old show a slight female predominance (M:F = 0.8). Approximately 80% of patients present with painless adenopathy, most commonly involving the supraclavicular or cervical areas. Involvement of the anterior mediastinum, often asymptomatic, is present in about 75% of adolescents and young adults, yet only 35% of young children.[46]

H/RS cells nearly always express CD30, with CD15 also expressed in approximately 70%. Other B-cell antigens, such as CD45, CD19, and CD79A, are generally not expressed on the H/RS cell.[47] CD20 is expressed in approximately 6% to 10% of cHL, which is further subdivided into 4 main histologic subtypes: (1) lymphocyte-rich: H/RS cells exist in a background predominantly of lymphocytes; (2) mixed cellularity: H/RS cells are frequent in a background of abundant normal reactive cells; (3) nodular sclerosis: most common subtype in adolescents (77%) and young adults (72%) compared with younger children (44%).[48] Collagenous bands divide the lymph node into nodules that often contain an H/RS cell variant called the lacunar cell; and (4) lymphocyte-depleted: rarely observed in children and adolescents and more commonly confused with ALCL, often presents as disseminated disease and associated with a poorer prognosis. EBV-positive cHL is frequently associated with the mixed cellularity subtype and is generally more common in male patients. EBV+ cHL is especially notable for a high incidence in developing countries.[49] EBV is identified in H-RS cells by the presence of EBV-encoded RNA in situ hybridization and/or latent membrane protein by immunohistochemistry.

Nodular lymphocyte predominant Hodgkin lymphoma

NLPHL accounts for 5% to 10% of childhood HL.[50] The characteristic lymphocyte and histiocytic cells express CD20, and rarely, CD30 and CD15. A prognostic score incorporating variant histologic patterns (diffuse and T-cell-rich) along with gender and serum albumin has been recently reported.[51] NLPHL tends to be indolent with a lengthy time to diagnosis and propensity for multiple late relapses. Although the overall prognosis is favorable, a higher risk for transformation or development of DLBCL is observed.[52] It is more common in children less than 10 years old, wherein it commonly involves a single peripheral lymph node region and infrequently involves the mediastinum.[50] Expression of EBV is rarely reported.[53]

The risk of both cHL and NLPHL is increased in individuals with an underlying or acquired immunodeficiency disorder, although the overall risk is not as high as that observed for NHL. However, specific defects, such as seen in those individuals with fas mutation–associated autoimmune lymphoproliferative syndrome, have a 51-fold increased risk for all types of HL and 14-fold increased risk for NHL.[54] HL associated with HIV infection is more common with moderate rather than severe immunosuppression, especially with the advent of highly active antiretroviral therapy.[55] Mixed cellularity subtype and presence of extranodal involvement are typical.

Staging for Childhood Hodgkin Lymphoma

Physical examination and diagnostic imaging evaluations (upright posteroanterior and lateral thoracic radiographs; CT of the neck, chest, abdomen, and pelvis with intravenous and oral contrast; and functional nuclear imaging studies with FDG-PET) are used to designate a clinical stage. Data from retrospective studies suggest that FDG-PET may replace the need for bone marrow biopsies in patients with clinical stage III to IV disease or B symptoms; however, this has not been prospectively validated.[56] Staging laparotomy is rarely appropriate with the imaging modalities available today, but biopsy of specific sites with equivocal findings by clinical staging should be considered when results will alter therapy.

The most widely used staging scheme for both childhood and adult HL is that of the Ann Arbor Staging,[57] a system primarily developed to facilitate delivery of radiotherapy. Following the identification of the prognostic importance of bulky disease (>10 cm in maximum dimension on CT), this factor was incorporated with the Cotswolds modification.[58] However, as shown in **Table 5**, treatment allocation is based on several prognostic factors, other than just stage, and varies considerably across different clinical trials consortia.

Stage I: involvement of a single lymph node region (I) or of a single extralymphatic organ or site (IE)

Stage II: involvement of 2 or more lymph node regions on the same side of the diaphragm (II) or localized involvement of extralymphatic organ or site and of 1 or more lymph node regions on the same side of the diaphragm (IIE)

Stage III: involvement of lymph node regions on both sides of the diaphragm (III), which may also be accompanied by localized involvement of extralymphatic organ or site (IIIE) or by involvement of the spleen (IIIS), or both (IIISE)

Stage IV: diffuse or disseminated involvement of 1 or more extralymphatic organs or tissues (eg, bone marrow, liver, lungs) with or without associated lymph node enlargement.

Each stage is further subdivided into A and B categories, with B denoting those with constitutional symptoms, present in approximately 26% to 38% of childhood HL.[59,60] B symptoms include (1) unexplained weight loss of more than 10% of the body weight in the 6 months before diagnosis; (2) unexplained fever with temperatures greater than 38°C; and (3) drenching night sweats. Pruritus alone is not considered a B symptom. Short, febrile illness associated with a known infection similarly does not qualify for B classification.

General Treatment Considerations

Management goals
Risk stratification With the high cure rates observed in children and adolescents with HL, the ongoing focus has been on the development of less toxic therapy. Recent pediatric HL trials have investigated titration of therapy because of risk group stratification using clinical prognostic factors, with further refinement through assessment of interim or end of chemotherapy response in most cases. Presenting features at diagnosis, including B symptoms, mediastinal and peripheral lymph node bulk, extranodal extension of disease to contiguous structures, number of involved nodal regions, Ann Arbor stage, serum markers of inflammation, and gender, as well as response to initial chemotherapy, are used for risk stratification. Stage IV disease, fever, low serum

Table 5
Variability in risk stratification across pediatric Hodgkin lymphoma clinical trials consortia

	Risk	IA	IB	IIA	IIB	IIIA	IIIB	IVA	IVB
EuroNet C1	Low								
	Int	E	E	E					
	High				E	E			
COG	Low								
	Int	E		E					
		X		X					
	High								
St Jude	Low								
Stanford	Int	E		E					
DFCI		mX		mX					
				>2					
	High								

Abbreviations: E, extranodal extension; Int, intermediate; mX, mediastinal bulk; X, bulky disease (peripheral >6 cm and mediastinal).

albumin, and bulky mediastinal mass, along with early response measured by CT and to a lesser extent FDG-PET, were strong predictors of EFS in a COG study.[46] Unfortunately, there is no uniform risk stratification algorithm in pediatric HL (see **Table 5**).

Role of radiographic imaging in childhood Hodgkin lymphoma Functional imaging has a larger role in the management of HL as compared with NHL. Similar to NHL, stage migration occurs; however, despite this limitation, its use is now routine.[61] As is the case for HL in adults, interim assessment of response by FDG-PET is incorporated into contemporary treatment approaches; however, the optimum time point for assessment and the criteria for response have not been defined. Continued surveillance for relapse with FDG-PET in the after-treatment period is not recommended because of its low positive predictive value.[62]

Pharmacologic and novel targeted strategies
Classical Hodgkin lymphoma Recent trials (summarized in **Tables 6, 7**) have used chemotherapy regimens of varying dose intensity and have significant differences in the criteria for omission of radiotherapy. The European consortium has investigated OEPA (vincristine, etoposide, prednisone, doxorubicin) for low risk, and OEPA with COPDac (cyclophosphamide, vincristine, prednisone, dacarbazine) for intermediate-risk and high-risk groups. In North America, the COG has primarily evaluated ABVE-PC (doxorubicin, bleomycin, vincristine, etoposide, prednisone, cyclophosphamide) and its derivatives across the risk groups.

Radiotherapy usage varies considerably. The COG recently reported that radiotherapy may be safely omitted in intermediate-risk patients who have a rapid reduction in tumor dimensions by CT after 2 cycles of chemotherapy.[46,63] The European Consortium has omitted radiotherapy for low-risk patients achieving a complete response after 2 cycles of OEPA.[60] In general, pediatric radiotherapy approaches use lower doses (15–25 Gy) and fields (involved field or node).[64]

Bv, a murine/human chimeric monoclonal conjugate linked to monomethyl auristatin E (vedotin) that targets the CD30 antigen expressed on H/RS cells, is approved for relapsed/refractory HL, after results from a pivotal phase 2 trial in adults with relapsed HL following autologous stem cell transplant demonstrated a 34% complete response and 40% partial response with a median duration of response of 6.7 months.[65] Bv in conjunction with doxorubicin, vinblastine, and dacarbazine is safe and associated with

Table 6
Results of recent trials for pediatric low-risk Hodgkin lymphoma

Group	Study	n	LR Definition	Chemotherapy	RT (Dose, Field)	EFS or DFS, OS (y)
Europe						
French Society of Pediatric Oncology[119]	MDH90	202	IA, IB, IIA, IIB	VBVP × 4 (+OPPA × 1-2 if PR after cycle 4)	20–40 Gy IF	91.1%, 97.5% (5 y)
German Society of Pediatric Oncology and Hematology	GPOH-HD-95[120]	328	IA, IB, IIA	OPPA (F); OEPA (M) × 2	CR after cycle 2: no RT PR after cycle 2: 20–30 Gy IF	93.2%, 98.8% (10 y)
	GPOH-HD-2002[60]	195	IA, IB, IIA	OPPA (F); OEPA (M) × 2	CR after cycle 2: no RT PR after cycle 2: 20–30 Gy IF	92%, 99.5% (5 y)
North America						
Stanford, Dana Farber, St Jude consortium	[121]	110	IA, IB, IIA, IIB no bulk, no E	VAMP × 4	15–22.5 Gy IF	89.4%, 96.1% (10 y)
	[122]	88	IA, IIA, <3 nodal sites, no bulk, no E	VAMP × 4	CR after cycle 2: no RT PR after cycle 2: 25.5 Gy IF	EFS: 90.8% (2 y)
CCG, POG, and COG	CCG 5942[59]	294	IA, IB, IIA without adverse features[a]	COPP/ABV × 4	CR after cycle 4: randomized to 21 Gy IFRT vs no RT PR: 21 Gy IF	10 y EFS IFRT: 100% No RT: 89.1% (P = .001) 10 y OS: RT: 97.1% No RT: 95.9% (P = .5)
	P9426[123]	294	IA, IB, IIA, IIIA	DBVE × 2-4 (based on response after cycle 2)		86.2% 97.4% (8 y)
	AHOD0431[46]	287	IA, IIA, no bulk	AV-PC × 3	CR after cycle 3: no RT PR after cycle 3: 21 Gy IF	79.8% 99.6% (4 y)

Abbreviations: AV-PC, doxorubicin, vincristine, prednisone, cyclophosphamide; COPP/ABV, cyclophosphamide, vincristine, procarbazine, prednisone, doxorubicin, bleomycin, vinblastine; CR, complete response; DBVE, doxorubicin, bleomycin, vincristine, etoposide; DFS, disease-free survival: EFS, event-free survival; F, female; IF, involved field; LR, low risk; M, male; OEPA, vincristine, etoposide, prednisone, doxorubicin; OPPA, vincristine, procarbazine, prednisone, doxorubicin; OS, overall survival; PR, partial response; RT, radiation therapy; VAMP, vinblastine, doxorubicin, methotrexate, prednisone; VBVP, vinblastine, bleomycin, etoposide, prednisone.

[a] Adverse features = hilar disease, bulk, ≥4 nodal regions, mediastinal tumor.

Table 7
Results of recent trials for pediatric intermediate and high-risk Hodgkin lymphoma

Group	Study	N	Definition	Chemotherapy	RT (Dose, Field)	EFS or DFS, OS (y)
Europe						
German Society of Pediatric Oncology and Hematology	GPOH-HD-95[120]	341	Intermediate: I_EA/B; II_EA; IIB; IIIA High: II_EB; III_EA/B; IIIB; IV	2 OPPA/OEPA + 4 COPP.	CR after cycle 2: no RT PR after cycle 2: 20–35 Gy IF	84.5%, 93.2% (10 y)
	GPOH-HD-2002[60]	Intermediate: 139 High: 239	Intermediate: I_EA/B; II_EA; IIIA High: II_EB; III_EA/B; IIIB; IV	OPPA (F); OEPA (M) × 2 Intermediate: COPDAC × 2 High: COPDAC × 4	19.8–35 Gy IF	Intermediate: 88.3%, 99.5% High: 86.9%, 94.9% (5 y)
North America						
CCG, POG, and COG	CCG 5942[59]	Intermediate: 394 High: 141	Intermediate: IA, IB, IIA with adverse features[a], IIB, III High: IV	Intermediate: COPP/ABV × 6 High: COPP/ABV, CHOP, Etoposide/Cytarabine × 2	CR after cycle 6: randomized to 21 Gy IFRT vs no RT PR: 21 Gy IF	Intermediate: RT: 87%, 95% No RT: 83%, 100% High: RT: 90%, 100% No RT: 81%, 94% (EFS P<.05)
	P9425[123]	Intermediate: 53 High: 163	Intermediate: IB, IIA$_{LMA}$, IIIA High: IIB, IIIB, IV	DBVE-PC × 3-5 (based on response after cycle 3)	PR: 21 Gy IF	Intermediate: 84%, OS NR High: 85%, OS NR (5 y)
	C59704[124]	99	IIB/IIIB + bulk, IV	BEACOPP × 4 M RER: ABVD × 2 F RER: COPP/ABV × 4 SER: BEACOPP × 4	M RER: 21 Gy IF F RER: No RT SER: 21 Gy IF	94%, 97% (5 y)
	AHOD0031[46]	1712	IA, IIA + bulk, IB, IIB, IIIA, IVA	ABVE-PC × 4 SER: randomized DECA × 2	Randomized RER after cycle 2 and CR after cycle 4: no RT All others: 21 Gy IF	85.6%, 98.2% (3 y)

Abbreviations: ABVE-PC, doxorubicin, bleomycin, vincristine, etoposide, prednisone, cyclophosphamide; BEACOPP, bleomycin, etoposide, doxorubicin, cyclophosphamide, vincristine, prednisone, procarbazine; CHOP, cyclophosphamide, doxorubicin, vincristine, prednisone; COPDac, cyclophosphamide, vincristine, prednisone, dacarbazine; COPP/ABV, cyclophosphamide, vincristine, procarbazine, prednisone, doxorubicin, bleomycin, vinblastine; CR, complete response; DBVE-PC, doxorubicin, bleomycin, vincristine, etoposide, prednisone, cyclophosphamide; DECA, dexamethasone, etoposide, cisplatin, cytarabine; F, female; IF, involved field; M, male; OEPA, vincristine, etoposide, prednisone, doxorubicin; OPPA, vincristine, procarbazine, prednisone, doxorubicin; PR, partial response; RER, rapid early responder; RT, radiation therapy; SER, slow early responder.

[a] Adverse features = hilar disease, bulk, ≥4 nodal regions, mediastinal tumor.

a very high complete response rate.[66] Its efficacy is being evaluated in a large international phase 3 trial in adults (clinicaltrials.gov # NCT01777152). In COG, Bv will be incorporated into a slightly modified version of ABVE-PC, termed Bv-AVEPC, in a phase 3 trial for high-risk HL (clinicaltrials.gov # NCT02166463). Sensory peripheral neuropathy has been observed in adults receiving Bv for HL and will be carefully monitored in the upcoming trial.

The focus on balancing efficacy with long-term toxicities continues into the management of patients with relapsed HL. In contrast to NHL, the prognosis for relapsed HL is generally favorable. Although high-dose chemotherapy and autologous hematopoietic stem cell transplantation (AHSCT) are still considered the standard approach for most patients with relapsed/refractory HL, a subset of children with low-risk relapse do not require AHSCT to be cured. A proposed retrieval therapy stratification algorithm has recently been reported.[67]

Nodular lymphocyte predominant Hodgkin lymphoma Adult guidelines have included surgery only for limited disease, radiation with doses of 30 to 36 Gy, chemotherapy only, combined modality therapy, and the anti-CD20 monoclonal antibody rituximab. Given the recognition that late complications of treatment such as secondary malignancies or cardiopulmonary toxicity, or transformation to aggressive B-cell lymphoma, account for most adverse fatal events, pediatric approaches have diverged from those used in adults.[50] A recent COG trial (AHOD03P1) evaluated a reduced intensity strategy for early-stage pediatric NLPHL. Among patients with a completely resected single node, greater than 80% did not recur at 4 years. Among all other early-stage patients, 3 cycles of a low-intensity chemotherapy regimen (doxorubicin, vincristine, prednisone, and cyclophoshamide) was associated with a 4-year EFS of 88.1% with greater than 90% avoiding radiotherapy.[46]

HISTIOCYTIC DISORDERS
Langerhans Cell Histiocytosis

LCH is a disease characterized by lesions that include pathologic CD207+ dendritic cells (DCs) with phenotypic similarity to epidermal Langerhans cells in a background of inflammatory cells that may include lymphocytes, eosinophils, and macrophages (**Table 8**). Clinical manifestations of LCH range from relatively trivial single lesions to potentially life-threatening disseminated disease. Historically, the pediatric oncology community has not fully embraced LCH, likely because of the unresolved biological ambiguity of LCH as a malignancy versus inflammatory disorder. More recently, identification of recurrent somatic mutations in *BRAF-V600E* in hematopoietic precursor cells more clearly define LCH as a true myeloid neoplasia.

Epidemiology
The incidence of LCH is approximately 5 cases per 1 million children younger than 15 years of age. There are roughly equal numbers of boys and girls affected, and the median age of presentation is 30 months, although new disease may develop throughout adulthood.[68–71] LCH may arise concurrently in identical twins. There are occasional reports of affected nonidentical siblings, although it is not clear if this is a higher rate than would occur by chance.[72] The role of inherited risk of LCH therefore remains uncertain.

Pathobiology
Until recently, research of the cause of LCH has been challenged by typical issues of rare disease research, including lack of access to viable tissue, compounded by heterogeneity of the LCH lesions and lack of reliable in vitro or animal models. For

Table 8
Differentiating characteristics of histiocytes

Histologic Features	LCH	Malignant Histiocytosis	ECD/JXG	HLH	RDD
HLA-DR	++	+	+/−	+	+
CD1a	++	+/−	−	−	−
CD14	−	+/−	++	++	++
CD68	+/−	+/−	++	++	++
CD163	−	−	+	++	++
CD 207 (Langerin)	+++	+/−	−	−	−
Factor XIIIa	−	−	++	−	−
Fascin	−	+/−	++	+/−	+
Birbeck granules	+	+/−	−	−	−
Hemophagocytosis	+/−	+/−	−	+/−	−
Emperipolesis	−	−	−	−	+

Adapted from Refs.[125–127]

decades, LCH has been assumed to arise from neoplastic transformation or inappropriate immune activation of epidermal Langerhans cells.[73] However, gene expression analysis of purified CD207+ cells from LCH lesions revealed a transcriptional profile more consistent with less differentiated myeloid DCs.[74] Next-generation sequencing strategies further revealed that DCs purified from archived biopsy specimens had high frequency of the *BRAF-V600E* somatic mutation.[75] Recurrent *BRAF-V600E* mutations have subsequently been validated in subsequent LCH cohorts.[76–79] Interestingly, the state of differentiation in which *BRAF-V600E* mutations arise is associated with anatomic distribution of lesions and severity of disease in patients with LCH. The functional significance of acquisition of *BRAF-V600E* in specific myeloid lineages is supported by the ability to recapitulate LCH-like phenotype in mice.[79] In the authors' opinion, these data support reclassification of LCH as a myeloid neoplasia.

Clinical manifestations
LCH is a classic "morning report" disease with protean manifestations from a single skin or bone lesion to acute myelogenous leukemia-like disseminated disease with multisystem organ failure. LCH lesions can involve almost any organ system: clinical "high-risk" LCH is defined by infiltration of liver, spleen, and/or bone marrow with lesions; clinical "low-risk" LCH is defined by lesions anywhere else. The most common symptoms are skin rash or painful bone lesions. Less frequent manifestations include diabetes insipidus (DI) with pituitary involvement or back pain with vertebra plana. Late effects are a significant problem for patients and may be caused by disease or therapy; progressive neurodegeneration and sclerosing cholangitis associated with LCH are particularly devastating.

Differential diagnosis
Because of the infrequent occurrence of LCH and similar appearance to candidiasis, seborrhea, eczema, and other common rashes, many infants with LCH skin lesions have symptoms for more than 1 year before diagnostic biopsy.[80] Mastoid LCH in toddlers may resemble chronic otitis media with chronic discharge. In older patients, skin lesions may resemble sexually transmitted diseases or viral infections. Lytic bone lesions require biopsy to differentiate from other primary or metastatic malignancies or infections. Patients with intestinal involvement may have symptoms and imaging

also consistent with inflammatory bowel disease. Liver, spleen, and bone marrow infiltration may resemble acute leukemia. Isolated DI may be caused by hypophysitis, germinoma, or lymphoma. Once LCH is suspected, definitive diagnosis is relatively straightforward with biopsy.

Prognosis (staging)

Patients with high-risk LCH have greater than 85% long-term survival, and patients with low-risk LCH have nearly 100% survival.[81] However, refractory or relapsed LCH is a problem for more than 50% of patients with both high-risk and low-risk multifocal disease,[82] and long-term morbidity is associated with uncontrolled LCH.[83] Although there is no standard approach to staging, a combination of imaging and laboratory tests is typically used to identify lesions and potential organ damage. In the case of infants with skin LCH, patients are often incorrectly assumed to have skin-limited disease, delaying timely diagnosis and therapy for potentially fatal occult multisystem high-risk disease.[80] In one study, PET scan was the most sensitive imaging modality for LCH. Complete evaluation is important because lesions in more than one site impact the need for systemic chemotherapy.[84]

Therapy

Optimal therapy has not yet been completely defined with clinical trials. However, standard practice bases therapy on extent of disease. Patients with proven skin-limited disease may be observed and do not require therapy unless they are symptomatic. Single bone lesions may be cured by curettage. It is contraindicated to perform resections with surgical margins because this impairs bone remodeling, which typically occurs with resolution of LCH. Patients with multisystem disease are treated with systemic chemotherapy. The authors consider therapy based on LCHIII, the most recent Histiocyte Society trial, to be standard of care for children, which is basically 1 year of vinblastine and prednisone. In LCHIII, patients treated for 1 year had significantly fewer recurrences than patients treated for 6 months.[81] Patients with single bone lesions in sinuses, orbit, or pituitary are treated with chemotherapy because of reports of decreased risk of subsequent development of neurodegenerative disease. In an institutional study, adults with LCH had nearly universal toxicity to vinblastine and prednisone, although some were effectively treated with cytarabine chemotherapy.[85]

There is no standard for treating a patient with recurrent disease, although strategies with nucleoside analogues, cladribine and cytarabine, have been effective.[86–88] For patients refractory to other nucleoside analogues, clofarabine has been effective. In rare cases of disease refractory to any chemotherapy, stem cell transplant with reduced intensity conditioning has been curative. An early report described promising responses to vemurafanib in adults who had both ECD and LCH lesions with the *BRAF-V600E* mutation.[89] The significant rate of toxicities associated with first-generation BRAF inhibitors makes it difficult to determine the optimal patient in whom to use these drugs, and clinical trials are ongoing in adults and children.[90]

The Histiocyte Society trial LCH-IV is currently open and accruing with observational and/or therapeutic arms for patients with all manifestations of LCH (clinicaltrials.gov # NCT02205762). Additional local and cooperative clinical trial efforts are required to identify effective novel agents and more rapidly determine optimal up-front and salvage therapy strategies for patients with LCH.

Non-Langerhans Cell Histiocytic Disorders

Juvenile xanthogranuloma

JXG has many similarities to LCH, but has a distinct pattern of presentation and histology. The precise incidence is not known, but registry data estimate it to be 5 times less common than LCH[91]; there are reported associations with juvenile myelomono-cytic leukemia and neurofibromatosis, diseases characterized by hyperactive Ras pathway signaling (reviewed in[92]).

The most common clinical manifestation is limited skin disease, as either a single lesion or multiple lesions. Less frequently, lesions may also arise in soft tissue, internal organs, brain, or eye.[91,93,94] Diagnosis is made by biopsy with characteristic histiocytes that stain with macrophage markers, including CD68, factor XIIIa, and fascin. "Touton giant cells," vacuolated, foamy histiocytes with multiple nuclei, are classic but not uni-versally present. Biopsies may also include spindle-shaped cells resembling benign fibrous histiocytoma with foamy histiocytes.[91] Physical examination and laboratory and imaging studies are required to differentiate skin-limited from systemic JXG.

In most cases, patients with skin-limited disease do not require therapy and lesions resolve over time. Systemic JXG, like high-risk LCH, may be lethal. Strategies effective in LCH have been reported as effective in JXG.[95] Cladrabine and clofarabine have been reported as effective in patients with refractory or recurrent disease in case re-ports and case series.[88,96]

Erdheim-Chester disease

ECD is an extremely rare disease that is histologically indistinguishable from JXG but arises in characteristic clinical patterns in adults. Lesions may arise in virtually any organ system, but osteosclerosis of the leg bones, perirenal infiltration resulting in a "hairy" rind on kidneys on MRI, and formation of fibrotic sheath around the aorta are characteristic. The mean survival of ECD patients remains less than 3 years. As in LCH, somatic mutations in *BRAF-V600E* are common in ECD.[78] Therapies have included interferon-α, blocking of inflammatory signals with targeted agents, and more recently, vemurafenib in patients with the *BRAF-V600E* mutation.[89,97]

Malignant histiocytosis

Malignant histiocytosis (also described as histiocytic sarcomas) describes a group of conditions with cells resembling macrophages or DCs that have biological and histo-logic features of malignant cells. This diagnosis is largely a diagnosis of exclusion, with ALCL and other T-lineage and B-lineage large cell lymphomas ruled out.[98] Increasing cases of "transdifferentiation" between lymphoid malignancies and malignant histio-cytic diagnoses are being reported, which likely reflect parallel differentiation from a common transformed precursor cell.[99–101]

Rosai-Dorfman disease

Rosai-Dorfman disease (RDD), also known as sinus histiocytosis with massive lymph-adenopathy, is an intriguing and still poorly understood phenomenon of apparently nonmalignant proliferation of histiocytes generally restricted to lymph nodes.[102] How-ever, extranodal lesions may also be observed, most often as subcutaneous nodules, sinus lesions, or bone lesions. The classic clinical presentation, as noted by disease nomenclature, is massive painless bilateral cervical lymphadenopathy. Biopsies demonstrate infiltration of lymph nodes with histiocytes with emperipolesis, the traf-ficking of viable lymphocytes through the phagocyte. The histiocytes stain for typical macrophage markers including CD68 and CD14.[103] Most cases are self-limiting, but lymphadenopathy may cause potential harm through mass effect on vital structures. Many agents used in lymphoma and LCH have been reported to have temporizing effects on RDD lesions, although the lymph nodes typically rebound after discontinu-ation of therapy. Some patients with refractory bone and CNS lesions were effectively treated with clofarabine.[88] It should be noted that the frequent nonspecific histologic description of lymph nodes having "sinus histiocytosis" is distinct from RDD.

Hemophagocytic lymphohistiocytosis

Hemophagocytic lymphohistiocytosis (HLH) is a syndrome of pathologic activation of macrophages and T cells that results in end-organ damage. There are numerous causes that lead to this phenomenon, including inherited defects of cytotoxic lymphocyte function, infections, persistent antigen stimulation in the setting of autoimmune disease, malignancies with antigen-presenting function, and iatrogenic derangement of normal immune function due to chemotherapy or bone marrow transplant (reviewed in[104]). Germline mutations in genes encoding proteins involved in cytotoxic function of NK cells and lymphocytes, including PRF1, MUNC13-4, AP3, LYST, Rab27a, STX11, and STXBP2, can cause "familial" HLH and typically arises in young children (reviewed in[105]). "Secondary" HLH is a term used to describe pathologic inflammation associated with an antigen trigger, such as malignancy or autoimmune disease, and may occur at any age. However, the line between presumed familial and secondary or acquired HLH is becoming increasingly blurred with the discovery of hypomorphic, heterozygous, or compound heterozygous mutations in HLH-associated genes in patients with "secondary" HLH.[106–108]

The finding of "hemophagocytosis" or engulfment of erythrocytes (and leukocytes) by activated macrophages for which HLH is named is neither sensitive nor specific for HLH. Diagnosis is made by a series of clinical criteria,[104,109] followed by investigations for the causes of the pathologic inflammation. When unrecognized and untreated, HLH is generally fatal. Therapy consists of immune suppression, and in cases of fixed immune defects or intractable pathologic inflammation, HSCT. Outcomes for patients with presumed familial or secondary HLH were not different in the HLH-94 clinical trial. Immune suppression with etoposide and dexamethasone, according to HLH-94, is generally considered the standard of care for initial treatment of patients with HLH.[110] Although differentiating stochastic immune challenges from inherited, fixed immune defects is important in determining whether a patient ultimately requires stem cell transplant, this distinction is not as significant in managing inflammation in the acute setting. In contrast to the other histiocytic diseases discussed with the possible exception of RDD, HLH is not a neoplastic condition, rather it represents induced pathologic function in histiocytes (macrophages).

SUMMARY

Although there have been dramatic improvements in the treatment of children with lymphoma, approximately 25% of children will still relapse or fail to respond to initial therapy. In addition, late effects remain a concern. The identification of both clinical and biologic features at the time of diagnosis that predict treatment failure will enable investigators to refine existing risk-adapted therapeutic approaches. Strategies to be considered for children at high risk for treatment failure include the intensification of existing regimens and the incorporation of new active or novel agents. Novel approaches include the incorporation of immunotherapeutic agents into multi-agent chemotherapy regimens. For example, there is increasing experience with the anti-CD20 and anti-CD30 antibodies,[28] including radiolabeled forms. Novel immunotherapeutic approaches using cytotoxic T lymphocytes for EBV-associated lymphomas as well as gene-modified T cells using the CAR-CD19 are also entering advanced phase trials.[111–113] Finally, agents targeting specific molecular lesions (eg, the ALK inhibitor for ALCL) are promising and being studied in combination with standard chemotherapy. Comprehensive molecular characterization of childhood lymphomas is also essential and may help to further refine disease classification, provide a means of detecting minimal residual disease during clinical remission, and enhance the assessment of early response. Recognition of the long-term toxicities of therapy is still a major driving principle for the development of new approaches.

Progress in improving outcomes for patients with histiocytic disorders has been challenged by ambiguous classification of the diseases as inflammatory versus malignant as well as organizational and biological obstacles to translational research efforts. Recent advances in understanding the pathogenesis of LCH include identification of recurrent mutations in *BRAF-V600E* and localization of somatic mutations to hematopoietic stem cells in patients with high-risk disease.[75,79] The functional importance of activation of MAPK pathway by *BRAF-V600E* is supported by the ability to recapitulate a high-risk LCH-like phenotype in mice in which BRAF-V600E expression is enforced in early myeloid lineages, as well as by promising responses in early case series of patients with combined LCH/ECD treated with vemerafanib (BRAF inhibition).[78,88] Together, these findings have philosophic significance in supporting reclassification of LCH (and by extension JXG and ECD) as myeloid neoplastic diseases. Practically, these advances support further investigation of novel approaches to diagnosis, risk-stratification, and therapy. The pace of improvements for patients with histiocytic disorders will be accelerated by enhanced support for preclinical translational research as well as cooperative clinical trials.

REFERENCES

1. Castellino SM, Geiger AM, Mertens AC, et al. Morbidity and mortality in long-term survivors of Hodgkin lymphoma: a report from the Childhood Cancer Survivor Study. Blood 2011;117(6):1806–16.
2. Gurney JG, Severson RK, Davis S, et al. Incidence of cancer in children in the United States. Cancer 1995;75(8):2186–95.
3. Sandlund JT, Downing JR, Crist WM. Non-Hodgkin's lymphoma in childhood. N Engl J Med 1996;334(19):1238–48.
4. Jaffe ES, Harris NL, Stein H, et al. Classification of lymphoid neoplasms: the microscope as a tool for disease discovery. Blood 2008;112(12):4384–99.
5. Swerdlow SH, Webber SA, Chadburn A, et al. Post transplant lymphoproliferative disorders. In: Swerdlow SH, Campo E, Harris NL, et al, editors. WHO Classification of Tumours of Haematopoietic and Lymphoid Tissues. Lyon, France: IARC; 2008. p. 343–9.
6. Mbulaiteye SM, Biggar RJ, Bhatia K, et al. Sporadic childhood Burkitt lymphoma incidence in the United States during 1992-2005. Pediatr Blood Cancer 2009; 53(3):366–70.
7. Klapper W, Szczepanowski M, Burkhardt B, et al. Molecular profiling of pediatric mature B-cell lymphoma treated in population-based prospective clinical trials. Blood 2008;112(4):1374–81.
8. Dave SS, Fu K, Wright GW, et al. Molecular diagnosis of Burkitt's lymphoma. N Engl J Med 2006;354(23):2431–42.
9. Sevilla DW, Gong JZ, Goodman BK, et al. Clinicopathologic findings in high-grade B-cell lymphomas with typical Burkitt morphologic features but lacking the MYC translocation. Am J Clin Pathol 2007;128(6):981–91.
10. Woessmann W, Seidemann K, Mann G, et al. The impact of the methotrexate administration schedule and dose in the treatment of children and adolescents with B-cell neoplasms: a report of the BFM Group Study NHL-BFM95. Blood 2005;105(3):948–58.
11. Reiter A, Klapper W. Recent advances in the understanding and management of diffuse large B-cell lymphoma in children. Br J Haematol 2008;142(3):329–47.

12. Burkhardt B, Zimmermann M, Oschlies I, et al. The impact of age and gender on biology, clinical features and treatment outcome of non-Hodgkin lymphoma in childhood and adolescence. Br J Haematol 2005;131(1):39–49.
13. Oschlies I, Burkhardt B, Salaverria I, et al. Clinical, pathological and genetic features of primary mediastinal large B-cell lymphomas and mediastinal gray zone lymphomas in children. Haematologica 2011;96(2):262–8.
14. Savage KJ, Monti S, Kutok JL, et al. The molecular signature of mediastinal large B-cell lymphoma differs from that of other diffuse large B-cell lymphomas and shares features with classical Hodgkin lymphoma. Blood 2003;102(12): 3871–9.
15. Oschlies I, Klapper W, Zimmermann M, et al. Diffuse large B-cell lymphoma in pediatric patients belongs predominantly to the germinal-center type B-cell lymphomas: a clinicopathologic analysis of cases included in the German BFM (Berlin-Frankfurt-Munster) Multicenter Trial. Blood 2006;107(10):4047–52.
16. Loren AW, Porter DL, Stadtmauer EA, et al. Post-transplant lymphoproliferative disorder: a review. Bone Marrow Transplant 2003;31(3):145–55.
17. Savage KJ, Harris NL, Vose JM, et al. ALK- anaplastic large-cell lymphoma is clinically and immunophenotypically different from both ALK+ ALCL and peripheral T-cell lymphoma, not otherwise specified: report from the International Peripheral T-Cell Lymphoma Project. Blood 2008;111(12):5496–504.
18. Murphy SB. Classification, staging and end results of treatment of childhood non-Hodgkin's lymphomas: dissimilarities from lymphomas in adults. Semin Oncol 1980;7(3):332–9.
19. King DR, Patrick LE, Ginn-Pease ME, et al. Pulmonary function is compromised in children with mediastinal lymphoma. J Pediatr Surg 1997;32(2):294–9.
20. Azizkhan RG, Dudgeon DL, Buck JR, et al. Life-threatening airway obstruction as a complication to the management of mediastinal masses in children. J Pediatr Surg 1985;20(6):816–22.
21. Cairo MS, Coiffier B, Reiter A, et al. Recommendations for the evaluation of risk and prophylaxis of tumour lysis syndrome (TLS) in adults and children with malignant diseases: an expert TLS panel consensus. Br J Haematol 2010;149(4): 578–86.
22. Galardy PJ, Hochberg J, Perkins SL, et al. Rasburicase in the prevention of laboratory/clinical tumour lysis syndrome in children with advanced mature B-NHL: a Children's Oncology Group Report. Br J Haematol 2013;163(3):365–72.
23. Cheng G, Servaes S, Zhuang H. Value of (18)F-fluoro-2-deoxy-D-glucose positron emission tomography/computed tomography scan versus diagnostic contrast computed tomography in initial staging of pediatric patients with lymphoma. Leuk Lymphoma 2013;54(4):737–42.
24. Eissa HM, Allen CE, Kamdar K, et al. Pediatric Burkitt's lymphoma and diffuse B-cell lymphoma: are surveillance scans required? Pediatr Hematol Oncol 2014;31(3):253–7.
25. Meadows AT, Sposto R, Jenkin RD, et al. Similar efficacy of 6 and 18 months of therapy with four drugs (COMP) for localized non-Hodgkin's lymphoma of children: a report from the Childrens Cancer Study Group. J Clin Oncol 1989;7(1):92–9.
26. Link MP, Shuster JJ, Donaldson SS, et al. Treatment of children and young adults with early-stage non-Hodgkin's lymphoma. N Engl J Med 1997;337(18):1259–66.
27. Wilson WH, Jung SH, Porcu P, et al. A Cancer and Leukemia Group B multicenter study of DA-EPOCH-rituximab in untreated diffuse large B-cell lymphoma with analysis of outcome by molecular subtype. Haematologica 2012;97(5): 758–65.

28. Meinhardt A, Burkhardt B, Zimmermann M, et al. Phase II window study on rituximab in newly diagnosed pediatric mature B-cell non-Hodgkin's lymphoma and Burkitt leukemia. J Clin Oncol 2010;28(19):3115–21.

29. Goldman S, Smith L, Anderson JR, et al. Rituximab and FAB/LMB 96 chemotherapy in children with Stage III/IV B-cell Non-Hodgkin lymphoma: a Children's Oncology Group report. Leukemia 2013;27:1174–7.

30. Patte C, Auperin A, Gerrard M, et al. Results of the randomized international FAB/LMB96 trial for intermediate risk B-cell non-Hodgkin lymphoma in children and adolescents: it is possible to reduce treatment for the early responding patients. Blood 2007;109(7):2773–80.

31. Dunleavy K, Pittaluga S, Maeda LS, et al. Dose-adjusted EPOCH-rituximab therapy in primary mediastinal B-cell lymphoma. N Engl J Med 2013;368(15): 1408–16.

32. Wilson WH, Grant C, Dunleavy K. Therapy in primary mediastinal B-cell lymphoma. N Engl J Med 2013;369(3):283–4.

33. Lowe EJ, Sposto R, Perkins SL, et al. Intensive chemotherapy for systemic anaplastic large cell lymphoma in children and adolescents: final results of Children's Cancer Group Study 5941. Pediatr Blood Cancer 2009;52(3):335–9.

34. Le Deley MC, Reiter A, Williams D, et al. Prognostic factors in childhood anaplastic large cell lymphoma: results of a large European intergroup study. Blood 2008;111(3):1560–6.

35. Brugieres L, Pacquement H, Le Deley MC, et al. Single-drug vinblastine as salvage treatment for refractory or relapsed anaplastic large-cell lymphoma: a report from the French Society of Pediatric Oncology. J Clin Oncol 2009; 27(30):5056–61.

36. Alexander S, Kraveka JM, Weitzman S, et al. Advanced stage anaplastic large cell lymphoma in children and adolescents: results of ANHL0131, a randomized phase III trial of APO versus a modified regimen with vinblastine: A report from the children's oncology group. Pediatr Blood Cancer 2014. [Epub ahead of print].

37. Le Deley MC, Rosolen A, Williams DM, et al. Vinblastine in children and adolescents with high-risk anaplastic large-cell lymphoma: results of the randomized ALCL99-vinblastine trial. J Clin Oncol 2010;28(25):3987–93.

38. Wrobel G, Mauguen A, Rosolen A, et al. Safety assessment of intensive induction therapy in childhood anaplastic large cell lymphoma: report of the ALCL99 randomised trial. Pediatr Blood Cancer 2011;56(7):1071–7.

39. Pro B, Advani R, Brice P, et al. Brentuximab vedotin (SGN-35) in patients with relapsed or refractory systemic anaplastic large-cell lymphoma: results of a phase II study. J Clin Oncol 2012;30(18):2190–6.

40. Mosse YP, Balis FM, Lim MS, et al. Efficacy of crizotinib in children with relapsed/refractory ALK-driven tumors including anaplastic large cell lymphoma and neuroblastoma: a Children's Oncology Group phase I consortium study [abstract]. J Clin Oncol 2012;30(Suppl 15):6–30.

41. Gross TG, Bucuvalas JC, Park JR, et al. Low-dose chemotherapy for Epstein-Barr virus-positive post-transplantation lymphoproliferative disease in children after solid organ transplantation. J Clin Oncol 2005;23(27):6481–8.

42. Leen AM, Bollard CM, Mendizabal AM, et al. Multicenter study of banked third-party virus-specific T cells to treat severe viral infections after hematopoietic stem cell transplantation. Blood 2013;121(26):5113–23.

43. Morton LM, Wang SS, Devesa SS, et al. Lymphoma incidence patterns by WHO subtype in the United States, 1992-2001. Blood 2006;107(1):265–76.

44. Kanzler H, Kuppers R, Hansmann ML, et al. Hodgkin and Reed-Sternberg cells in Hodgkin's disease represent the outgrowth of a dominant tumor clone derived from (crippled) germinal center B cells. J Exp Med 1996;184(4):1495–505.

45. Swerdlow SH, Webber SA, Chadburn A, et al. Classification of tumours of haematopoietic and lymphoid tissues. Lyon (France): International Agency for Research on Cancer; 2008. p. 342–9.

46. Kelly KM, Hodgson D, Appel B, et al. Children's Oncology Group's 2013 blueprint for research: Hodgkin lymphoma. Pediatr Blood Cancer 2013;60(6):972–8.

47. Tzankov A, Zimpfer A, Pehrs AC, et al. Expression of B-cell markers in classical Hodgkin lymphoma: a tissue microarray analysis of 330 cases. Mod Pathol 2003;16(11):1141–7.

48. Cleary SF, Link MP, Donaldson SS. Hodgkin's disease in the very young. Int J Radiat Oncol Biol Phys 1994;28(1):77–83.

49. Lee JH, Kim Y, Choi JW, et al. Prevalence and prognostic significance of Epstein-Barr virus infection in classical Hodgkin's lymphoma: a meta-analysis. Arch Med Res 2014;45(5):417–31.

50. Shankar A, Daw S. Nodular lymphocyte predominant Hodgkin lymphoma in children and adolescents–a comprehensive review of biology, clinical course and treatment options. Br J Haematol 2012;159(3):288–98.

51. Hartmann S, Eichenauer DA, Plutschow A, et al. The prognostic impact of variant histology in nodular lymphocyte-predominant Hodgkin lymphoma: a report from the German Hodgkin Study Group (GHSG). Blood 2013;122(26): 4246–52.

52. Biasoli I, Stamatoullas A, Meignin V, et al. Nodular, lymphocyte-predominant Hodgkin lymphoma: a long-term study and analysis of transformation to diffuse large B-cell lymphoma in a cohort of 164 patients from the Adult Lymphoma Study Group. Cancer 2010;116(3):631–9.

53. Huppmann AR, Nicolae A, Slack GW, et al. EBV may be expressed in the LP cells of nodular lymphocyte-predominant Hodgkin lymphoma (NLPHL) in both children and adults. Am J Surg Pathol 2014;38(3):316–24.

54. Straus DJ, Portlock CS, Qin J, et al. Results of a prospective randomized clinical trial of doxorubicin, bleomycin, vinblastine, and dacarbazine (ABVD) followed by radiation therapy (RT) versus ABVD alone for stages I, II, and IIIA nonbulky Hodgkin disease. Blood 2004;104(12):3483–9.

55. Biggar RJ, Jaffe ES, Goedert JJ, et al. Hodgkin lymphoma and immunodeficiency in persons with HIV/AIDS. Blood 2006;108(12):3786–91.

56. Adams HJ, Kwee TC, de KB, et al. Systematic review and meta-analysis on the diagnostic performance of FDG-PET/CT in detecting bone marrow involvement in newly diagnosed Hodgkin lymphoma: is bone marrow biopsy still necessary? Ann Oncol 2014;25(5):921–7.

57. Carbone PP, Kaplan HS, Musshoff K, et al. Report of the Committee on Hodgkin's disease staging classification. Cancer Res 1971;31(11):1860–1.

58. Lister TA, Crowther D, Sutcliffe SB, et al. Report of a committee convened to discuss the evaluation and staging of patients with Hodgkin's disease: Cotswolds meeting. J Clin Oncol 1989;7(11):1630–6.

59. Nachman JB, Sposto R, Herzog P, et al. Randomized comparison of low-dose involved-field radiotherapy and no radiotherapy for children with Hodgkin's disease who achieve a complete response to chemotherapy. J Clin Oncol 2002;20(18):3765–71.

60. Mauz-Korholz C, Hasenclever D, Dorffel W, et al. Procarbazine-free OEPA-COPDAC chemotherapy in boys and standard OPPA-COPP in girls have

comparable effectiveness in pediatric Hodgkin's lymphoma: the GPOH-HD-2002 study. J Clin Oncol 2010;28(23):3680–6.

61. Sioka C. The utility of FDG PET in diagnosis and follow-up of lymphoma in childhood. Eur J Pediatr 2013;172(6):733–8.

62. Levine JM, Weiner M, Kelly KM. Routine use of PET scans after completion of therapy in pediatric Hodgkin disease results in a high false positive rate. J Pediatr Hematol Oncol 2006;28(11):711–4.

63. Friedman DL, Chen L, Wolden S, et al. Dose-Intensive Response-Based Chemotherapy and Radiation Therapy for Children and Adolescents With Newly Diagnosed Intermediate-Risk Hodgkin Lymphoma: A Report From the Children's Oncology Group Study AHOD0031. Schwartz J Clin Oncol 2014. [Epub ahead of print].

64. Hodgson DC, Hudson MM, Constine LS. Pediatric Hodgkin lymphoma: maximizing efficacy and minimizing toxicity. Semin Radiat Oncol 2007;17(3):230–42.

65. Younes A, Bartlett NL, Leonard JP, et al. Brentuximab vedotin (SGN-35) for relapsed CD30-positive lymphomas. N Engl J Med 2010;363(19):1812–21.

66. Younes A, Connors JM, Park SI, et al. Brentuximab vedotin combined with ABVD or AVD for patients with newly diagnosed Hodgkin's lymphoma: a phase 1, open-label, dose-escalation study. Lancet Oncol 2013;14(13):1348–56.

67. Harker-Murray PD, Drachtman RA, Hodgson DC, et al. Stratification of treatment intensity in relapsed pediatric Hodgkin lymphoma. Pediatr Blood Cancer 2014; 61(4):579–86.

68. Arico M, Girschikofsky M, Genereau T, et al. Langerhans cell histiocytosis in adults. Report from the International Registry of the Histiocyte Society. Eur J Cancer 2003;39(16):2341–8.

69. Guyot-Goubin A, Donadieu J, Barkaoui M, et al. Descriptive epidemiology of childhood Langerhans cell histiocytosis in France, 2000-2004. Pediatr Blood Cancer 2008;51(1):71–5.

70. Salotti JA, Nanduri V, Pearce MS, et al. Incidence and clinical features of Langerhans cell histiocytosis in the UK and Ireland. Arch Dis Child 2009;94(5):376–80.

71. Stalemark H, Laurencikas E, Karis J, et al. Incidence of Langerhans cell histiocytosis in children: a population-based study. Pediatr Blood Cancer 2008;51(1): 76–81.

72. Arico M, Nichols K, Whitlock JA, et al. Familial clustering of Langerhans cell histiocytosis. Br J Haematol 1999;107(4):883–8.

73. Nezelof C, Basset F, Rousseau MF. Histiocytosis X histogenetic arguments for a Langerhans cell origin. Biomedicine 1973;18(5):365–71.

74. Allen CE, Li L, Peters TL, et al. Cell-specific gene expression in Langerhans cell histiocytosis lesions reveals a distinct profile compared with epidermal Langerhans cells. J Immunol 2010;184(8):4557–67.

75. Badalian-Very G, Vergilio JA, Degar BA, et al. Recurrent BRAF mutations in Langerhans cell histiocytosis. Blood 2010;116(11):1919–23.

76. Satoh T, Smith A, Sarde A, et al. B-RAF mutant alleles associated with Langerhans cell histiocytosis, a granulomatous pediatric disease. PLoS One 2012;7(4): e33891.

77. Sahm F, Capper D, Preusser M, et al. BRAFV600E mutant protein is expressed in cells of variable maturation in Langerhans cell histiocytosis. Blood 2012; 120(12):e28–34.

78. Haroche J, Charlotte F, Arnaud L, et al. High prevalence of BRAF V600E mutations in Erdheim-Chester disease but not in other non-Langerhans cell histiocytoses. Blood 2012;120(13):2700–3.

79. Berres ML, Lim KP, Peters T, et al. BRAF-V600E expression in precursor versus differentiated dendritic cells defines clinically distinct LCH risk groups. J Exp Med 2014;211:669–83.
80. Simko SJ, Garmezy B, Abhyankar H, et al. Differentiating skin-limited and multi-system Langerhans cell histiocytosis. J Pediatr, in press.
81. Gadner H, Minkov M, Grois N, et al. Therapy prolongation improves outcome in multi-system Langerhans cell histiocytosis. Blood 2013;121:5006–14.
82. Minkov M, Steiner M, Potschger U, et al. Reactivations in multisystem Langerhans cell histiocytosis: data of the international LCH registry. J Pediatr 2008; 153(5):700–5, 705.
83. Haupt R, Nanduri V, Calevo MG, et al. Permanent consequences in Langerhans cell histiocytosis patients: a pilot study from the Histiocyte Society-Late Effects Study Group. Pediatr Blood Cancer 2004;42(5):438–44.
84. Phillips M, Allen C, Gerson P, et al. Comparison of FDG-PET scans to conventional radiography and bone scans in management of Langerhans cell histiocytosis. Pediatr Blood Cancer 2009;52(1):97–101.
85. Cantu MA, Lupo PJ, Bilgi M, et al. Optimal therapy for adults with Langerhans cell histiocytosis bone lesions. PLoS One 2012;7(8):e43257.
86. Rodriguez-Galindo C, Jeng M, Khuu P, et al. Clofarabine in refractory Langerhans cell histiocytosis. Pediatr Blood Cancer 2008;51(5):703–6.
87. Abraham A, Alsultan A, Jeng M, et al. Clofarabine salvage therapy for refractory high-risk langerhans cell histiocytosis. Pediatr Blood Cancer 2013;60(6):E19–22.
88. Simko SJ, Tran HD, Jones J, et al. Clofarabine salvage therapy in refractory multifocal histiocytic disorders, including Langerhans cell histiocytosis, juvenile xanthogranuloma and Rosai-Dorfman disease. Pediatr Blood Cancer 2014; 61(3):479–87.
89. Haroche J, Cohen-Aubart F, Emile JF, et al. Dramatic efficacy of vemurafenib in both multisystemic and refractory Erdheim-Chester disease and Langerhans cell histiocytosis harboring the BRAF V600E mutation. Blood 2013;121(9):1495–500.
90. Pratilas CA, Xing F, Solit DB. Targeting oncogenic BRAF in human cancer. Curr Top Microbiol Immunol 2012;355:83–98.
91. Janssen D, Harms D. Juvenile xanthogranuloma in childhood and adolescence: a clinicopathologic study of 129 patients from the kiel pediatric tumor registry. Am J Surg Pathol 2005;29(1):21–8.
92. Berres ML, Allen CE, Merad M. Pathological consequence of misguided dendritic cell differentiation in histiocytic diseases. Adv Immunol 2013;120:127–61.
93. Dehner LP. Juvenile xanthogranulomas in the first two decades of life: a clinicopathologic study of 174 cases with cutaneous and extracutaneous manifestations. Am J Surg Pathol 2003;27(5):579–93.
94. Freyer DR, Kennedy R, Bostrom BC, et al. Juvenile xanthogranuloma: forms of systemic disease and their clinical implications. J Pediatr 1996;129(2):227–37.
95. Stover DG, Alapati S, Regueira O, et al. Treatment of juvenile xanthogranuloma. Pediatr Blood Cancer 2008;51(1):130–3.
96. Rajendra B, Duncan A, Parslew R, et al. Successful treatment of central nervous system juvenile xanthogranulomatosis with cladribine. Pediatr Blood Cancer 2009;52(3):413–5.
97. Diamond EL, Dagna L, Hyman DM, et al. Consensus guidelines for the diagnosis and clinical management of Erdheim-Chester disease. Blood 2014; 124(4):483–92.
98. Favara BE, Feller AC, Pauli M, et al. Contemporary classification of histiocytic disorders. The WHO Committee On Histiocytic/Reticulum Cell Proliferations.

Reclassification Working Group of the Histiocyte Society. Med Pediatr Oncol 1997;29(3):157–66.

99. Chen W, Jaffe R, Zhang L, et al. Langerhans cell sarcoma arising from chronic lymphocytic lymphoma/small lymphocytic leukemia: lineage analysis and BRAF V600E Mutation Study. N Am J Med Sci 2013;5(6):386–91.

100. West DS, Dogan A, Quint PS, et al. Clonally related follicular lymphomas and Langerhans cell neoplasms: expanding the spectrum of transdifferentiation. Am J Surg Pathol 2013;37(7):978–86.

101. Yohe SL, Chenault CB, Torlakovic EE, et al. Langerhans cell histiocytosis in acute leukemias of ambiguous or myeloid lineage in adult patients: support for a possible clonal relationship. Mod Pathol 2014;27(5):651–6.

102. Rosai J, Dorfman RF. Sinus histiocytosis with massive lymphadenopathy. A newly recognized benign clinicopathological entity. Arch Pathol 1969;87(1):63–70.

103. McClain KL, Natkunam Y, Swerdlow SH. Atypical cellular disorders. Hematology Am Soc Hematol Educ Program 2004;283–96.

104. Jordan MB, Allen CE, Weitzman S, et al. How I treat hemophagocytic lymphohistiocytosis. Blood 2011;118(15):4041–52.

105. Meeths M, Chiang SC, Lofstedt A, et al. Pathophysiology and spectrum of diseases caused by defects in lymphocyte cytotoxicity. Exp Cell Res 2014; 325(1):10–7.

106. Zhang K, Biroschak J, Glass DN, et al. Macrophage activation syndrome in patients with systemic juvenile idiopathic arthritis is associated with MUNC13-4 polymorphisms. Arthritis Rheum 2008;58(9):2892–6.

107. Zhang K, Jordan MB, Marsh RA, et al. Hypomorphic mutations in PRF1, MUNC13-4, and STXBP2 are associated with adult-onset familial HLH. Blood 2011;118(22):5794–8.

108. Zhang K, Chandrakasan S, Chapman H, et al. Synergistic defects of different molecules in the cytotoxic pathway lead to clinical familial hemophagocytic lymphohistiocytosis. Blood 2014;124:1331–4.

109. Henter JI, Horne A, Arico M, et al. HLH-2004: diagnostic and therapeutic guidelines for hemophagocytic lymphohistiocytosis. Pediatr Blood Cancer 2007; 48(2):124–31.

110. Henter JI, Samuelsson-Horne A, Arico M, et al. Treatment of hemophagocytic lymphohistiocytosis with HLH-94 immunochemotherapy and bone marrow transplantation. Blood 2002;100(7):2367–73.

111. Bollard CM, Gottschalk S, Leen AM, et al. Complete responses of relapsed lymphoma following genetic modification of tumor-antigen presenting cells and T-lymphocyte transfer. Blood 2007;110(8):2838–45.

112. Heslop HE, Slobod KS, Pule MA, et al. Long-term outcome of EBV-specific T-cell infusions to prevent or treat EBV-related lymphoproliferative disease in transplant recipients. Blood 2010;115(5):925–35.

113. Bollard CM, Gottschalk S, Torrano V, et al. Sustained complete responses in patients with lymphoma receiving autologous cytotoxic T lymphocytes targeting Epstein-Barr virus latent membrane proteins. J Clin Oncol 2014;32(8): 798–808.

114. Cairo MS, Gerrard M, Sposto R, et al. Results of a randomized international study of high-risk central nervous system B non-Hodgkin lymphoma and B acute lymphoblastic leukemia in children and adolescents. Blood 2007; 109(7):2736–43.

115. Gerrard M, Cairo MS, Weston C, et al. Excellent survival following two courses of COPAD chemotherapy in children and adolescents with resected localized

B-cell non-Hodgkin's lymphoma: results of the FAB/LMB 96 international study. Br J Haematol 2008;141(6):840–7.

116. Seidemann K, Tiemann M, Schrappe M, et al. Short-pulse B-non-Hodgkin lymphoma-type chemotherapy is efficacious treatment for pediatric anaplastic large cell lymphoma: a report of the Berlin-Frankfurt-Munster Group Trial NHL-BFM 90. Blood 2001;97(12):3699–706.

117. Attarbaschi A, Mann G, Rosolen A, et al. Limited stage I disease is not necessarily indicative of an excellent prognosis in childhood anaplastic large cell lymphoma. Blood 2011;117(21):5616–9.

118. Reiter A, Schrappe M, Tiemann M, et al. Improved treatment results in childhood B-cell neoplasms with tailored intensification of therapy: a report of the Berlin-Frankfurt-Munster Group Trial NHL-BFM 90. Blood 1999;94(10): 3294–306.

119. Landman-Parker J, Pacquement H, Leblanc T, et al. Localized childhood Hodgkin's disease: response-adapted chemotherapy with etoposide, bleomycin, vinblastine, and prednisone before low-dose radiation therapy-results of the French Society of Pediatric Oncology Study MDH90. J Clin Oncol 2000;18(7): 1500–7.

120. Dorffel W, Ruhl U, Luders H, et al. Treatment of children and adolescents with Hodgkin lymphoma without radiotherapy for patients in complete remission after chemotherapy: final results of the multinational trial GPOH-HD95. J Clin Oncol 2013;31(12):1562–8.

121. Donaldson SS, Link MP, Weinstein HJ, et al. Final results of a prospective clinical trial with VAMP and low-dose involved-field radiation for children with low-risk Hodgkin's disease. J Clin Oncol 2007;25(3):332–7.

122. Metzger ML, Weinstein HJ, Hudson MM, et al. Association between radiotherapy vs no radiotherapy based on early response to VAMP chemotherapy and survival among children with favorable-risk Hodgkin lymphoma. JAMA 2012;307(24):2609–16.

123. Tebbi CK, Mendenhall NP, London WB, et al. Response-dependent and reduced treatment in lower risk Hodgkin lymphoma in children and adolescents, results of P9426: a report from the Children's Oncology Group. Pediatr Blood Cancer 2012; 59(7):1259–65.

124. Kelly KM, Sposto R, Hutchinson R, et al. BEACOPP chemotherapy is a highly effective regimen in children and adolescents with high-risk Hodgkin lymphoma: a report from the Children's Oncology Group. Blood 2011;117(9):2596–603.

125. Jaffe R. The diagnostic histopathology of Lanerhans cell histiocytosis. In: Weitzman S, Egeler RM, editors. Histiocytic disorders of children and adults. Basic Science, Clinical Features, and Therapy. Cambridge: Cambridge University Press; 2005. p. 14–39.

126. Chikwava K, Jaffe R. Langerin (CD207) staining in normal pediatric tissues, reactive lymph nodes, and childhood histiocytic disorders. Pediatr Dev Pathol 2004;7(6):607–14.

127. Lau SK, Chu PG, Weiss LM. Immunohistochemical expression of Langerin in Langerhans cell histiocytosis and non-Langerhans cell histiocytic disorders. Am J Surg Pathol 2008;32(4):615–9.

Brain Tumors

Murali Chintagumpala, MD[a],*, Amar Gajjar, MD[b]

KEYWORDS

- Medulloblastoma • Glioblastoma • Anaplastic astrocytoma
- Diffuse intrinsic pontine glioma • Ependymoma

KEY POINTS

- The past 2 decades have witnessed a revolution in the management of childhood brain tumors, with the establishment of multidisciplinary teams and national and international consortiums.
- Unprecedented cooperation within the pediatric neuro-oncology community and sophisticated rapidly evolving technology have led to advances that are likely to revolutionize treatment strategies and improve outcomes.

Brain tumors in children represent the second most common malignancy in children. The number of children, adolescents, and young adults (0–19 years) with a diagnosis of a brain tumor is approximately 4350 per year.[1] The cause for most of these tumors is unknown, but there are some predisposing conditions that give rise to certain types of brain tumors. Turcot syndrome, Li-Fraumeni syndrome, and Gorlin syndrome are examples that can give rise to high-grade glioma (HGG) and medulloblastoma.[2–4]

Management of children with brain tumors requires a multidisciplinary approach, and these children are best served at pediatric hospitals, which are equipped with the necessary resources and personnel. Pediatric neurosurgeon, oncologist, neuropathologist, neuroradiologist, radiation oncologist, endocrinologist, and physical rehabilitation services among others should be available.

These children present most commonly with symptoms related to increased intracranial pressure or one or several of the following: cranial nerve palsies, incoordination, seizures, loss of vision, and short stature.

A few of the more common brain tumors and recent advances in their management are discussed in the following sections.

a Texas Children's Cancer Center, Baylor College of Medicine, 6701 Fannin Street, CC1510.15, Houston, TX 77030, USA; b Department of Oncology, St Jude Children's Research Hospital, Room 6024, 262 Danny Thomas Place, Memphis, TN 38105, USA
* Corresponding author.
E-mail address: mxchinta@txch.org

Pediatr Clin N Am 62 (2015) 167–178
http://dx.doi.org/10.1016/j.pcl.2014.09.011
0031-3955/15/$ – see front matter © 2015 Elsevier Inc. All rights reserved.

MEDULLOBLASTOMA

Medulloblastoma is the most common malignancy in children and represents approximately 20% of all malignant brain tumors that affect children between the ages of 0 and 14 years.[5,6] There is a bimodal distribution peak between 3 and 4 years and again between 8 and 10 years of age. It can occur in teenagers and young adults, but less frequently.

The cause of medulloblastoma is unknown. However several familial syndromes like Gorlin syndrome, Turcot syndrome, and Li-Fraumeni syndrome, which have a genetic predisposition to development of medulloblastoma, offer clues to the molecular pathologic mechanisms that can lead to growth of medulloblastoma. About 3% to 5% of children with Gorlin syndrome develop medulloblastoma. Gorlin syndrome is characterized by an inherited germline mutation of the PATCHED1 gene on chromosome 9, which encodes the sonic hedgehog (SHH) receptor PTCH1 and normally suppresses SHH signaling by inhibiting the SMO receptor.[2,7] Approximately 40% of medulloblastomas show evidence of mutations in the PTCH1, and these tumors are mostly associated with the desmoplastic variant of medulloblastoma.[2,8,9] Children with Turcot syndrome have mutations in the adenomatosis polyposis coli gene (type 2) or mutations in the DNA mismatch repair genes HPS2 and MLH1 (type 1). Patients with type 2 disease are at increased risk for developing medulloblastoma.[2,10] Approximately 10% of children with medulloblastoma have a favorable prognosis and have abnormalities in the WNT molecular pathway, which is also aberrant in Turcot syndrome. Patients with Li-Fraumeni syndrome with germline mutations in the TP53 gene can develop medulloblastoma, particularly of the SHH subtype, although gliomas are more common in this syndrome.[2,11]

Clinical Presentation

The symptoms at presentation caused by medulloblastoma are related to obstruction of cerebrospinal fluid (CSF) pathways and direct involvement of the cerebellum or the brainstem. Headaches and vomiting as a result of raised intracranial pressure, constant features later in the course of the disease, are often nonspecific in the early stages. Unsteadiness, mostly truncal, is present in about 50% to 80% of children with medulloblastoma. Esotropia in 1 or both eyes and papilledema are common. Clumsiness, dropping things frequently, and declining academic performance are other symptoms that can indicate the presence of a cerebellar lesion like medulloblastoma. Macrocephaly, unexplained lethargy, and head tilt are more common in infants.

Diagnosis

The diagnosis of medulloblastoma is initially suspected based on imaging studies, which include MRI of the brain. A typical radiographic presentation is the presence of a solid midline posterior fossa mass that seems to arise from the cerebellum and occupies the fourth ventricle. It shows variable and heterogeneous enhancement pattern. Occasionally, it may arise from the lateral aspect of either cerebellar hemisphere and often indicates a specific subtype of medulloblastoma that shows activation of the SHH pathway. The differential diagnosis of a midline posterior fossa mass includes ependymoma and pilocytic astrocytoma. The former is a solid tumor, which tends to spread toward the cerebellopontine angle via the foramen of Luschka or toward the spinal cord via the foramen of Magendie. The latter consists of solid and cystic components, with often a uniform enhancement of the solid component. In the younger child, the differential diagnosis includes atypical teratoid rhabdoid tumor, which may show involvement of the cerebellopontine angle. A complete MRI evaluation of the full length of the spinal cord and the thecal sac is strongly recommended before surgical intervention for the primary tumor. A lumbar puncture to assess the involvement of CSF should be performed at least 2 weeks after surgical removal of the primary tumor.[12] Attempts at lumbar puncture at the time of diagnosis before alleviation of increased intracranial pressure are strongly contraindicated. In the absence of peripheral blood count abnormalities, bone marrow evaluation is not indicated. It is rare for bone metastases to be present at the time of diagnosis.

Clinical Staging

Most treatment strategies have used the modified Chang system for classification of medulloblastoma into standard-risk (average-risk) or high-risk categories.[13] A gross total resection (GTR) or near total resection of the primary (with ≤ 1.5 cm^2 of residual tumor) and the absence of metastases renders a patient as having average-risk disease. Residual tumor greater than 1.5 cm^2 or evidence of metastases indicates high-risk disease.

Management of Medulloblastoma

A multidisciplinary team is essential for optimal management of a child with medulloblastoma. Primary intervention consists of complete removal of the primary tumor and is commonly achieved at most pediatric centers in the United States. Postoperatively, one of the main complications of surgery is the appearance of posterior fossa syndrome or cerebellar mutism, which occurs approximately 72 hours after surgery. This complication is characterized by inability to speak with or without accompanying neurologic deficits. The cause of this complication is unclear. Disruption of long white matter tracts is implicated. There is no evidence that this complication can be avoided by modifying surgical technique. In 1 retrospective study of more than 400 patients,[14] approximately 25% of patients were affected by posterior fossa syndrome. Most of these patients suffer long-term severe to moderate neurocognitive deficits. There is no evidence that the course of this syndrome can be modified by medical intervention.

Radiation therapy is an important component of adjuvant therapy and was the mainstay of therapy after surgery until the early 1990s. After early reports of increased failures after radiation volumes that did not include the whole craniospinal axis, improved outcomes of approximately 70% were achieved using a standard CSI dose of 36 Gy with a posterior fossa boost to 54 Gy in patients with average-risk disease. To reduce the long-term adverse neurocognitive effects of a craniospinal radiation dose of 36 Gy, a randomized trial was initiated within the Children's Cancer Group (CCG) and Pediatric Oncology Group (POG) comparing 36 Gy to 23.4 Gy for craniospinal irradiation (CSI) with a posterior fossa boost up to 54 Gy.[15] The results of this intergroup trial showed a trend toward a better outcome with those who received 36 Gy to CSI. However in the interim, a multi-institutional study clearly showed a benefit with the use of multiagent chemotherapy (chloroethylnitrosourea [CCNU], cisplatin, and vincristine) after radiation therapy (23.4 Gy to CSI) in patients with average-risk disease.[16] The sequence of surgery followed by reduced dose of CSI and multiagent chemotherapy became the standard of care for children with medulloblastoma with average-risk disease, with an expected 5-year event-free survival (EFS) of approximately 80%. Variation of this treatment schema with decrease in duration and an increase in dose intensity of chemotherapy agents produced similar results.[17] Substitution of CCNU with cyclophosphamide in the multiagent regimen yielded similar results.[18] Tumors with anaplastic histology have a poorer outcome, especially those that have either MYC or MYCN amplification.[17] Success in improving outcomes in average-risk disease comes at a price. Significant neurocognitive effects have been described, even with CSI dose of 23.4 Gy. Ninety percent of patients develop growth hormone deficiency, and many develop deficiencies of other hormones, requiring lifelong supplementation, which carries its own risks as a result of lack of adherence, especially in the teenage years.[18] Sensorineural deafness as a result of radiation therapy and cisplatin can also be debilitating. The current Children's Oncology Group (COG) trial is testing whether the use of 18 Gy to CSI can achieve the same outcome as 23.4 Gy and decrease the severity and incidence of long-term effects mentioned earlier.

The role of chemotherapy after radiation therapy in patients with medulloblastoma with high-risk disease was clearly established, with a 5-year EFS of 46% with chemotherapy.[19] Data from POG trial 9031 showed that patients with high-risk disease had a 5-year EFS of 70% with higher doses of radiation therapy and chemotherapy, including cyclophosphamide and cisplatin.[20] Similar results were obtained with more intensive chemotherapy with stem cell rescue.[17] A current trial within the COG is testing whether the use of carboplatin as a radiosensitizer and a differentiating agent (retinoic acid) can further improve the outcome in patients with high-risk disease.

Children younger than 3 years present a unique challenge. The developing brain is highly susceptible to devastating effects of radiation therapy, and therefore, clinical trials had centered on the use of chemotherapy alone and delaying the use of CSI until the patient is 3 years of age. This strategy had resulted in a poor outcome in infants, except in those infants who have nonmetastatic disease, undergo GTR, and have a particular type of histopathology, described as nodular desmoplastic or medulloblastoma with extensive nodularity. The use of higher doses of systemic methotrexate and concomitant use of intrathecal methotrexate has obviated radiation therapy in infants but still resulted in leukoencephalopathy in 19 of 23 patients tested; this could lead to long-term significant neurocognitive deficits.[21]

Recent Advances

Until recently, medulloblastoma was considered one disease and was treated uniformly with the same regimen. Northcott and colleagues,[22] along with others, showed that medulloblastoma can be categorized into 4 groups. Tumors displaying WNT pathway activation with resultant nuclear accumulation of β-catenin and monosomy 6 constitute about 10% of all children with medulloblastoma and have a favorable prognosis. Efforts are under way to significantly reduce radiation therapy or chemotherapy or both for this subtype. Approximately 30% of patients with medulloblastoma have evidence of activation of the SHH pathway as a result of mutations in the *PTCH1* or the *SMO* genes. Survival rate in this subgroup is approximately 75%. SMO inhibitors are in clinical trials, and one such trial was recently published.[23] Group 3 constitutes tumors that have a poor prognosis, with survival rate of approximately 50%; survival rate of group 4 is approximately 70%. Newer and more effective agents are needed to improve outcomes in these groups. Genomic sequencing data offer further clues to the biology of these tumors and potentially new targets. With the burgeoning data, there is increased hope for more effective and targeted therapies, which could lead to improved outcomes with lesser toxicities.

HIGH-GRADE GLIOMA AND DIFFUSE INTRINSIC PONTINE GLIOMA

Glioblastoma, anaplastic astrocytoma, and diffuse intrinsic pontine glioma (DIPG) represent the most common high-grade glial tumors in childhood, and together, up to 0.8 per 100,000 children younger than 19 years are estimated to develop HGGs each year. Therefore, along with embryonal tumors, these tumors constitute the most common malignant neoplasms of the brain in children. DIPGs are midline tumors, and among the other HGGs, 25% occur in the deep midline structures of the cerebrum, 15% in the posterior fossa, and the rest in cerebral hemispheres.[24,25] The median age at diagnosis is 9 to 10 years for HGG and 6 to 7 years for DIPGs.

Symptoms and signs of disease manifest rapidly after a short clinical history and can be related to increased intracranial pressure characterized by headaches, seizures, or weakness on the opposite side. Children with DIPGs can present with gait imbalance and lower cranial nerve paresis, after a short prodromal phase.

HGGs are heterogeneous on computed tomography and MRI with ill-defined margins, usually with marked surrounding edema, hemorrhage, necrosis, mass effect, and irregular enhancement. These tumors show restricted diffusion on apparent diffusion coefficient maps on MRI and a marked increase in choline levels with a reduction in N-acetyl aspartate on magnetic resonance spectroscopy. On perfusion imaging, these tumors tend to have high relative cerebral blood volume values. MRI findings in DIPGs are similar and are characterized by a diffuse expansion of the pons which is isointense or hypointense on T1 and bright on T2 sequences.

HGGs show several histologic features of malignancy, including hypercellularity, cytologic and nuclear atypia, mitoses, necrosis with or without pseudopalisading, and vascular proliferation with endothelial hyperplasia. The most common malignant glial neoplasms are anaplastic astrocytoma and glioblastoma multiforme, which may alternatively be termed grade III and grade IV astrocytomas, respectively.

HGGs often show a histologically heterogeneous nature, and areas of low-grade histology may be seen particularly in small biopsies taken from the more superficial areas of tumor. Therefore, more generous sampling is recommended to avoid confusion about the true nature of the HGG. The pathologic features may vary in DIPGs. There could be regions with low-grade, diffuse, fibrillary-type, World Health Organization (WHO) grade II histopathology, or, more often, high-grade anaplastic astrocytoma (WHO grade III) or glioblastoma multiforme (WHO grade IV).

Treatment

Surgery
Removal of more than 90% of the tumor confers a favorable prognosis in HGG.[25] The infiltrative nature of the tumor does not render itself to complete resection. Local progression therefore is common, thus resulting in a poor prognosis.

Radiation therapy and chemotherapy
Postoperative radiation therapy is the mainstay of therapy in children with HGG. Although rarely curative, the addition of radiation alone had shown improved survival in children, with higher rates of 1-year to 3-year disease control. Postoperative therapy incorporates wide local irradiation. The radiation field typically includes enhancing tumor on T1 and the perilesional infiltration estimated by findings on T2 or fluid-attenuated inversion recovery sequences. Typical dose is 54 to 60 Gy in pediatrics. The role of chemotherapy in addition to postoperative radiotherapy is still unclear. Initial encouraging results with a chemotherapy regimen consisting of prednisone, vincristine, and CCNU (pCV regimen) showed that progression-free survival (PFS) for children receiving postradiation chemotherapy was significantly higher (46%) than for those receiving radiation therapy alone (16%; $P = .026$).[26] A subsequent trial conducted by CCG (CCG-945), which is one of the largest pediatric trials in children with HGG, randomized patients to receive adjuvant chemotherapy with an 8-in-1 regimen or PCV (P, procarbazine). No difference was observed between the 2 chemotherapy arms, and 5-year PFS rates were 33% and 36% for 8-in-1 chemotherapy and

PCV, respectively.[25] Thus, there seemed to be little benefit from addition of chemotherapy, when compared with surgery and radiation therapy alone. A recent COG trial, ACNS0126, combined radiation therapy with temozolomide, 90 mg/m^2/d, daily for 42 days, followed by 10 cycles of adjuvant temozolomide, 200 mg/m^2/d × 5 days given every 28 days.[27] EFS for 99 eligible patients with HGG on ACNS0126 was compared with a similar cohort of 122 patients from CCG-945, which was open to accrual between 1985 and 1992. Outcome for ACNS0126 did not significantly differ from historical controls, with 1-year EFS of 39% ± 5% for ACNS0126 compared with 42% ± 4.5% for CCG-945 (logrank P = .14). Patients with low/absent methyl guanine methyl transferase expression had longer EFS and overall survival, and therefore, temozolomide may be useful as part of a chemotherapy regimen for future studies in this subgroup of patients. Another approach to circumventing temozolomide resistance is through inhibition of PARP (poly-ADP ribose polymerase), a critical nuclear enzyme that activates proteins in the base excision repair and other DNA repair pathways. Inhibition of this enzymatic activity with a PARP inhibitor such as ABT-888 may overcome temozolomide resistance. Trials with ABT-888 and temozolomide are in progress. The use of concurrent radiation and temozolomide followed by temozolomide and lomustine for pediatric HGGs was evaluated in a COG trial (ACNS0423) and the results are yet to be published. A COG trial with involved-field radiation with concurrent vorinostat or temozolomide or bevacizumab followed by maintenance with bevacizumab and temozolomide was recently completed.

In the management of children with DIPG, radiation therapy is the mainstay of treatment. Improvement in symptoms, signs, and neuroimaging occurs in most children, although the duration of benefit is measured in months, with few long-term survivors.[28,29] Variations in the delivery and total dose of radiation therapy were attempted. Hyperfractionated delivery consisting of twice-daily irradiation with fractions of 1.0 to 1.25 Gy to total doses ranging from 64.8 to 78.0 Gy showed no significant improvement.[29–32] A randomized trial comparing hyperfractionated radiation at dose level of 70.2 Gy with conventional fractionation (1.8 Gy once daily to 55.8 Gy) showed no difference, leading North American centers to consider conventional fractionation as the standard for current management and trials.[33]

Attempts at radiosensitization using cis-platinum concurrently with radiation seemed to show similar or marginally inferior outcome for children with brainstem tumors when compared with radiation alone.[34] Various agents have been used with radiation therapy to improve outcome in these patients, with little benefit.

The Pediatric Brain Tumor Consortium conducted a phase 1 trial with radiation therapy and capecitabine.[35,36] It was well tolerated, and a phase 2 trial is in progress. Radiation therapy is a potent inducer of thymidine phosphorylase (TP), which converts capecitabine to 5-fluorouracil within the tumor. Capecitabine antitumor activity is correlated with intratumoral TP; therefore, this combination may be more effective than radiotherapy alone for brainstem gliomas.

Advances in the management of DIPG have been hindered by the lack of tissue specimens to gain insights into the biology of these tumors. Recent data from autopsy specimens have provided much information, as discussed later. Also, current protocols, which require a biopsy of these tumors before initiation of therapy, are likely to shed more light on the pathways leading to tumor formation.

Recent advances in high-grade glioma and diffuse intrinsic pontine glioma

Recently, rapid advances in molecular biology have generated detailed catalogs of genomic and epigenomic alterations in HGG and DIPG in children. Using many samples from children with HGG and DIPG, sequencing studies showed recurrent heterozygous mutations in histone H3F3A, with amino acid substitutions at positions K27 or G34. K27 was also found to be mutated in the H3.1 histone genes *HIST1H3B* and *HIST1H3C*.[37,38] These mutations directly or indirectly target important sites on the histone tail for posttranslational modifications. H3 mutations occur exclusively in approximately 38% of childhood, and young adult patients with HGG and are mutually exclusive with respect to mutations in IDH1.[37,39] Mutations in H3F3A, which result in amino acid changes at K27, occur in 70% to 80% of midline glioblastoma multiforme and DIPG in younger children.[38,40,41] Mutations in H3F3A that result in amino acid changes at G34 occur in adolescents at around the age of 20 years who have disease exclusively located in hemispheric regions. Mutations at K27 seem to confer a dismal prognosis, whereas G34 mutations seem to be associated with slightly prolonged overall survival.[40,41] Novel activating mutations in ACVR1 are identified in approximately 20% of children with DIPG. Taken together, these data raise the possibility of developing targeted therapies against these known mutations and thereby improve outcomes in these children, who collectively have a dismal prognosis with the current therapies.

EPENDYMOMA

Ependymomas represent approximately 10% of all primary tumors of the central nervous system in children. These tumors arise from the ependymal lining of the ventricular system or the central canal of the spinal cord. Ninety percent of the tumors are intracranial, and up to two-thirds of these occur in the posterior fossa. There are 2 peaks in incidence: one in the first 7 years of life and the second in the third to fifth decades of life.[42] The ratio of male to female is between 1.3 and 2.0.

Within the posterior fossa, ependymomas represent the fourth most common posterior fossa tumor in children, after medulloblastoma, cerebellar astrocytoma, and brainstem glioma. They usually grow out of the fourth ventricle via the foramina of Luschka and Magendie toward the cerebellopontine angle and through the foramen magnum into the upper cervical canal around the spinal cord. On MRI, these tumors are heterogeneous, containing cysts, calcification, and occasional hemorrhage, as well as irregular, heterogeneous enhancement with gadolinium.

Ependymomas vary from well-differentiated tumors with no anaplasia, rare or absent mitoses, and mild pleomorphism to highly cellular lesions with brisk mitotic activity, anaplasia, microvascular proliferation, and pseudopalisading necrosis. The former are low-grade tumors (WHO grade II) and the latter are high-grade, anaplastic tumors (WHO grade III). Recent data[43,44] suggest a significant correlation between anaplastic histology and a higher rate of disease recurrence. Spinal subarachnoid dissemination has been estimated to be 7% to 12%, most commonly occurring in high-grade and posterior fossa tumors.[42,45]

Treatment

Surgery

The single most important prognostic factor in the management of ependymoma is the extent of tumor resection. The survival rate is higher after a GTR (66%–75%) versus a less complete resection (0%–11%). However, in most series, only approximately 60% to 70% of patients undergo a GTR. GTRs are generally more difficult for posterior fossa ependymomas than for supratentorial ependymomas, because of the propensity for infratentorial lesions to infiltrate the brainstem and to surround cranial nerves and vessels lateral and ventral to the brainstem. Infants are particularly likely to have large infratentorial ependymomas, and this is one of the reasons why they have a less favorable prognosis.[46–48] Aggressive surgical procedures to confer a good prognosis can result in multiple lower cranial nerve palsies, which often necessitate a tracheostomy and gastric feeding device. Recent treatment protocols have allowed for second-look surgery to be performed after initial chemotherapy to make complete resections safe.

Radiation therapy

Local postoperative radiation therapy has increased the overall survival rates of patients with ependymoma from approximately 60% to 85%.[49] There are data to suggest that radiation therapy may not be necessary in patients with well-differentiated supratentorial ependymomas and intramedullary spinal cord or cauda equina.[50,51]

In a large prospective study of 153 children with localized ependymomas, GTR and conformal, high-dose, postoperative radiation (59.4 Gy with a 1-cm margin around the target volume) resulted in a 7-year local control, EFS, and overall survival rates of 87.3%, 69.1%, and 81.0%, respectively.[49] However, local failure continues to be the greatest obstacle to improving clinical outcome in children with ependymoma, with local failures occurring in 59% to 97% of recurrent cases, and isolated local failure accounting for 39% of failures in the large series reported by Merchant and colleagues.

The recently closed COG trial ACNS 0121 used a 1-cm margin, which most consider the standard of care. However, the most recent COG prospective study incorporates further reduction in treatment volume, with only a 0.5-cm margin around the target volume to 54 Gy and no clinical target volume expansion for the final boost to 59.4 Gy.

Although chemotherapy is considered to be active in this disease, with good response rates to various chemotherapeutic agents, their contribution to overall survival is still not proved. The recently completed COG ACNS0121 trial will provide data as to whether 2 cycles of multiagent chemotherapy in patients with subtotal resections make their tumors more amenable to a GTR before the initiation of conformal radiation therapy, and the ongoing ACNS0831 study will examine the contribution of postradiation chemotherapy to improve outcome compared with patients who undergo radiation therapy alone in patients who have a GTR. The chemotherapy regimen is based on a recently reported study that showed similar EFS in patients with subtotal resection who received chemotherapy in addition to radiation therapy compared with those with complete resection and who received radiation therapy alone.

Future treatment strategies in ependymoma will be based on the advances made in the biology of these tumors. Recent advances, as discussed in the following section, clearly indicate that all intracranial ependymomas are not the same. Furthermore, these advances have given us potential target, which can lead to innovative therapies, which are likely to improve outcomes with less morbidity.

Recent advances

Location of the tumor and molecular data define 4 subtypes of ependymoma-supratentorial, posterior fossa type A (PFA), posterior fossa type B (PFB) and spinal cord ependymoma. PFA and PFB also differ in age of onset and prognosis.[52] The PFA subtype is found predominantly in infants and is associated with a poor prognosis, despite maximally aggressive therapy. The PFB subtype occurs in older children and adults and carries a good prognosis.

Among supratentorial tumors, Parker and colleagues[53] found frequent cases in which translocation of a region of chromosome 11 caused the fusion of 2 genes, RELA and C11orf95. Wild-type RELA is located in the cytoplasm, but the C11orf95-RELA hybrid protein spontaneously translocates to the nucleus, where it activates the expression of target genes. The sequencing of posterior fossa tumors did not show any recurrently mutated gene or translocation. It has been suspected that defective epigenetic modifications might also be oncogenic. These modifications include methylation or acetylation of DNA or DNA-associated chromatin proteins. Mack and colleagues[54] did find increased DNA methylation of specific genes, as well as silencing of their expression, in PFA, but not PFB, ependymomas. PFB differs from PFA in that it is associated with gains and losses of entire chromosomes or large chromosomal fragments. Therefore, it will be challenging to test whether chromosomal gains and losses or epigenetic modifications without gene mutations can drive cancer development. The clinical implications of these alternative oncogenic routes can be far reaching, because most research has focused on drugs that target gene mutations.

SUMMARY

The past 2 decades have witnessed a revolution in the management of childhood brain tumors, with the establishment of multidisciplinary teams and national and international consortiums. Unprecedented cooperation within the pediatric neuro-oncology community and sophisticated rapidly evolving technology have led to advances that are likely to revolutionize treatment strategies and improve outcomes.

REFERENCES

1. Central Brain Tumor Registry of the United States (CBTRUS). Fact sheet. Stromberg Allen; 2013. Available at: www.cbtrus.org.
2. Taylor MD, Mainprize TG, Rutka JT. Molecular insight into medulloblastoma and central nervous system primitive neuroectodermal tumor biology from hereditary syndromes: a review. Neurosurgery 2000;47:888–901.
3. Malkin D, Li FP, Strong LC, et al. Germ line p53 mutations in a familial syndrome of breast cancer, sarcomas, and other neoplasms. Science 1990;250:1233–8.
4. Liaw D, Marsh DJ, Li J, et al. Germline mutations of the PTEN gene in Cowden disease, an inherited breast and thyroid cancer syndrome. Nat Genet 1997;16: 64–7.
5. Louis DN, Ohgaki H, Wiestler OD, et al, editors. WHO classification of tumors of the central nervous system. Lyon (France): IARC; 2007.
6. Ostrom QT, Gittleman H, Liao P et al. Central Brain Tumor Registry of the United States. Statistical report, primary brain and central nervous system tumors diagnosed in the United States, 2007–2011. Central Brain Tumor Registry of the United States. Neuro-oncology 2014; 16(Suppl 4).
7. Amlash SF, Riffaud L, Brassier G, et al. Nevoid basal cell carcinoma syndrome: relation with desmoplastic medulloblastoma in infancy. Cancer 2003;98:618–24.
8. Thompson MC, Fuller C, Hogg TL, et al. Genomics identifies medulloblastoma subgroups that are enriched for specific genetic alterations. J Clin Oncol 2006; 24:1924–31.
9. Eberhart CG, Kepner JL, Goldthwaite PT, et al. Histopathologic grading of medulloblastomas: a Pediatric Oncology Group study. Cancer 2002;94:552–60.
10. Clifford SB, Lusher MR, Lindsey JC, et al. Wnt/wingless pathway activation and chromosome 6 loss characterize a distinct molecular sub-group of medulloblastomas associated with a favorable prognosis. Cell Cycle 2006;5:2666–70.
11. Srivastava S, Zou ZQ, Pirollo K, et al. Germ-line transmission of a mutated p53 gene in a cancer-prone family with Li-Fraumeni syndrome. Nature 1990;348: 747–9.

12. Gajjar A, Fouladi M, Walter AW, et al. Comparison of lumbar and shunt cerebrospinal fluid specimens for cytologic detection of leptomeningeal disease in pediatric patients with brain tumors. J Clin Oncol 1999;17(6):1825–8.

13. Bartlett F, Kortmann R, Saran F. Medulloblastoma. Clin Oncol (R Coll Radiol) 2013;25(1):36–45.

14. Robertson PL, Muraszko KM, Holmes EJ, et al. Incidence and severity of postoperative cerebellar mutism syndrome in children with medulloblastoma: a prospective study by the Children's Oncology Group. J Neurosurg 2006;105(6 Suppl):444–51.

15. Thomas PR, Deutsch M, Kepner JL, et al. Low-stage medulloblastoma: final analysis of trial comparing standard-dose with reduced-dose neuraxis irradiation. J Clin Oncol 2000;18:3004–11.

16. Packer RJ, Goldwein J, Nicholson HS, et al. Treatment of children with medulloblastomas with reduced-dose craniospinal radiation therapy and adjuvant chemotherapy: a Children's Cancer Group Study. J Clin Oncol 1999;17:2127–36.

17. Gajjar A, Chintagumpala M, Ashley D, et al. Risk-adapted craniospinal radiotherapy followed by high-dose chemotherapy and stem-cell rescue in children with newly diagnosed medulloblastoma (St Jude Medulloblastoma-96): long-term results from a prospective, multicentre trial. Lancet Oncol 2006;7(10):813–20.

18. Packer RJ, Gajjar A, Vezina G, et al. Phase III study of craniospinal radiation therapy followed by adjuvant chemotherapy for newly diagnosed average-risk medulloblastoma. J Clin Oncol 2006;24(25):4202–8.

19. Zeltzer PM, Boyett JM, Finlay JL, et al. Metastasis stage, adjuvant treatment, and residual tumor are prognostic factors for medulloblastoma in children: conclusions from the Children's Cancer group 921 randomized phase III study. J Clin Oncol 1999;17:8322–45.

20. Tarbell NJ, Friedman H, Polkinghorn WR, et al. High-risk medulloblastoma: a Pediatric Oncology Group randomized trial of chemotherapy before or after radiation therapy (POG 9031). J Clin Oncol 2013;31(23):2936–41.

21. Rutkowski S, Bode U, Deinlein F, et al. Treatment of early childhood medulloblastoma by postoperative chemotherapy alone. N Engl J Med 2005;352:978–86.

22. Northcott PA, Korshunov A, Witt H, et al. Medulloblastoma comprises four distinct molecular variants. J Clin Oncol 2011;29(11):1408–14.

23. Gajjar A, Stewart CF, Ellison DW, et al. Phase I study of vismodegib in children with recurrent or refractory medulloblastoma: a pediatric brain tumor consortium study. Clin Cancer Res 2013;19(22):6305–12.

24. Heideman RL, Kuttesch J Jr, Gajjar AJ, et al. Supratentorial malignant gliomas in childhood: a single institution perspective. Cancer 1997;80:497–504.

25. Finlay JL, Boyett JM, Yates AJ, et al. Randomized phase III trial in childhood high-grade astrocytoma comparing vincristine, lomustine, and prednisone with the eight-drugs-in-1-day regimen. Children's Cancer Group. J Clin Oncol 1995;13:112–23.

26. Sposto R, Ertel IJ, Jenkin RD, et al. The effectiveness of chemotherapy for treatment of high grade astrocytoma in children: results of a randomized trial. A report from the Children's Cancer Study Group. J Neurooncol 1989;7:165–77.

27. Cohen KJ, Pollack IF, Zhou T. Temozolomide in the treatment of high-grade gliomas in children: a report from the Children's Oncology Group. Neuro Oncol 2011;13(3):317–23.

28. Freeman CR, Farmer JP. Pediatric brain stem gliomas: a review. Int J Radiat Oncol Biol Phys 1998;40:265–71.

29. Packer RJ, Boyett JM, Zimmerman RA, et al. Hyperfractionated radiation therapy (72 Gy) for children with brain stem gliomas. A Children's Cancer Group Phase I/II Trial. Cancer 1993;72:1414–21.
30. Freeman CR, Krischer JP, Sanford RA, et al. Final results of a study of escalating doses of hyperfractionated radiotherapy in brain stem tumors in children: a Pediatric Oncology Group study. Int J Radiat Oncol Biol Phys 1993;27:197–206.
31. Shrieve DC, Wara WM, Edwards MS, et al. Hyperfractionated radiation therapy for gliomas of the brainstem in children and in adults. Int J Radiat Oncol Biol Phys 1992;24:599–610.
32. Packer RJ, Boyett JM, Zimmerman RA, et al. Outcome of children with brain stem gliomas after treatment with 7800 cGy of hyperfractionated radiotherapy. A Children's Cancer Group phase I/II trial. Cancer 1994;74:1827–34.
33. Mandell LR, Kadota R, Freeman C, et al. There is no role for hyperfractionated radiotherapy in the management of children with newly diagnosed diffuse intrinsic brainstem tumors: results of a Pediatric Oncology Group phase III trial comparing conventional vs. hyperfractionated radiotherapy. Int J Radiat Oncol Biol Phys 1999;43:959–64.
34. Freeman CR, Kepner J, Kun LE, et al. A detrimental effect of a combined chemotherapy-radiotherapy approach in children with diffuse intrinsic brain stem gliomas? Int J Radiat Oncol Biol Phys 2000;47:561–4.
35. Kilburn LB, Kocak M, Schaedeli Stark F, et al. Phase I trial of capecitabine rapidly disintegrating tablets and concomitant radiation therapy in children with newly diagnosed brainstem gliomas and high-grade gliomas. Neuro Oncol 2013;15(6):759–66.
36. Sawada N, Ishikawa T, Sekiguchi F, et al. X-ray irradiation induces thymidine phosphorylase and enhances the efficacy of capecitabine (Xeloda) in human cancer xenografts. Clin Cancer Res 1999;5:2948–53.
37. Schwartzentruber J, Korshunov A, Liu XY, et al. Driver mutations in histone H3.3 and chromatin remodelling genes in paediatric glioblastoma. Nature 2012;482:226–31.
38. Wu G, Broniscer A, McEachron TA, et al. Somatic histone H3 alterations in pediatric diffuse intrinsic pontine gliomas and non-brainstem glioblastomas. Nat Genet 2012;44:251–3.
39. Downing J, Wilson RK, Zhang J, et al. The Pediatric Cancer Genome Project. Nat Genet 2012;44:619–22.
40. Khuong-Quang DA, Buczkowicz P, Rakopoulos P, et al. K27M mutation in histone H3.3 defines clinically and biologically distinct subgroups of pediatric diffuse intrinsic pontine gliomas. Acta Neuropathol 2012;124:439–47.
41. Sturm D, Witt H, Hovestadt V, et al. Hotspot mutations in H3F3A and IDH1 define distinct epigenetic and biological subgroups of glioblastoma. Cancer Cell 2012;22:425–37.
42. Kun LE, Kovnar EH, Sanford RA. Ependymomas in children. Pediatr Neurosci 1988;14:57–63.
43. Tihan T, Zhou T, Holmes E, et al. The prognostic value of histological grading of posterior fossa ependymomas in children: a Children's Oncology Group study and a review of prognostic factors. Mod Pathol 2008;21:165–77.
44. Merchant TE, Jenkins JJ, Burger PC, et al. Influence of tumor grade on time to progression after irradiation for localized ependymoma in children. Int J Radiat Oncol Biol Phys 2002;53:52–7.
45. Vanuytsel L, Brada M. The role of prophylactic spinal irradiation in localized intracranial ependymoma. Int J Radiat Oncol Biol Phys 1991;21:825–30.

46. Duffner PK, Horowitz ME, Krischer JP, et al. The treatment of malignant brain tumors in infants and very young children: an update of the Pediatric Oncology Group experience. Neuro Oncol 1999;1:152–61.
47. Nagib MG, O'Fallon MT. Posterior fossa lateral ependymoma in childhood. Pediatr Neurosurg 1996;24:299–305.
48. Sanford RA, Kun LE, Heideman RL, et al. Cerebellar pontine angle ependymoma in infants. Pediatr Neurosurg 1997;27:84–91.
49. Merchant TE, Li C, Xiong X, et al. Conformal radiotherapy after surgery for paediatric ependymoma: a prospective study. Lancet Oncol 2009;10:258–66.
50. Hukin J, Epstein F, Lefton D, et al. Treatment of intracranial ependymoma by surgery alone. Pediatr Neurosurg 1998;29:40–5.
51. Wallner KE, Wara WM, Sheline GE, et al. Intracranial ependymomas: results of treatment with partial or whole brain irradiation without spinal irradiation. Int J Radiat Oncol Biol Phys 1986;12:1937–41.
52. Witt H, Mack SC, Ryzhova M, et al. Delineation of two clinically and molecularly distinct subgroups of posterior fossa ependymoma. Cancer Cell 2011;20(2): 143–57.
53. Parker M, Mohankumar KM, Punchihewa C, et al. C11orf95-RELA fusions drive oncogenic NF-κB signalling in ependymoma. Nature 2014;506(7489):451–5.
54. Mack SC, Witt H, Piro RM, et al. Epigenomic alterations define lethal CIMP-positive ependymomas of infancy. Nature 2014;506(7489):445–50.

Sarcomas

Josephine H. HaDuong, MD[a], Andrew A. Martin, MD[b],
Stephen X. Skapek, MD[b], Leo Mascarenhas, MD, MS[a],*

KEYWORDS

- Soft-tissue sarcoma • Rhabdomyosarcoma • Nonrhabdomyosarcoma • Bone
- Ewing's • Osteosarcoma

KEY POINTS

- Osteosarcoma and Ewing sarcoma are the 2 most common malignant bone tumors of pediatrics, with peak incidence during the adolescent years.
- Rhabdomyosarcoma is the most common soft-tissue sarcoma of childhood, with a bimodal age distribution of 2 to 6 years and 15 to 19 years of age.
- Sarcomas are best treated with multimodality treatment that often includes chemotherapy, surgery, and/or radiation therapy.
- Children with localized sarcoma fare well with multimodality treatment, whereas those with metastatic or recurrent disease have poor outcomes.
- Improved molecular understanding of these diseases has led to the possibility of using new molecular targeted agents in the setting of clinical trials.

INTRODUCTION

Osteosarcoma (OS) and Ewing sarcoma (EWS) are the 2 most common malignant bone tumors in children and adolescents, and make up approximately 6% of all childhood malignancies. Rhabdomyosarcoma (RMS) and nonrhabdomyosarcoma soft-tissue sarcomas (NRSTS), the 2 major classes of soft-tissue sarcoma, account for another 7% of all childhood malignancies. Optimal comprehensive care of patients with either bone or soft-tissue sarcoma requires a multidisciplinary team, which includes an oncologist, a surgeon, a radiation oncologist, a pathologist, and a radiologist. Treatment is multimodal, with the overall goal being to achieve local control with surgery and/or

[a] Division of Hematology, Oncology, and Blood & Marrow Transplantation, Department of Pediatrics, Children's Center for Cancer and Blood Diseases, Children's Hospital Los Angeles, University of Southern California Keck School of Medicine, 4650 Sunset Boulevard, MS 54, Los Angeles, CA 90027, USA; [b] Division of Hematology/Oncology, Department of Pediatrics, Pauline Allen Gill Center for Cancer and Blood Disorders, Children's Medical Center, University of Texas Southwestern Medical Center, 5323 Harry Hines Boulevard, MC 9063, Dallas, TX 75390, USA
* Corrresponding author.
E-mail address: lmascarenhas@chla.usc.edu

Pediatr Clin N Am 62 (2015) 179–200
http://dx.doi.org/10.1016/j.pcl.2014.09.012
0031-3955/15/$ – see front matter © 2015 Elsevier Inc. All rights reserved.
pediatric.theclinics.com

radiation and to use chemotherapy to control metastatic disease, even though it may not be clinically detectable. Over the last 4 decades improvements in chemotherapy regimens, surgery, radiation, and the use of collaborative group clinical trials have led to significant improvements in outcome for patients with sarcoma; this is particularly true for patients with localized tumors, most of whom now survive their disease. However, patients with metastatic and recurrent disease continue to have poor prognoses despite various attempts at intensifying chemotherapy. Furthermore, sarcoma patients who survive have one of the highest risks of developing long-term treatment effects, many of which can be life-threatening. Better treatments are therefore still needed to improve the outcomes of patients with sarcomas, especially for those with metastatic and recurrent disease, and to limit long-term complications for those who survive. Uncovering the key vulnerabilities, developing ways to target these key molecular pathways, and improving the risk stratification to better predict outcome are developing areas that it is hoped will improve the outcome for children with these diseases.

PATHOLOGY AND BIOLOGY
Osteosarcoma

OS is a malignancy that derives its origin from mesenchymal cells. The pathologic hallmark is the production of malignant osteoid by pleomorphic malignant cells within a connective tissue matrix. OS can be divided into several subsets defined by location (appendicular vs axial, central vs surface), histologic grade (low, intermediate, or high), and the predominant matrix type.[1] Most OS tumors are conventional OS, a high-grade OS made up of 3 major subtypes based on the predominant mix of cartilage matrix and fibrous tissue: osteoblastic, chrondroblastic, and fibroblastic. The remainder includes low-grade OS, parosteal OS, periosteal OS, and telangiectatic OS, which are less common (**Box 1**). Although the presence of malignant osteoid is necessary to confirm a diagnosis of OS (**Fig. 1**A), radiographic appearance of the tumor is helpful in arriving at the diagnosis. Immunohistochemistry and cytogenetics are not diagnostic of OS. There are no consistent chromosomal or gene abnormalities described in OS; however, several genes have been implicated in OS pathogenesis following the observations of increased frequency of OS seen in patients with cancer predisposition syndromes, including Rothmund-Thomson syndrome, Bloom syndrome, Werner syndrome, Li-Fraumeni syndrome, and hereditary retinoblastoma (**Box 2**).[2,3]

Box 1
Pathologic subtypes of osteosarcoma

Conventional

  Osteoblastic

  Chondroblastic

  Fibroblastic

Secondary

Telangiectatic

Small cell

Periosteal

High-grade surface

Low-grade intramedullary

Parosteal

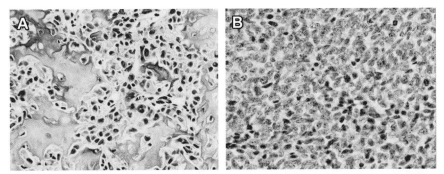

Fig. 1. Pathology of osteosarcoma (OS) and Ewing sarcoma (EWS). (*A*) Conventional, high-grade OS showing malignant cells and their production of a lace-like neoplastic osteoid matrix. (*B*) EWS showing a sheet of small, round, blue cell tumors. Hematoxylin and eosin (H&E) stain. 40X magnification. (*Courtesy of* Shengmei Zhou, Department of Pathology and Laboratory Medicine, Children's Hospital Los Angeles, Los Angeles, California.)

Ewing sarcoma

EWS arises most commonly in the bone but can also originate in extraosseous soft tissues, and lacks the matrix of malignant osteoid that characterizes OS. EWS is part of a larger family of tumors that includes peripheral primitive neuroectodermal tumors (PNET) as part of the spectrum; however, EWS tumors are characterized by sheets of small, round, blue cell tumors that do not form pseudorosettes, have no evidence of neural differentiation, and tend to lack distinct nucleoli (see **Fig. 1**B). Unlike OS, EWS is immunohistochemically distinct, with the vast majority expressing CD99 in a membranous pattern and FLI1 nuclear staining.[4] More than 85% of EWS tumors are also characterized by the pathognomonic t(11;22)(q24;q12) EWSR1-FLI1 translocation, while the remaining tumors (10%) consist primarily of the t(21;22)(q22;q12) EWSR1-ERG translocation followed by other, very rare translocations involving chromosomes 2 or 16.[5] The EWSR1 breakpoint can be detected by fluorescence in situ hybridization (FISH) (**Fig. 2**) or reverse transcriptase–polymerase chain reaction (RT-PCR), and is often used to confirm the diagnosis of EWS.

Rhabdomyosarcoma

RMS represents a malignant neoplasm composed of cells reminiscent of immature, skeletal myoblasts based on morphologic and molecular features.[6] Although the cell of origin is not clear, certain experimental models indicate that it can arise from immature myoblast-like cells.[7,8] RMS can be divided into 2 major histologic subtypes: alveolar and embryonal RMS (ARMS and ERMS, respectively). Approximately 80% of the ARMS cases contain a balanced translocation involving either the *PAX3* or *PAX7* genes

Box 2	
Cancer predisposition syndromes associated with increased incidence of osteosarcoma	
Syndrome	**Gene**
Hereditary retinoblastoma	RB1
Li-Fraumeni syndrome	TP53
Rothmund-Thomson syndrome	RECQL4
Bloom syndrome	RECQL2
Werner syndrome	WRN

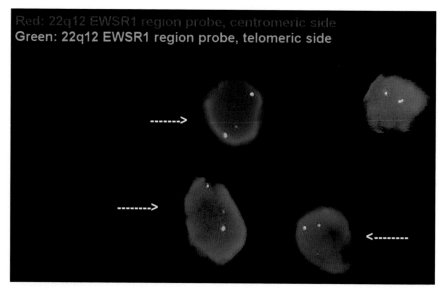

Red: 22q12 EWSR1 region probe, centromeric side
Green: 22q12 EWSR1 region probe, telomeric side

Fig. 2. Cytogenetics of EWS. Fluorescence in situ hybridization using the EWSR1 dual-color break-apart probe located on chromosome 22q12 to detect a t(11;22)(q24;q12) translocation in EWS, showing split red and green signals in 3 Ewing sarcoma cells (*arrows*). These cells were obtained from the primary proximal humerus lesion from a 12-year-old patient with EWS. (*Courtesy of* Shi-Qi Wu, Department of Pathology and Laboratory Medicine, Children's Hospital Los Angeles, Los Angeles, California.)

on chromosomes 2 or 1, respectively, and the *FOXO1* gene found on chromosome 13.[9] Elegant studies with genetically engineered animal models prove that the expression of this so-called fusion gene is sufficient to cause ARMS, but additional tumor-suppressor genes must be inactivated in the process.[7] By contrast, ERMS notably lacks a defining molecular genetic abnormality. Indeed, recent DNA sequencing studies show that this class of tumors can contain a variety of genomic abnormalities that somehow contribute to the malignant features of the disease.[10,11]

Nonrhabdomyosarcoma Soft-Tissue Sarcoma

NRSTS in children represents a relatively large and heterogeneous group of soft-tissue neoplasms that are essentially unified based on their proven or suspected origin from mesenchymal cells. Nomenclature is largely based on cellular morphology gleaned from light microscopy. The most common forms of NRSTS in children are dermatofibrosarcoma protuberans, synovial sarcoma, malignant peripheral nerve sheath tumor, and fibrosarcoma, which has infantile and adult forms.[12] The distribution of histologic subtypes of NRSTS is shown in **Fig. 3**.[13,14] NRSTS can also be generally classified into 2 biologically distinct classes. One class is driven by tumor histology–specific, chromosomal translocations that often generate novel fusion proteins, much like ARMS already described.[12] The translocation involving chromosomes X and 18 to generate the SS18/SYT-SSX fusion protein in synovial sarcoma is a representative example.[15] The other group, similar to ERMS, is generally marked by more widespread chromosomal rearrangements (such as smaller insertions, deletions, or gains or losses of all or parts of chromosomes).[16] The biological behavior of NRSTS is largely driven by more subtle histologic features that are used to define an individual tumor as low, intermediate, or high grade (see later discussion).

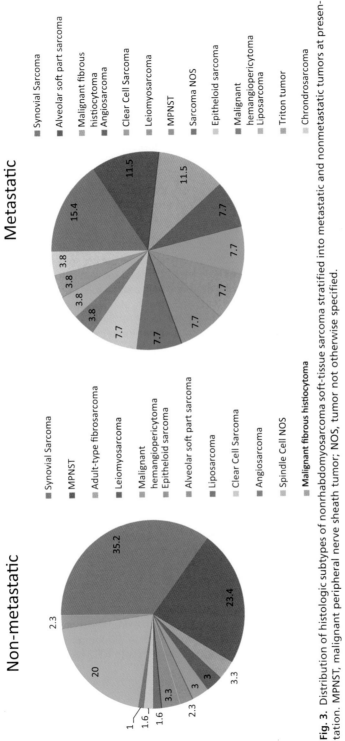

Fig. 3. Distribution of histologic subtypes of nonrhabdomyosarcoma soft-tissue sarcoma stratified into metastatic and nonmetastatic tumors at presentation. MPNST, malignant peripheral nerve sheath tumor; NOS, tumor not otherwise specified.

EPIDEMIOLOGY

OS is the most common malignant bone tumor in pediatrics, with an incidence of approximately 4.5 cases per 1 million children in the developed world.[17] EWS is the second most common malignant bone tumor in pediatrics, with an incidence of nearly 3 cases per 1 million children, a slight predilection for males over females, and a markedly lower incidence in individuals of African descent.[17,18] Both OS and EWS peak in the second decade of life, but whereas OS is very rare in young children, EWS can occur in this age group. Furthermore, prior radiation therapy is a well-described risk factor for the development of OS, whereas no such association has been described with EWS.[19] About 500 children in the United States are diagnosed with NRSTS each year, and approximately 350 with RMS, with 60% of those having ERMS.[20] Although most cases of RMS and NRSTS are sporadic, the incidence increases in certain cancer susceptibility syndromes such as Li-Fraumeni syndrome, Costello syndrome, and neurofibromatosis type 1, among others.[21–23]

CLINICAL FEATURES

Both OS and EWS, when they occur as primary bone tumors, most commonly present with locoregional pain and swelling, which often last for weeks to months before presentation. In the appendicular skeleton, the pain can be followed by a palpable mass. In the case of OS, fevers, weight loss, and other systemic complaints are uncommon. In EWS, where there may be bone marrow involvement in advanced disease, systemic symptoms may be present. Because these symptoms can be nonspecific and occur most commonly in the active, adolescent age group, symptoms are often mistaken for activity-related or sports-related injuries, which can delay diagnosis and treatment. In addition to OS and EWS, the differential diagnosis of a primary bone tumor can include osteomyelitis, benign bone lesions, trauma, bone cysts, Langerhans cell histiocytosis, giant-cell tumor of the bone, chondrosarcoma, or other malignancies that can have bone involvement, such as lymphoma or neuroblastoma.

OS and EWS both most commonly arise in the long bones around the knee, although they have predilections for different locations. EWS tends to arise from the diaphysis, whereas OS tends to arise from the metaphysis. Nearly half of EWS tumors arise from the axial skeleton, particularly the pelvis but also the ribs or spine. The remaining OS tumors are more likely to arise in the proximal humerus or the pelvis.[17] The most common sites of disease for each tumor are shown in **Fig. 4**.

In much the same way, both NRSTS and RMS typically present as a palpable soft-tissue mass, or from symptoms (eg, abdominal pain, swelling, proptosis) directly referable to the mass.[12] The mass may or may not be painful, often depending on impingement of adjacent structures. Primary tumor sites for RMS are often grouped as head/neck sites (eg, parameningeal, orbital, head/neck), genitourinary (eg, prostate, vaginal tract, bladder, paratesticular), extremity, and "other." NRSTS primary sites are also widely distributed, with approximately 60% of children with unresected, nonmetastatic disease having primary sites in an extremity or head/neck.[24] The distribution of primary tumor sites seen in soft-tissue sarcomas is shown in **Fig. 5**.[25] Systemic symptoms are notably rare for children with NRSTS.

DIAGNOSTIC WORKUP

Although the initial evaluation of a child or adolescent with a suspected bone or soft-tissue tumor often starts with radiography in the primary care setting, the importance of referral to a pediatric tertiary care center must be emphasized. A multidisciplinary

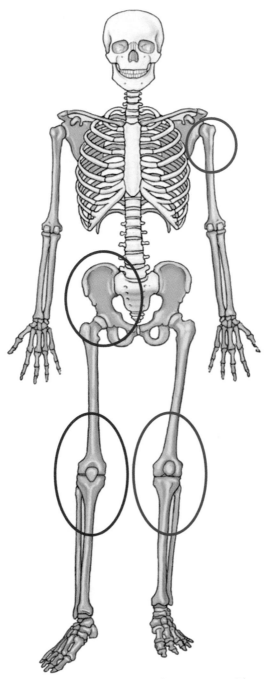

Fig. 4. Most common primary tumor sites in EWS and osteosarcoma. Blue = OS and Red = EWS. (*Adapted from* Steinsultz KA. General anatomy, terminology and positioning principles. In: Bontrager KL, Lampignano JP, editors. Textbook of radiographic positioning and related anatomy. St. Louis: Elsevier/Mosby, 2010; with permission.)

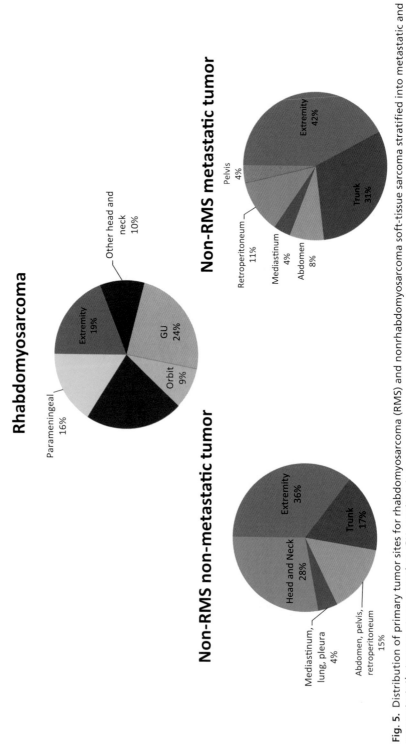

Fig. 5. Distribution of primary tumor sites for rhabdomyosarcoma (RMS) and nonrhabdomyosarcoma soft-tissue sarcoma stratified into metastatic and nonmetastatic tumors at presentation. GU, genitourinary.

team including pediatric general and orthopedic surgery, oncology, radiology, and pathology is critical for accurate diagnosis, staging, and initial therapy (**Figs. 6** and **7**).

Plain radiographs are often helpful for discriminating OS or EWS from other lesions. Both OS tumors and EWS tumors can have sclerotic and lytic lesions, but OS tumors may also have significant calcification secondary to the deposition of malignant osteoid. Cortical destruction and a periosteal reaction are not uncommon in both tumor types. The classically described findings on plain radiograph are the Codman triangle and the sunburst pattern, both of which can be seen in either OS or EWS. Codman triangle is the triangular area created when a mass breaks through and raises the periosteum away from the bone. The sunburst pattern describes the "hair on end" periosteal reaction that occurs in rapidly enlarging tumors when the periosteum does not have time to lay down a new shell of bone. Typical radiographs, MRI, and bone scans are shown in **Figs. 4** and **5** for an OS tumor and 2 EWS tumors, respectively.

Complete primary tumor evaluation for bone or soft-tissue sarcoma includes MRI and/or computed tomography (CT). For extremity lesions, the imaging should include the entire long bone involved and should capture adjacent joints. Imaging and other evaluations for metastatic disease include a whole-body nuclear bone scan and CT of the chest for patients with any bone or soft-tissue sarcoma. Additional imaging of the abdomen/pelvis should be conducted for those with RMS involving the abdomen or pelvis. Imaging of the head/neck and cerebrospinal fluid cytology should be considered for those with RMS at parameningeal or orbital sites. Bone marrow aspirate/biopsy should be performed for those with EWS and RMS. Finally, surgical regional lymph node evaluation should be undertaken for those with RMS involving the extremity or paratesticular sites, or if the node is clinically enlarged.

A biopsy is required for the diagnosis of bone or soft-tissue sarcoma. For those with OS or EWS, this should be done in coordination with the orthopedic surgeon who will ultimately resect the primary tumor following neoadjuvant chemotherapy. Blood tests in OS and EWS can show an elevated lactate dehydrogenase or alkaline phosphatase, but these are neither specific nor sensitive for disease and are reflective of disease burden. Diagnosis of RMS or NRSTS is made by incisional or excisional biopsy, also typically performed by a pediatric general or orthopedic surgeon with expertise

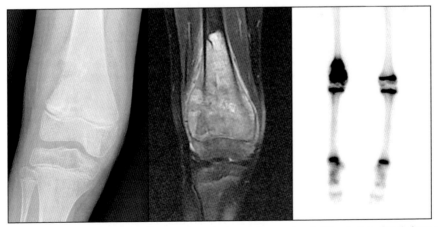

Fig. 6. Radiology of OS. (*Left*) Anteroposterior radiograph of OS of the distal femur showing a mixed pattern of bone lysis and sclerosis, with cortical destruction and a soft-tissue tumor component. (*Middle*) Coronal T2-weighted magnetic resonance image. (*Right*) Nuclear bone scan showing uptake in the right distal femur.

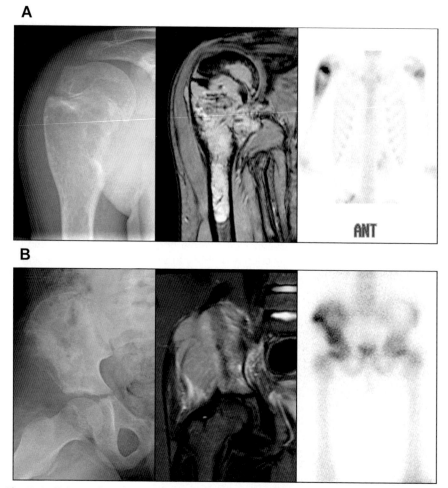

Fig. 7. Radiology of EWS. (*A*) Left, anteroposterior radiograph of EWS of the proximal humerus showing lytic lesion with cortical destruction. Middle, coronal T2-weighted magnetic resonance image. Right, nuclear bone scan showing uptake in the right proximal humerus. (*B*) Left, anteroposterior radiograph of EWS in the pelvis. Middle, coronal short-tau inversion recovery magnetic resonance image. Right, nuclear bone scan showing uptake in the right ilium.

in surgical oncology. In general, fine-needle aspiration is not sufficient for diagnosis of soft-tissue sarcoma. It should be noted that the detection of a sarcoma-specific fusion transcript (such as EWS-FLI1, PAX3-FOXO1, or SS18/SYT-SSX1) by RT-PCR or a chromosomal translocation by FISH can confirm a diagnosis even in the face of ambiguous pathologic features.

STAGING

For both EWS and OS, conventional TNM (Tumor, Lymph Node, Metastases) staging is not used. Patients with OS and EWS rarely metastasize to the lymph nodes. Instead, tumors are considered either localized or metastatic. In OS, although patients are generally considered to have either localized or metastatic disease, the Enneking staging system exists, which incorporates tumor grade in addition to the presence or absence of metastatic disease to account for those rare low-grade OS tumors such as parosteal or low-grade intramedullary OS. In this staging system all high-grade tumors, whether metastatic or localized, require chemotherapy in addition to surgical resection. However, for low-grade tumors surgical resection alone is sufficient unless there is metastatic disease. In OS, approximately 20% of patients present with metastatic disease at diagnosis, with the lung being the most common site of metastases, followed by bone. In EWS, approximately 25% of patients present with metastatic disease, with the most common sites of metastatic disease being lung, bone, and bone marrow, in descending order.[26] RMS staging is accomplished by using a system that incorporates anatomic site and features of primary disease with the presence of regional and distant metastases (essentially, a modified TNM system) to assign a clinical "stage" of 1 to 4.[27] This staging system is unusual in that it recognizes that certain anatomic sites are more favorable than others. The tumor stage is complemented by a clinical "group" assignment, which incorporates the initial surgical interventions. Group assignments range from I, in which the tumor is localized and completely resected, to IV, in which distant metastatic disease is present. There is no standard staging system for NRSTS, although several staging systems have been developed for adult NRSTS.[12] Metastatic disease is evident in 15% to 20% of children with NRSTS or RMS.[20] Lung metastasis is common for children with NRSTS, whereas lymph node metastasis is distinctly unusual. RMS can metastasize widely, including to the bone marrow.

PROGNOSTIC FACTORS
Osteosarcoma and Ewing Sarcoma

The most important adverse prognostic factor in OS and EWS is the presence or absence of metastatic disease. Patients with localized disease at diagnosis have a 5-year overall survival of about 75% compared with patients with metastatic disease at diagnosis, who have a 5-year overall survival of approximately 20% to 25%.[26,28] Since complete surgical resection of macroscopic disease is essential for cure in OS, surgical resectability is also an important prognostic factor; therefore, tumors arising from the axial skeleton portend a poorer prognosis than those arising from the appendicular skeleton.[29] An additional important prognostic indicator in OS is the tumor response to neoadjuvant chemotherapy, described by the degree of necrosis present at the time of surgical resection after the completion of neoadjuvant chemotherapy. Patients who have greater than 90% necrosis of their tumors are considered good histologic responders, whereas those who have 90% or less necrosis are considered poor histologic responders. Five-year survival for good responders is approximately 75%, compared with 50% for poor responders.[29–31] Additional adverse prognostic factors in EWS include axial location, older age at diagnosis, larger size of primary tumor, and histologic response to therapy.[32] Just as in OS, the fact that a tumor in the axial location is an adverse prognostic indicator is likely related to the surgical resectability of the tumor.

Nonrhabdomyosarcoma Soft-Tissue Sarcoma and Rhabdomyosarcoma

Both NRSTS and RMS can be grouped into low-, intermediate-, and high-risk groups, with survival rates approaching 90% for the low-risk groups and 10% to 25% for the high-risk groups. RMS risk group assignment is accomplished by merging these clinical stage and group assignments with histologic features: historically, whether the tumor had embryonal or alveolar histology features.[27] Emerging evidence indicates that molecular features, that is, the presence or absence of a PAX3(7)-FOXO1 fusion, is more robust than alveolar histology in risk group stratification.[33] In much the same way, NRSTS risk groups are largely based on extent of disease at diagnosis (eg, localized vs metastatic disease; small vs large primary tumor), initial surgical intervention (eg, resected vs unresected), and tumor-specific histologic features (eg, low vs high grade).[13]

MANAGEMENT GOALS

The care of a child or adolescent with a malignant bone or soft-tissue sarcoma requires a multidisciplinary approach to achieve successful multimodality care. The overarching goals are to achieve local disease control with wide surgical resection and/or radiation therapy and distant disease control, typically through the use of systemic chemotherapy. Surgical approaches, the use of radiation therapy, and specific chemotherapy regimens are unique to the sarcoma subtypes, as outlined next.

Osteosarcoma

Chemotherapy

Before the advent of chemotherapy for patients with OS, surgical resection alone achieved dismal survival rates of approximately 20%.[34–36] It is now understood that clinically undetectable micrometastatic disease likely exists at the time of diagnosis, and surgery and the addition of chemotherapy aims to eradicate this micrometastatic disease. The standard chemotherapy drugs used in the upfront treatment of OS include high-dose methotrexate, doxorubicin, and cisplatin (MAP) (**Table 1**).

Although no differences in outcome are reported with the addition of neoadjuvant chemotherapy versus upfront surgery,[37] neoadjuvant chemotherapy does provide several potential advantages, including improved surgical planning and endoprosthetic customization, improved resectability if there is tumor shrinkage, immediate treatment of micrometastatic disease, and, perhaps most importantly, the ability to measure tumor response to chemotherapy, the only validated surrogate predictor of outcome in patients with OS.

Additional agents that have led to tumor response include ifosfamide and etoposide, and these agents were part of a recent international collaborative study (EURAMOS), which randomized children with poor histologic responses to either MAP with or without the addition of high-dose ifosfamide and etoposide, and those with good histologic responses to MAP versus pegylated interferon-α2b. The results of the randomization for good responders were recently presented and did not improve outcomes.[38] The results of the poor responder randomization are pending, and reflect the first randomized, international, collaborative study examining intensification of chemotherapy based on response.

Table 1
Standard chemotherapy for children with osteosarcoma

Week	1	2	3	4	5	6	7	8	9	10	11
Chemotherapy	AP			M	M	AP			M	M	Surgery

Week	12	13	14	15	16	17	18	19	20	21	22	23	24	25	26	27	28	29
Chemotherapy	AP			M	M	AP			M	M	A		M	M	A		M	M

Surgery indication wide resection of gross tumor.
Abbreviations: A, adriamycin/doxorubicin; M, high-dose methotrexate; P, cisplatin.

Surgery

Complete surgical resection of macroscopic disease remains a requirement for the successful treatment of OS. The goal of surgery is to achieve adequate primary tumor control and the best possible functional outcome. Definitive surgery consists of both resection of the bulk tumor en bloc and reconstruction of the limb if amputation can be avoided. The risk of local recurrence is increased when resection margins are inadequate or histologic response to chemotherapy is poor.[39,40] Similarly, in metastatic disease, wide resection of any gross metastatic disease is seen as mandatory for potential cure. As long as adequate margins can be achieved, there are no significant differences in outcome between patients who undergo amputation and those who undergo limb-sparing surgeries.[41]

Advances in surgical technique and endoprosthetic technologies, in addition to improvements in surgical planning and resectability related to neoadjuvant chemotherapy, have led to an increase in limb-salvage surgery over amputation. Limb-salvage surgeries can include allografts and/or endoprostheses, which may be fixed or expandable to account for the continued growth of a child or adolescent. In children and adolescents for who limb salvage is not the best surgical option (because of concern for adequacy of margins, poor endoprosthetic quality for the joint, or significant anticipated growth), amputation is the mainstay. In the case of patients with tumors in the area of the knee, rotationplasty can provide wide resection without compromising oncologic outcome while allowing for excellent function. An intraoperative and postoperative example of a patient with a proximal tibia OS who has undergone rotationplasty is shown in **Fig. 8**.

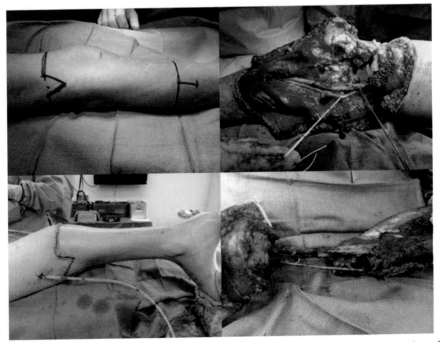

Fig. 8. Rotationplasty of a proximal tibial tumor. Clockwise, from upper left: Amputation of proximal tibia osteosarcoma followed by rotationplasty whereby the ankle joint subsequently serves as a functional knee. (*Courtesy of* Alexandre Arkader, Children's Orthopaedic Center at Children's Hospital Los Angeles, Los Angeles, CA; with permission.)

Radiation

The role of radiation in OS has typically been considered palliative because of the very high doses required for adequate local control and the associated morbidity. However, the use of proton therapy, which limits the radiation exit dose and therefore decreases toxicity, has recently been described in patients with unresectable or incompletely resected OS involving the axial skeleton.[42] Although not part of standard of care, proton therapy may provide an additional means of local control in patients for whom wide surgical resection is not feasible. At present, radiation therapy is recommended adjuvantly following primary local tumor surgery for microscopically involved surgical margins, typically delivered at the completion of planned chemotherapy.

Emerging therapy

At this time there is no agent with sufficient clinical information able to test in a randomized fashion for newly diagnosed patients. Some agents of particular interest in the relapsed population include the anti-GD2 antibody and the RANKL (receptor activator of nuclear factor κB ligand) antibody denosumab. Anti-GD2 has been used with success in patients with neuroblastoma, and most OS tumors express GD2, making it a potential therapeutic target.[43] Further work is needed to elucidate potential molecular targets in OS.

Ewing Sarcoma

Chemotherapy

Although nearly three-quarters of children presenting with a new diagnosis of EWS have localized disease, primary tumor control alone without chemotherapy is insufficient, and most of these children will develop metastatic disease. The standard of care for both localized and metastatic disease in North America starts with neoadjuvant chemotherapy, which includes vincristine, doxorubicin, and cyclophosphamide (VDC) alternating with ifosfamide and etoposide (IE). Doxorubicin was established early on as a key agent in treating EWS,[44] and the addition of ifosfamide and etoposide, particularly for those with localized disease, was subsequently found to significantly increase both event-free survival and overall survival.[45] Recently a Children's Oncology Group (COG) study examined the role of interval compression in standard chemotherapy, and found that alternating cycles of VDC and IE given every 2 weeks was more effective than when given every 3 weeks, with no additional toxicity.[46] The standard regimen for treatment of EWS is shown in **Table 2**. Interval compression with VDC/IE has increased 5-year event-free survival to nearly 75% in patients with localized EWS.

Although the addition of IE and the compressed regimen has not been proved to increase survival in patients with metastatic disease, the standard of care in North America remains the same for patients with localized or metastatic disease. Attempts at incorporating myeloablative chemotherapy with high-dose chemotherapy followed by autologous stem cell rescue have not significantly improved OS, with rates around 35%,[47] leaving the role of dose intensification with autologous stem cell rescue controversial at best. In progressive and relapsed disease, outcomes are dismal and there is no standard, effective chemotherapy regimen for these patients.

Surgery

Surgery remains the preferred method of local control in North America if wide resection is feasible with an associated loss of function that is acceptable to the patient and family. However, in cases where complete surgical resection is not possible, adjuvant radiotherapy remains the treatment of choice for primary tumor control given the radiosensitivity of EWS. The unique challenge of EWS is that a large percentage of these tumors occur in the axial skeleton, making complete surgical resection challenging at best and often not feasible without unacceptable morbidity. Primary tumor

Table 2
Current North American standard of chemotherapy for patients with Ewing Sarcoma

Week	Cycle	Treatment
1	1	VDC
2		
3	2	IE
4		
5	3	VDC
6		
7	4	IE
8		
9	5	VDC
10		
11	6	IE
12		
13–14	n/a	Surgery
15	7	VDC[a]
16		
17	8	IE
18		
19	9	VDC
20		
21	10	IE
22		
23	11	VC
24		
25	12	IE
26		
27	13	VC
28		
29	14	IE
30		

Abbreviations: C, cyclophosphamide; D, doxorubicin/adriamycin; E, etoposide; I, ifosfamide; n/a, not available; V, vincristine.
[a] If radiation is required for local control, it is started with cycle 7 and cycle 9 doxorubicin is omitted and administered later at cycle 11 after the completion of radiation therapy.

control of pelvic EWS is particularly difficult, but there is no definitive evidence that any one modality (surgery vs radiation vs surgery + radiation) is superior in providing local control.[48] In patients with metastatic disease, local control of metastatic sites is also important in providing a chance at survival. In patients with pulmonary metastatic disease, the value of whole-lung irradiation has been shown,[49] whereas the role of surgery (metastasectomy), even in the case of resectable pulmonary disease, is more controversial. In patients with extrapulmonary metastatic disease, local control of metastatic sites in addition to the primary site can result in improved survival.[50] Furthermore, the modality of local control matters, and combined modalities that include both surgery and radiation appear to affect survival favorably.

Radiation
EWS is very radiosensitive and, in fact, radiation therapy alone can provide sufficient local control. The local control rates of radiation therapy alone vary between 60% and

90%, with the recommended doses typically between 50 and 60 Gy.[51] Although historically radiation therapy was the sole method of local control, the improvement in surgical techniques, including limb salvage, and the description of late effects of radiation therapy have led to an increase in the use of surgical resection for local control. Radiation therapy for local control in North America is now usually reserved for patients with unresectable tumors (usually axial), those with residual disease following surgery, or those who refuse the loss of function that may accompany adequate surgical resection (see **Table 2**). It is not clear, however, that surgical resection provides superior rates of local control in comparison with radiation therapy, as tumors amenable to surgical resection are often those which carry favorable prognostic factors.[32,52] However, when residual disease is present or surgery is not a feasible option, radiation therapy is a requirement for the successful treatment of EWS.

Emerging therapy

The addition of topotecan/cyclophosphamide in an interval-compressed regimen is being investigated by COG in a phase III randomized trial in patients with newly diagnosed localized EWS following demonstration of feasibility in a pilot clinical trial.[53] The IGF-1R antibody has been shown to cause some objective responses in multiple early-phase trials looking at various IGF-1R inhibitors in adults. Therefore, for patients with metastatic disease, the addition of an antibody against IGF-1R added to the intensified VDC/IE backbone will be investigated.[54] Additional strategies are needed to improve the outcome of patients with EWS, particularly those with metastatic and recurrent disease.

Rhabdomyosarcoma

Surgery

The importance of surgical resection in the treatment of children with RMS is best evidenced by survival being better for those with localized disease in Group I (completely resected) than for those in Groups II or III.[55,56] Nonetheless, the fact that RMS is also responsive to ionizing radiation and chemotherapy must be emphasized. As such, the North American Intergroup Rhabdomyosarcoma Study Group and the Soft Tissue Sarcoma Committee of the COG developed and maintain the philosophy that surgical resection of RMS should not compromise form or function.

In situations where initial resection is not possible, some have advocated for delayed, primary resection after 12 weeks or more of chemotherapy. The value of delayed resection is not clear. Indeed, a recent report demonstrated that the survival of children with Group III RMS (ie, gross residual primary without metastasis at the initiation of therapy) was the same regardless of the presence or absence of gross disease at the end of therapy.[57] Similarly, there is no general role for the resection of metastatic disease.

Radiation

Standard accepted approaches call for ionizing radiation to be administered to the primary tumor or operative site for nearly all children with RMS. Notable exceptions are the rare cases whereby amputation is performed, and for children with Group I (ie, completely resected), nonalveolar tumors that are not metastatic. Radiation has most often been recommended during the first 12 weeks of therapy, and a recent COG study (ARST0531) used radiation at week 4 for those with intermediate-risk disease. In rare situations, such as spinal cord compression, loss of vision, or other imminently organ-compromising situations, emergency radiation should be considered.

Chemotherapy

RMS represents a sarcoma that generally displays sensitivity to cytotoxic chemotherapy. A series of multicenter, prospective clinical trials conducted under the aegis of the Intergroup Rhabdomyosarcoma Study Group and the COG spanning almost 4 decades has done much to optimize chemotherapeutic approaches for children with RMS. These studies have helped to define dose-intensive combination chemotherapy with vincristine, actinomycin-D, and cyclophosphamide (VAC) as the historical standard of care for most children with RMS. More recent studies have defined certain subsets of children with low-risk disease who can be effectively treated with vincristine and actinomycin alone or with a low dose of cyclophosphamide, thus limiting certain late effects of that drug.[20] Recent attempts to further intensify therapy for those with metastatic disease have found that the addition of other active agents, including irinotecan and doxorubicin, may improve failure-free survival, but whether this translates into improved overall survival remains to be seen.[20] It is hoped that insight gleaned from next-generation DNA sequencing studies of RMS will unmask vulnerabilities that can guide the application of molecularly targeted drugs, but this potential is yet to be realized.

Nonrhabdomyosarcoma Soft-Tissue Sarcoma

Surgery
NRSTS has been viewed as a cancer that is resistant to cytotoxic chemotherapy. As such, surgical resection of the primary tumor represents a key element in effective therapy. The survival of children with localized NRSTS that are widely excised dramatically exceeds the survival for those with unresected disease ($\sim$80% vs $\sim$40%, respectively, at 5 years).[13] In general wide surgical resection is required, although postoperative radiation therapy can help to achieve primary tumor control in cases where surgical resection is incomplete (see later discussion). Amputation is typically reserved for those patients in whom the tumor cannot otherwise be resected or for whom functional outcome will be poor after limb-sparing surgery. Surgical resection has typically been performed before any additional therapy; however, a recent COG trial evaluated delayed surgical resection following a phase of combined chemotherapy and radiation in an attempt to make surgical resection more feasible. Outcomes from this study are not yet available.

Although surgery is typically focused on the primary tumor, given the general resistance of NRSTS to chemotherapy, surgical resection of metastatic disease may be beneficial in some cases.

Radiation
Although unresected NRSTS is unlikely to be controlled by radiation therapy alone, the application of ionizing radiation can improve local control rates for those with microscopic residual disease following surgical resection. High doses (63–70 Gy) are typically prescribed for adult patients with NRSTS.[12] A recent COG NRSTS trial evaluated doses ranging from 45 Gy for those in the intermediate-risk group receiving preoperative radiation followed by a surgical resection with negative margins, to 64.8 Gy for those with high-risk disease in which macroscopic residual disease follows the definitive surgical resection.

Chemotherapy
The role for standard, cytotoxic chemotherapy in childhood NRSTS is somewhat controversial and is evolving with the advent of newer, molecularly targeted agents. A pooled analysis of European and North American patients showed major responses to chemotherapy including alkylating agents and anthracyclines approached 40%.[13] It is not known whether chemotherapy provides a survival advantage, but this conclusion is clouded by one important fact: individual NRSTS subtypes are biologically distinct and, therefore, likely to have different response rates to chemotherapy.

However, because individual subtypes are rare, the capacity to systematically study them is limited.

Given these problems, a recent COG study tested the use of ifosfamide and doxo-rubicin, largely accepted as the 2 most active chemotherapy agents in this disease, in a prospective study that ultimately accrued more than 500 children. Chemotherapy was recommended for several groups: those with localized but unresectable disease, which could become more curable if preoperative chemotherapy could render the disease resectable; those with high-grade tumors larger than 5 cm, in which case microscopic metastatic disease is more likely; and those with metastatic disease.

As alluded to earlier, improved understanding of NRSTS biology is beginning to transform how the disease can be managed using chemotherapy. Perhaps the best example for NRSTS stems from the finding that dermatofibrosarcoma protuberans (DFSP) is often associated with a chromosomal translocation that essentially activates platelet-derived growth factor signaling.[12] Indeed, selective targeting of that growth factor receptor using imatinib mesylate shows activity against DFSP.[58]

SUMMARY

The outcome for patients with localized sarcoma has improved dramatically with the addition of systemic, combination chemotherapy in conjunction with local control us-ing surgery and/or radiation. Improvements in surgical technique and the ability to salvage functional limbs have led to greater use of surgery for local control with satis-factory function. However, patients with metastatic and recurrent disease continue to have dismal outcomes despite the use of intensive chemotherapy, surgery, and/or ra-diation therapy. It seems that a plateau for cures has been reached with presently available treatment. A better understanding of the molecular mechanisms underlying the biology of sarcomas will be essential for further advances in therapy, and interna-tional collaboration may be necessary to improve outcomes in patients with bone and soft-tissue sarcomas.

REFERENCES

1. Klein MJ, Siegal GP. Osteosarcoma: anatomic and histologic variants. Am J Clin Pathol 2006;125(4):555–81. http://dx.doi.org/10.1309/UC6K-QHLD-9LV2-KENN.
2. Gorlick R. Current concepts on the molecular biology of osteosarcoma. Cancer Treat Res 2009;152:467–78. http://dx.doi.org/10.1007/978-1-4419-0284-9_27.
3. Ragland BD, Bell WC, Lopez RR, et al. Cytogenetics and molecular biology of osteosarcoma. Lab Invest 2002;82(4):365–73.
4. Folpe AL, Goldblum JR, Rubin BP, et al. Morphologic and immunophenotypic diversity in Ewing family tumors: a study of 66 genetically confirmed cases. Am J Surg Pathol 2005;29(8):1025–33.
5. Hattinger CM, Potschger U, Tarkkanen M, et al. Prognostic impact of chromo-somal aberrations in Ewing tumours. Br J Cancer 2002;86(11):1763–9. http://dx.doi.org/10.1038/sj.bjc.6600332.
6. Saab R, Spunt SL, Skapek SX. Myogenesis and rhabdomyosarcoma the Jekyll and Hyde of skeletal muscle. Curr Top Dev Biol 2011;94:197–234.
7. Keller C, Arenkiel BR, Coffin CM, et al. Alveolar rhabdomyosarcomas in condi-tional Pax3:Fkhr mice: cooperativity of Ink4a/ARF and Trp53 loss of function. Genes Dev 2004;18:2614–26.
8. Galindo RL, Allport JA, Olson EN. A Drosophila model of the rhabdomyosarcoma initiator PAX7-FKHR. Proc Natl Acad Sci U S A 2006;103(36):13439–44.

9. Sorensen PH, Lynch JC, Qualman SJ, et al. PAX3-FKHR and PAX7-FKHR gene fusions are prognostic indicators in alveolar rhabdomyosarcoma: a report from the children's oncology group. J Clin Oncol 2002;20(11):2672–9.
10. Shern JF, Chen L, Chmielecki J, et al. Comprehensive genomic analysis of rhabdomyosarcoma reveals a landscape of alterations affecting a common genetic axis in fusion-positive and fusion-negative tumors. Cancer Discov 2014;4: 216–31. http://dx.doi.org/10.1158/2159-8290.CD-13-0639.
11. Chen X, Stewart E, Shelat AA, et al. Targeting oxidative stress in embryonal rhabdomyosarcoma. Cancer Cell 2013;24(6):710–24. http://dx.doi.org/10.1016/j.ccr. 2013.11.002.
12. Spunt SL, Skapek SX, Coffin CM. Pediatric nonrhabdomyosarcoma soft tissue sarcomas. Oncologist 2008;13(6):668–78.
13. Ferrari A, Miceli R, Rey A, et al. Non-metastatic unresected paediatric nonrhabdomyosarcoma soft tissue sarcomas: results of a pooled analysis from United States and European groups. Eur J Cancer 2011;47(5):724–31. http:// dx.doi.org/10.1016/j.ejca.2010.11.013.
14. Pappo AS, Rao BN, Jenkins JJ, et al. Metastatic nonrhabdomyosarcomatous soft-tissue sarcomas in children and adolescents: the St. Jude Children's Research Hospital experience. Med Pediatr Oncol 1999;33(2):76–82.
15. Storlazzi CT, Mertens F, Mandahl N, et al. A novel fusion gene, SS18L1/SSX1, in synovial sarcoma. Genes Chromosomes Cancer 2003;37(2):195–200.
16. Barretina J, Taylor BS, Banerji S, et al. Subtype-specific genomic alterations define new targets for soft-tissue sarcoma therapy. Nat Genet 2010;42(8): 715–21. http://dx.doi.org/10.1038/ng.619.
17. Ries LAG, Smith MA, Gurney JG, et al. editors. Cancer Incidence and Survival among Children and Adolescents: United States SEER Program 1975-1995, National Cancer Institute, SEER Program. NIH Pub. No. 99-4649. Bethesda, MD, 1999.
18. Wilkins RM, Pritchard DJ, Burgert EO Jr, et al. Ewing's sarcoma of bone. Experience with 140 patients. Cancer 1986;58(11):2551–5.
19. Burningham Z, Hashibe M, Spector L, et al. The epidemiology of sarcoma. Clin Sarcoma Res 2012;2(1):14. http://dx.doi.org/10.1186/2045-3329-2-14.
20. Hawkins DS, Spunt SL, Skapek SX. Children's Oncology Group's 2013 blueprint for research: soft tissue sarcomas. Pediatr Blood Cancer 2013;60(6):1001–8. http://dx.doi.org/10.1002/pbc.24435.
21. Malkin D, Li FP, Strong LC, et al. Germ line p53 mutations in a familial syndrome of breast cancer, sarcomas, and other neoplasms. Science 1990;250(4985):1233–8.
22. Smith AC, Squire JA, Thorner P, et al. Association of alveolar rhabdomyosarcoma with the Beckwith-Wiedemann syndrome. Pediatr Dev Pathol 2001;4(6):550–8.
23. Sung L, Anderson JR, Arndt C, et al. Neurofibromatosis in children with Rhabdomyosarcoma: a report from the Intergroup Rhabdomyosarcoma study IV. J Pediatr 2004;144(5):666–8. http://dx.doi.org/10.1016/j.jpeds.2004.02.026 pii: S0022-3476(04)00156-8.
24. Spunt SL, Hill DA, Motosue AM, et al. Clinical features and outcome of initially unresected nonmetastatic pediatric nonrhabdomyosarcoma soft tissue sarcoma. J Clin Oncol 2002;20(15):3225–35.
25. Meyer WH, Spunt SL. Soft tissue sarcomas of childhood. Cancer Treat Rev 2004; 30(3):269–80. http://dx.doi.org/10.1016/j.ctrv.2003.11.001.
26. Miser JS, Krailo MD, Tarbell NJ, et al. Treatment of metastatic Ewing's sarcoma or primitive neuroectodermal tumor of bone: evaluation of combination ifosfamide and etoposide—a Children's Cancer Group and Pediatric Oncology Group study. J Clin Oncol 2004;22(14):2873–6. http://dx.doi.org/10.1200/JCO.2004.01.041.

27. Raney RB, Maurer HM, Anderson JR, et al. The Intergroup Rhabdomyosarcoma Study Group (IRSG): major lessons from the IRS-I through IRS-IV studies as background for the current IRS-V treatment protocols. Sarcoma 2001;5(1):9–15.
28. Kager L, Zoubek A, Potschger U, et al, Cooperative German-Austrian-Swiss Osteosarcoma Study Group. Primary metastatic osteosarcoma: presentation and outcome of patients treated on neoadjuvant Cooperative Osteosarcoma Study Group protocols. J Clin Oncol 2003;21(10):2011–8. http://dx.doi.org/10.1200/JCO.2003.08.132.
29. Bielack SS, Kempf-Bielack B, Delling G, et al. Prognostic factors in high-grade osteosarcoma of the extremities or trunk: an analysis of 1,702 patients treated on neoadjuvant cooperative osteosarcoma study group protocols. J Clin Oncol 2002;20(3):776–90.
30. Davis AM, Bell RS, Goodwin PJ. Prognostic factors in osteosarcoma: a critical review. J Clin Oncol 1994;12(2):423–31.
31. Whelan JS, Jinks RC, McTiernan A, et al. Survival from high-grade localised extremity osteosarcoma: combined results and prognostic factors from three European Osteosarcoma Intergroup randomised controlled trials. Ann Oncol 2012; 23(6):1607–16. http://dx.doi.org/10.1093/annonc/mdr491.
32. Bacci G, Longhi A, Ferrari S, et al. Prognostic factors in non-metastatic Ewing's sarcoma tumor of bone: an analysis of 579 patients treated at a single institution with adjuvant or neoadjuvant chemotherapy between 1972 and 1998. Acta Oncol 2006;45(4):469–75. http://dx.doi.org/10.1080/02841860500519760.
33. Missiaglia E, Williamson D, Chisholm J, et al. PAX3/FOXO1 fusion gene status is the key prognostic molecular marker in rhabdomyosarcoma and significantly improves current risk stratification. J Clin Oncol 2012;30(14):1670–7. http://dx.doi.org/10.1200/JCO.2011.38.5591.
34. Whelan JS. Osteosarcoma. Eur J Cancer 1997;33(10):1611–8 [discussion: 1618–9].
35. Jaffe N. Historical perspective on the introduction and use of chemotherapy for the treatment of osteosarcoma. Adv Exp Med Biol 2014;804:1–30. http://dx.doi.org/10.1007/978-3-319-04843-7_1.
36. Jaffe N, Frei E 3rd, Traggis D, et al. Adjuvant methotrexate and citrovorum-factor treatment of osteogenic sarcoma. N Engl J Med 1974;291(19):994–7. http://dx.doi.org/10.1056/NEJM197411072911902.
37. Winkler K, Beron G, Delling G, et al. Neoadjuvant chemotherapy of osteosarcoma: results of a randomized cooperative trial (COSS-82) with salvage chemotherapy based on histological tumor response. J Clin Oncol 1988;6(2): 329–37.
38. Bielack SA, Marina N, Hook J, et al. MAP plus maintenance pegylated interferon α-2b (MPIfn) versus MAP alone in patients with resectable high-grade osteosarcoma and good histologic response to preoperative MAP: first results of the EURAMOS-1 "good response" randomization. 2013 ASCO Annual Meeting. J Clin Oncol 2013; 31(15). Abstract Number LBA10504.
39. Bacci G, Picci P, Gherlinzoni F, et al. Neoadjuvant chemotherapy for high grade osteosarcoma of the extremities: is a good response to preoperative treatment an indication to reduce postoperative chemotherapy? Chemioterapia 1986;5(2):140–3.
40. Grimer RJ, Taminiau AM, Cannon SR, Surgical Subcommittee of the European Osteosarcoma Intergroup. Surgical outcomes in osteosarcoma. J Bone Joint Surg Br 2002;84(3):395–400.
41. Marulanda GA, Henderson ER, Johnson DA, et al. Orthopedic surgery options for the treatment of primary osteosarcoma. Cancer Control 2008;15(1):13–20.

42. Ciernik IF, Niemierko A, Harmon DC, et al. Proton-based radiotherapy for unresectable or incompletely resected osteosarcoma. Cancer 2011;117(19): 4522–30. http://dx.doi.org/10.1002/cncr.26037.

43. Heiner JP, Miraldi F, Kallick S, et al. Localization of GD2-specific monoclonal antibody 3F8 in human osteosarcoma. Cancer Res 1987;47(20):5377–81.

44. Nesbit ME Jr, Gehan EA, Burgert EO Jr, et al. Multimodal therapy for the management of primary, nonmetastatic Ewing's sarcoma of bone: a long-term follow-up of the First Intergroup study. J Clin Oncol 1990;8(10):1664–74.

45. Grier HE, Krailo MD, Tarbell NJ, et al. Addition of ifosfamide and etoposide to standard chemotherapy for Ewing's sarcoma and primitive neuroectodermal tumor of bone. N Engl J Med 2003;348(8):694–701. http://dx.doi.org/10.1056/NEJMoa020890.

46. Womer RB, West DC, Krailo MD, et al. Randomized controlled trial of interval-compressed chemotherapy for the treatment of localized Ewing sarcoma: a report from the Children's Oncology Group. J Clin Oncol 2012;30(33):4148–54. http://dx.doi.org/10.1200/JCO.2011.41.5703.

47. Ladenstein R, Potschger U, Le Deley MC, et al. Primary disseminated multifocal Ewing sarcoma: results of the Euro-EWING 99 trial. J Clin Oncol 2010;28(20): 3284–91. http://dx.doi.org/10.1200/JCO.2009.22.9864.

48. Yock TI, Krailo M, Fryer CJ, et al, Children's Oncology Group. Local control in pelvic Ewing sarcoma: analysis from INT-0091—a report from the Children's Oncology Group. J Clin Oncol 2006;24(24):3838–43. http://dx.doi.org/10.1200/JCO.2006.05.9188.

49. Bolling T, Schuck A, Paulussen M, et al. Whole lung irradiation in patients with exclusively pulmonary metastases of Ewing tumors. Toxicity analysis and treatment results of the EICESS-92 trial. Strahlenther Onkol 2008;184(4):193–7. http://dx.doi.org/10.1007/s00066-008-1810-x.

50. Haeusler J, Ranft A, Boelling T, et al. The value of local treatment in patients with primary, disseminated, multifocal Ewing sarcoma (PDMES). Cancer 2010;116(2): 443–50. http://dx.doi.org/10.1002/cncr.24740.

51. Donaldson SS. Ewing sarcoma: radiation dose and target volume. Pediatr Blood Cancer 2004;42(5):471–6. http://dx.doi.org/10.1002/pbc.10472.

52. Bacci G, Longhi A, Briccoli A, et al. The role of surgical margins in treatment of Ewing's sarcoma family tumors: experience of a single institution with 512 patients treated with adjuvant and neoadjuvant chemotherapy. Int J Radiat Oncol Biol Phys 2006;65(3):766–72. http://dx.doi.org/10.1016/j.ijrobp.2006.01.019.

53. Mascarenhas L, Bond MC, Femino JD, et al. Pilot study of adding vincristine, topotecan, and cyclophosphamide to interval-compressed chemotherapy in newly diagnosed patients with localized Ewing sarcoma family of tumors: a children's oncology group trial. 2011 ASCO Annual Meeting. J Clin Oncol 2011;29(15). Abstract Number 9526.

54. Olmos D, Martins AS, Jones RL, et al. Targeting the insulin-like growth factor 1 receptor in Ewing's sarcoma: reality and expectations. Sarcoma 2011;2011: 402508. http://dx.doi.org/10.1155/2011/402508.

55. Crist W, Gehan EA, Ragab AH, et al. The Third Intergroup Rhabdomyosarcoma Study. J Clin Oncol 1995;13(3):610–30.

56. Malempati S, Hawkins DS. Rhabdomyosarcoma: review of the Children's Oncology Group (COG) Soft-Tissue Sarcoma Committee experience and rationale for current COG studies. Pediatr Blood Cancer 2012;59(1):5–10. http://dx.doi.org/10.1002/pbc.24118.

57. Rodeberg DA, Stoner JA, Hayes-Jordan A, et al. Prognostic significance of tumor response at the end of therapy in group III rhabdomyosarcoma: a report from the children's oncology group. J Clin Oncol 2009;27(22):3705–11.

58. Rubin BP, Schuetze SM, Eary JF, et al. Molecular targeting of platelet-derived growth factor B by imatinib mesylate in a patient with metastatic dermatofibrosarcoma protuberans. J Clin Oncol 2002;20(17):3586–91.

Retinoblastoma

Carlos Rodriguez-Galindo, MD[a],*, Darren B. Orbach, MD, PhD[b],
Deborah VanderVeen, MD[c]

KEYWORDS

- Retinoblastoma • Chemotherapy • Germline mutation
- Second malignant neoplasms

KEY POINTS

- Retinoblastoma is the most common cancer of the eye in children, accounting for 3% of all childhood malignancies. Retinoblastoma affects very young children: two-thirds of the cases are diagnosed before 2 years of age, and more than 90% before 5 years.
- Two clinical forms are identified: (1) unilateral retinoblastoma, which accounts for approximately 75% of the cases; and (2) bilateral retinoblastoma, which accounts for 25% of the cases. Patients with bilateral disease carry a germline mutation of the RB1 gene; this mutation is inherited from an affected parent in 25% of the cases, and results from a de novo mutation in utero in 75% of the cases.
- Treatment of retinoblastoma is risk adapted. Factors to be considered in the treatment decisions include intraocular and extraocular stage, laterality, and potential for vision. Ocular salvage treatments include systemic or intra-arterial chemotherapy, aggressive focal treatments (photocoagulation, thermotherapy, cryotherapy, and brachytherapy), and external beam radiation therapy.
- Children with bilateral disease are at high risk of developing second malignancies and therefore need to be followed closely. Radiation therapy is avoided whenever possible in this group of children.

INTRODUCTION

Retinoblastoma is the most common neoplasm of the eye in childhood, representing 2.5% to 4% of all pediatric cancers. The average age-adjusted incidence rate of retinoblastoma in the United States and Europe is 2 to 5 per million children (approximately 1 in 14,000–18,000 live births).[1,2] Retinoblastoma is a cancer of the very young; two-thirds are diagnosed before 2 years of age, and 95% before 5 years.[1]

Retinoblastoma presents in 2 distinct clinical forms: (1) a bilateral or multifocal, heritable form (25% of all cases), characterized by the presence of germline mutations of

[a] Department of Pediatric Oncology, Dana-Farber/Boston Children's Cancer and Blood Disorders Center, Harvard Medical School, 450 Brookline Avenue, D3-133, Boston, MA 02215, USA;
[b] Department of Radiology, Boston Children's Hospital, Harvard Medical School, 300 Longwood Avenue, Boston, MA 02215, USA; [c] Department of Ophthalmology, Boston Children's Hospital, Harvard Medical School, 300 Longwood Avenue, Boston, MA 02215, USA
* Corresponding author.
E-mail address: carlos_rodriguez-galindo@dfci.harvard.edu

Pediatr Clin N Am 62 (2015) 201–223
http://dx.doi.org/10.1016/j.pcl.2014.09.014
0031-3955/15/$ – see front matter © 2015 Elsevier Inc. All rights reserved.

the *RB1* gene and that may be inherited from an affected survivor (25%) or be the result of a new germline mutation (75%); and (2) a unilateral or unifocal form (75% of all cases), 90% of which are nonhereditary. About 10% of germline cases are unilateral and unifocal; however, in the absence of a positive family history, it is not possible without genetic screening to determine which unilateral cases involve the germ line and are thus capable of being transmitted to the next generation.

EPIDEMIOLOGY

The incidence of retinoblastoma is not distributed equally around the world. It seems to be higher (6–10 cases per million children) in Africa, India, and among children of Native American descent in the North American continent.[3] The increased incidence in those groups occurs primarily in unilateral cases. Whether these geographic variations are caused by ethnic or socioeconomic factors is not well known. Studies from Mexico and Brazil have documented an inverse correlation between the incidence of retinoblastoma and socioeconomic index,[4–6] and in more industrialized countries an increased incidence of retinoblastoma has also been associated with poverty and low levels of maternal education.[7]

On a perhaps related note, decreased dietary intake of vegetables and fruits during pregnancy, resulting in decreased intake of nutrients such as folate and carotenoids, which are necessary for DNA methylation and synthesis as well as for retinal formation, has also been associated with an increased risk of unilateral sporadic retinoblastoma.[8] In a case-control study, the risk of developing retinoblastoma was associated with a maternal polymorphism in dihydrofolate reductase (*DHFR*19bpdel), particularly in women taking prenatal synthetic folic acid supplements.[9]

Most germline mutations in sporadic heritable retinoblastoma are paternally derived,[10] and studies have suggested an association between paternal age and occupation and the occurrence of sporadic heritable retinoblastoma.[7,11–13] Reports have also suggested an association between retinoblastoma and increased sunlight exposure,[14,15] air toxics from gasoline and diesel combustion,[16] or in vitro fertilization.[17–19] In a case-control study of sporadic retinoblastoma, radiological studies of the abdomen leading to scattered radiation exposure of the gonads were associated with an increased risk of bilateral retinoblastoma in a subsequent child.[20]

BIOLOGY

In 1971, based on the mathematical analysis of the age at presentation of bilateral (hereditary) and unilateral (mostly nonhereditary) cases of retinoblastoma, Knudson[21] proposed the 2-hit hypothesis, in which 2 mutational events in a developing retinal cell lead to the development of retinoblastoma. This hypothesis was subsequently extended to suggest that the two events could be mutations of both alleles of the *RB1* gene. *RB1*, located in chromosome 13q14, was identified and cloned in 1986.[22,23] Its product, pRb, is a key substrate for G1 cyclin-cdk complexes, which phosphorylate target gene products required for the transition of the cell through the G1 phase of the cell cycle. The active pRb functions as a tumor suppressor and is the major gatekeeper to control this critical point in growth regulation. The lack of pRb, or its inactivation, removes the pRb constraint on cell cycle control, with the consequence of deregulated cell proliferation. Biallelic loss of *RB1* function is required for tumor development; this loss is germ line and somatic for patients with bilateral disease, and somatic in patients with unilateral disease. However, additional events are required for tumor progression. Approximately two-thirds of tumors have *MDM4/MDM2* amplification leading to inactivation of the *p53* pathway.[24] RB1 plays an important role in maintaining genomic stability[25–27] and thus inactivation of the *RB1* gene could lead to chromosome instability, allowing secondary and tertiary mutations in key cancer pathways to be rapidly acquired. RB1 has also been implicated in a variety of epigenetic processes; thus, it is also possible that perturbations in the epigenetic landscape may contribute to tumorigenesis in the retina. In support of an epigenetic mechanism, recent whole-genome sequencing and integrated epigenetic analysis of human retinoblastoma revealed that the tumors have stable genomes and several cancer genes were epigenetically deregulated.[28] At least 1 of those epigenetically deregulated genes (*SYK*) is required for retinoblastoma tumor cell survival in vivo (discussed later).[28] In addition, a small proportion of tumors seem to develop in the context of normal *RB1*; amplification of *N-MYC* has been described in those cases.[29,30]

PREVENTION, EARLY DETECTION, AND GENETIC COUNSELING

The successful management of retinoblastoma depends on the ability to detect the disease while it is still intraocular; disease stage correlates with delay in diagnosis.[31] In developing countries, late referrals are strongly associated with orbital and metastatic disease.[32] It is for this reason that eye assessment should be performed in all newborns and at all subsequent health supervision visits by the primary care provider.[33] Retinoblastoma is a unique neoplasm in that the genetic form imparts a predisposition to developing tumor in an autosomal dominant fashion with almost complete penetrance (85%–95%).[34] Most such children acquire the first mutation as a new germline mutation, with only 25% having a positive family history. Genetic counseling is critical to assist parents in understanding the genetic consequences of each form of retinoblastoma and to estimate the risk in relatives. Regardless of the clinical presentation, it is recommended that all patients undergo genetic testing. With the refinement in methods of mutational analysis over the last decade, detection rates have increased to greater than 90% at present.[35] Given the heterogeneity in the site and type of gene defects, no single technology is sensitive and effective, and a multistep approach must be taken. More than 80% of the mutations can be detected with sequencing of the 27 exons of the *RB1* using a quantitative multiplex polymerase chain reaction (QMPCR).[35,36] However, 10% to 20% of the defects are caused by large deletions[36] and therefore deletion scanning and Southern blotting is required for those cases with no detectable mutations by QMPCR. In addition, a small proportion of cases (probably <5%) may result from gene inactivation by promoter methylation, and therefore screening for constitutional[35,36] methylation should be considered if the other methods do not reveal a mutation.

CLINICAL MANIFESTATIONS, PATIENT EVALUATION, AND STAGING

Retinoblastoma is by definition a tumor of young children, and the age at presentation correlates with the risk of bilaterality. Patients with bilateral retinoblastoma tend to present at a younger age (usually before 1 year of age) than patients with unilateral disease (often in the second or third year of life).[34,37] In more than half of the cases, the presenting sign is leukocoria, which is occasionally first noticed after a flash photograph (**Fig. 1**). Strabismus is the second most common presenting sign, and usually correlates with macular involvement. Advanced intraocular tumors may become painful as a result of secondary glaucoma. The differential diagnosis of a child presenting with leukocoria includes persistent hyperplastic primary vitreous, retrolental fibrodysplasia, Coats disease, congenital cataracts, toxocariasis, and toxoplasmosis.

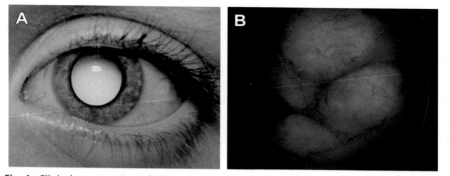

Fig. 1. Clinical presentation of retinoblastoma. (*A*) Leukocoria. (*B*) Maximally dilated pupil shows a large endophytic mass with massive vitreous seeding.

A small proportion of patients with bilateral disease (5%–6%) carry a deletion involving the 13q14 locus, which is large enough to be detected by karyotype analysis. In those cases, retinoblastoma is part of a more complex syndrome resulting from the loss of additional genetic material. Patients with the 13q syndrome are characterized by typical facial dysmorphic features, subtle skeletal abnormalities, and different degrees of mental retardation and motor impairment.[38] Dysmorphic features consistently found include thick anteverted ear lobes, high and broad forehead, prominent philtrum, and short nose. A proportion of patients also have overlapping fingers and toes, microcephaly, and delayed skeletal maturation.

Trilateral retinoblastoma refers to the association of bilateral retinoblastoma with an asynchronous intracranial tumor, which occurs in less than 10% of bilateral cases.[39] Tumors comprising trilateral retinoblastoma are primitive neuroectodermal tumors (PNETs) showing varying degrees of neuronal or photoreceptor differentiation, suggesting an origin from the germinal layer of primitive cells. Most of these tumors are pineal region PNETs (pineoblastomas), but in 20% to 25% of the cases the tumors are suprasellar or parasellar. Rare cases of quadrilateral retinoblastoma have been reported, in which bilateral retinoblastoma is associated with both pineal region and suprasellar intracranial primary PNETs.[40] The median age at diagnosis of trilateral retinoblastoma is 23 to 48 months and the interval between the diagnosis of bilateral retinoblastoma and the diagnosis of the brain tumor is usually more than 20 months.[41] Approximately 5% to 8% of patients with bilateral disease develop pineal cysts; these may be a forme fruste of trilateral retinoblastoma.[42,43]

The diagnosis of intraocular retinoblastoma is usually made without pathologic confirmation. An examination under anesthesia with a maximally dilated pupil and scleral indentation is required to examine the entire retina (see **Fig. 1**). Endophytic tumors are those that grow inward to the vitreous cavity. Because of its friability, endophytic retinoblastoma may seed the vitreous cavity. Exophytic retinoblastoma grows into the subretinal space, thus causing progressive retinal detachment and subretinal seeding. A detailed documentation must be performed of the number, location, and size of tumors; the presence of retinal detachment and subretinal fluid; and the presence of vitreous and subretinal seeds. Wide-angle real-time retinal imaging systems such as RetCam provide a 130° field of view and digital recording, facilitating diagnosis and monitoring.

Additional imaging studies that aid in the diagnosis include bidimensional ultrasonography, computed tomography (CT), and MRI. These imaging studies are particularly important to evaluate extraocular extension and to differentiate retinoblastoma from other causes of leukocoria. CT is helpful to detect calcifications, although its use is generally sparing, in order to limit radiation exposure, particularly in children with bilateral disease. MRI is helpful in working through the differential diagnosis, including Coats disease and other inflammatory conditions, as well as persistent fetal vasculature of hyperplastic primary vitreous.[44] MRI is not particularly useful in the work-up of microscopic or optic nerve involvement.[45–47] Ultrasonography is useful in the diagnosis of retinoblastoma because it can reveal highly reflective calcifications, when present, and it is used during the course of treatment to monitor tumor size with regard to growth or regression.

Metastatic disease occurs in approximately 10% to 15% of patients, and it usually occurs in association with distinct intraocular histologic features, such as deep choroidal and scleral invasion, or with involvement of the iris, ciliary body, or optic nerve beyond the lamina cribrosa. In these cases, additional staging procedures, including bone scintigraphy, bone marrow aspirates and biopsies, and lumbar puncture, must be performed. In up to one-third of high-risk patients, the synthase of ganglioside GD2 messenger RNA may be detected in the cerebrospinal fluid (CSF) by reverse transcriptase polymerase chain reaction, and it seems to correlate with massive involvement of the optic nerve, the presence of glaucoma at diagnosis, and a high risk of CSF relapse.[48] In general, in the absence of high-risk disorders in patients who have undergone enucleation, and in patients with intraocular disease undergoing ocular salvage therapies, metastatic work-up is usually not necessary. In patients with extraocular disease, the use of immunocytology with GD2 or CRX staining may increase the yield for detection of small clumps of metastatic cells.[49,50]

The Reese-Ellsworth (R-E) grouping system was the first classification scheme to be widely used to describe intraocular disease. This grouping system was designed to predict the outcome after external beam radiation therapy. It divides retinoblastoma-involved eyes into 5 groups by the size, location, and number of lesions, and by the presence of vitreous seeding (**Box 1**).[51] However, more recent developments in the conservative management of intraocular retinoblastoma have made the R-E grouping system less predictable of eye salvage, and less helpful in guiding treatment. A new staging system (International Classification of Intraocular Retinoblastoma) has been developed, with the goal of providing a simpler, user-friendly classification more applicable to current therapies. This new system is based on extent of tumor seeding within the vitreous cavity and subretinal space, rather than on tumor size and location, and seems to be a better predictor of treatment success (**Box 2, Fig. 2**).[52,53]

For patients undergoing enucleation, pathologic staging that incorporates other features that influence the choice of treatment modality and the prognosis, such as choroidal and scleral involvement, optic nerve extension, and presence of metastatic disease, are used. Different staging systems have classically been used, including the Grabowski-Adamson,[54] the St Jude Children's Research Hospital,[55] the American Joint Commission for Cancer (AJCC),[56] and the International Retinoblastoma Staging System (IRSS).[57] The IRSS is a newly proposed staging system developed by an international consortium of ophthalmologists and pediatric oncologists that incorporates the most important elements of the older systems (**Box 3**). The AJCC (**Box 4**) and the IRSS systems seem to be the most reliable for grouping patients according to their risk of extraocular relapse.[58]

PRINCIPLES OF TREATMENT

Treatment of retinoblastoma is designed to save life and preserve vision, and thus needs to be individualized. Factors that need to be considered include unilaterality

---

Box 1
Reese-Ellsworth grouping for suitability for treatment of retinoblastoma by radiation therapy

Group I. Very favorable

Ia: solitary tumor smaller than 4 dd at or behind the equator

Ib: multiple tumors, none larger than 4 dd, all at or behind equator

Group II. Favorable

IIa: solitary tumor 4 to 10 dd, at or behind equator

IIb: multiple tumors 4 to 10 dd, at or behind equator

Group III. Doubtful

IIIa: any lesion anterior to equator

IIIb: solitary tumor larger than 10 dd behind equator

Group IV. Unfavorable

IVa: multiple tumors, some larger than 10 dd

IVb: any lesion extending anteriorly to the ora serrata

Group V. Very unfavorable

Va: massive tumors involving more than half the retina

Vb: vitreous seeding

Abbreviation: dd, disk diameter (1.5 mm).
From Reese AB, Ellsworth RM. The evaluation and current concept of retinoblastoma therapy. Trans Am Acad Ophthalmol Otolaryngol 1963;67:164–72.

---

or bilaterality of the disease, potential for preserving vision, and intraocular and extraocular staging.[59]

Surgery

Enucleation is indicated for large tumors filling the vitreous, for which there is little or no likelihood of restoring vision, and in cases of tumor presence in the anterior chamber, or in the presence of neovascular glaucoma. Enucleation should be performed by an experienced ophthalmologist; the eye must be removed intact, without seeding the malignancy into the orbit, and avoiding globe perforation.[60] In addition, a long section (10–15 mm) of the optic nerve needs to be removed with the globe for optimal staging and best outcome when optic nerve involvement is present. An orbital implant is usually fitted during the same procedure, and the extraocular muscles can be attached to it. A prosthetic eye, usually made of a hard plastic, is later fitted in the orbital socket. For patients presenting with orbital disease, a judicious use of chemotherapy, surgery (enucleation), and radiation therapy results in good tumor control, avoiding the need for orbital exenteration.

Focal Therapies

Focal treatments are used for small tumors (<3–6 mm), usually in patients with bilateral disease, and in combination with chemotherapy.[61] Photocoagulation with argon laser is used for the treatment of tumors situated at or posterior to the equator of the eye, as well as for the treatment of retinal neovascularization caused by radiation therapy.[62] This technique is limited to tumors with a base no wider than 4.5 mm and no greater than 2.5 mm in thickness. The treatment is designed to coagulate all blood supply to

---

Box 2
International Classification for Intraocular Retinoblastoma

Group A

Small tumors away from foveola and disc

- Tumors less than or equal to 3 mm in greatest dimension confined to the retina, and
- Located at least 3 mm from the foveola and 1.5 mm from the optic disc

Group B

All remaining tumors confined to the retina

- All other tumors confined to the retina not in group A
- Subretinal fluid (without subretinal seeding) less than or equal to 3 mm from the base of the tumor

Group C

Local subretinal fluid or seeding

- Local subretinal fluid alone greater than 3 mm to less than or equal to 6 mm from the tumor
- Vitreous seeding or subretinal seeding less than or equal to 3 mm from the tumor

Group D

Diffuse subretinal fluid or seeding

- Subretinal fluid alone greater than 6 mm from the tumor
- Vitreous seeding or subretinal seeding greater than 3 mm from tumor

Group E

Presence of any of these poor prognosis features

- More than two-thirds of the globe filled with tumor
- Tumor in anterior segment
- Tumor in or on the ciliary body
- Iris neovascularization
- Neovascular glaucoma
- Opaque media from hemorrhage
- Tumor necrosis with aseptic orbital cellulitis
- Phthisis bulbi

From Linn Murphree A. Intraocular retinoblastoma: the case for a new group classification. Ophthalmol Clin North Am 2005;18:41–53; with permission.

---

the tumor. Cryotherapy is used for the treatment of small equatorial and peripheral lesions, measuring no more than 3.5 mm in base width and no more than 2 mm thickness.[63] One or 2 monthly sessions of triple freeze and thaw are performed, and tumor control rates are usually excellent. In addition, an important focal method is transpupillary thermotherapy, which applies focused heat at subphotocoagulation levels, usually with a diode laser.[64] In thermotherapy, the goal is to deliver a temperature of 42°C to 60°C for 5 to 20 minutes to the tumor, sparing retinal vessels from photocoagulation. The use of focal treatments is especially important in conjunction with chemotherapy, because the two treatment modalities seem to have a synergistic effect. In general, local control rates of 70% to 80% can be achieved. Complications of focal treatments

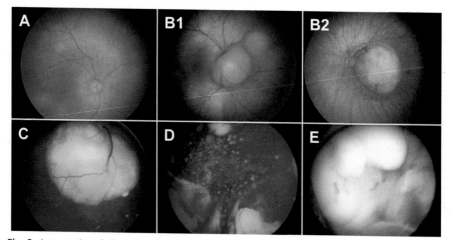

Fig. 2. International Classification for Intraocular Retinoblastoma. (*A*) Small tumor confined to the retina and distant from the foveola and the optic nerve (group A). (*B1*) Two small tumors confined to the retina but adjacent to the optic nerve (group B). (*B2*) Tumor with small amount of subretinal fluid and no subretinal seeding (group B). (*C*) Exophytic retinoblastoma with subretinal fluid and seeding (group C). (*D*) Endophytic retinoblastoma with massive vitreous seeding (group D). (*E*) Large retinoblastoma filling more than two-thirds of the globe (group E).

Box 3
IRSS

Stage 0. Patients treated conservatively.

Stage I. Eye enucleated, completely resected histologically.

Stage II. Eye enucleated, microscopic residual tumor.

Stage III. Regional extension.

a. Overt orbital disease

b. Preauricular or cervical lymph node extension

Stage IV. Metastatic disease

a. Hematogenous metastasis (without central nervous system [CNS] involvement)

   1. Single lesion

   2. Multiple lesions

b. CNS extension (with or without any other site of regional or metastatic disease)

   1. Prechiasmatic lesion

   2. CNS mass

   3. Leptomeningeal and CSF disease

From Chantada G, Doz F, Antonelli CB, et al. A proposal for an international retinoblastoma staging system. Pediatr Blood Cancer 2006;47:801–5; with permission.

Box 4
AJCC staging system

Clinical classification (tumor-node-metastasis staging by clinical examination [cTNM])

Primary tumor (T)

TX: primary tumor cannot be assessed.

T0: no evidence of primary tumor.

T1: tumors no more than two-thirds the volume of the eye with no vitreous or subretinal seeding.

T1a: no tumor in either eye is greater than 3 mm in largest dimension or located closer than 1.5 mm to the optic nerve or fovea.

T1b: at least 1 tumor is greater than 3 mm in largest dimension or located closer than 1.5 mm to the optic nerve or fovea. No retinal detachment or subretinal fluid beyond 5 mm from above the base of the tumor.

T1c: at least 1 tumor is greater than 3 mm in largest dimension or located closer than 1.5 mm to the optic nerve or fovea, with retinal detachment or subretinal fluid beyond 5 mm from the base of the tumor.

T2: tumors no more than two-thirds the volume of the eye with vitreous or subretinal seeding. Can have retinal detachment.

T2a: minimal tumor spread to vitreous and/or subretinal space. Focal vitreous and/or subretinal seeding of fine aggregates of tumor cells is present, but no large clumps or snowballs of tumor cells.

T2b: massive tumor spread to the vitreous and/or subretinal space. Massive vitreous and/or subretinal seeding is present, defined as diffuse clumps or snowballs of tumor cells.

T3: severe intraocular disease.

T3a: tumor fills more than two-thirds of the eye.

T3b: 1 or more complications present, which may include tumor-associated neovascular or angle closure glaucoma, tumor extension into the anterior segment, hyphema, vitreous hemorrhage, or orbital cellulitis.

T4: extraocular disease detected by imaging studies.

T4a: invasion of optic nerve.

T4b: invasion of the orbit.

T4c: intracranial extension not past chiasm.

T4d: intracranial extension past chiasm.

Regional lymph nodes (N)

NX: regional lymph nodes cannot be assessed.

N0: no regional lymph node involvement.

N1: regional lymph node involvement (preauricular, submandibular, or cervical).

N2: distant lymph node involvement.

Distant metastasis (M)

M0: no distant metastasis.

M1: systemic metastasis.

M1a: single lesion to sites other than CNS.

M1b: multiple lesions to sites other than CNS.

M1c: prechiasmatic CNS lesions.

M1d: postchiasmatic CNS lesions.

M1e: leptomeningeal and/or CSF involvement.

Pathologic classification (tumor-node-metastasis staging by pathology [pTNM])

Primary tumor (pT)

pTX: primary tumor cannot be assessed.

pT0: no evidence of primary tumor.

pT1: tumor confined to eye with no optic nerve or choroidal invasion.

pT2: tumor with minimal optic nerve and/or choroidal invasion.

  pT2a: tumor superficially invades optic nerve head but does not extend past lamina cribrosa or tumor shows focal choroidal invasion.

  pT2b: tumor superficially invades optic nerve head but does not extend past lamina cribrosa and shows focal choroidal invasion.

pT3: tumor with significant optic nerve and/or choroidal invasion.

  pT3a: tumor invades optic nerve past lamina cribrosa but not to surgical resection line or tumor shows massive choroidal invasion.

  pT3b: tumor invades optic nerve past lamina cribrosa but not to surgical resection line and shows massive choroidal invasion.

pT4: tumor invades optic nerve to resection line or shows extraocular extension elsewhere.

  pT4a: tumor invades optic nerve to resection line but no extraocular extension identified.

  pT4b: tumor invades optic nerve to resection line and extraocular extension identified.

Regional lymph nodes (pN)

pNX: regional lymph nodes cannot be assessed.

pN0: no regional lymph node involvement.

pN1: regional lymph node involvement (preauricular, cervical).

N2: distant lymph node involvement.

Distant metastasis (pM)

cM0: no metastasis.

pM1: metastasis to sites other than CNS.

  pM1a: single lesion.

  pM1b: multiple lesions.

  pM1c: CNS metastasis.

  pM1d: discrete masses without leptomeningeal and/or CSF involvement.

  pM1e: leptomeningeal and/or CSF involvement.

From AJCC. Retinoblastoma. In: Edge SB, Byrd DR, Compton CC, et al, editors. AJCC cancer staging manual. 7th edition. New York: Springer; 2010. p. 562–63; with permission.

include transient serous retinal detachment, retinal traction and tears, and localized fibrosis.

Chemotherapy

Chemotherapy is indicated in patients with extraocular disease, in the subgroup of patients with intraocular disease with high-risk histologic features after enucleation, and in patients with intraocular disease, in conjunction with aggressive focal therapies, for ocular preservation. Agents effective in the treatment of retinoblastoma include platinum compounds, etoposide, cyclophosphamide, doxorubicin, vincristine, and ifosfamide.[59] For ocular preservation, chemotherapy is given with the objective of attaining a maximal cytoreduction that can be further consolidated with focal treatments or radiation therapy. In this setting, chemotherapy has traditionally been administered intravenously, but in recent years direct ocular delivery via catheterization of the ophthalmic artery is becoming more popular (discussed later).

Radiotherapy

Retinoblastoma is a very radiosensitive tumor. Radiotherapy in combination with focal treatments can provide excellent tumor control.[65–67] However, because radiation therapy increases the risk of second malignancies, contemporary management of intraocular retinoblastoma is designed to avoid or delay its use; the role of irradiation is mainly as salvage management for eyes that have failed chemotherapy and focal treatments, usually because of progression of vitreous and subretinal seeding.[68] Radiation therapy can be delivered in the form of brachytherapy or external beam radiation. Brachytherapy is used for the control of small tumors, usually in conjunction with other therapies; implants of radioactive material are placed as episcleral plaques for a period of time to deliver high doses of radiation well focused to the tumor, sparing the normal structures. Most implants now use iodine-125 (^{125}I). Many other agents can be used, such as radioactive gold, cobalt, palladium, and ruthenium.[69–72] External beam technique is used for treatment of the entire eye globe for ocular salvage, or for the management of extraocular disease to the orbit, central nervous system (CNS), or metastatic sites. Several techniques can be used, usually through lateral or anterior fields.[65–67] Recommended total doses are 40 Gy to 45 Gy, in 180-cGy to 200-cGy fractions, although doses of 36 Gy and even lower may be effective in conjunction with other techniques.[73–76] Photons are commonly used; however, the use of proton therapy has significant advantages for patients with bilateral disease in terms of potentially lower risk of second malignancies.[77]

TREATMENT OF INTRAOCULAR RETINOBLASTOMA
Unilateral Retinoblastoma

In the absence of extraocular disease, enucleation alone is curative for 85% to 90% of children with unilateral retinoblastoma. The outcome for patients with unilateral disease that has been enucleated is excellent, with good functional results and minimal long-term effects.[78] In view of the apparent success in treating bilateral intraocular disease with chemoreduction, a conservative approach with systemic or intra-arterial chemotherapy and focal measures is increasingly being used. With the use of intra-arterial chemotherapy (discussed later), ocular salvage rates of more than 70% to 80% can be achieved.[79] For patients undergoing prior enucleation, a careful histologic evaluation is needed to assess high-risk conditions. Adjuvant treatment is indicated in those cases with trans-scleral invasion and in patients with positive tumor at the transection line of the optic nerve (discussed later). Adjuvant treatment of the remaining patients with intraocular disease is more debatable. In the absence of randomized studies, available information suggests that the use of adjuvant chemotherapy may be beneficial for the selected subgroup of patients with higher risk of extraocular dissemination, which includes involvement of the anterior chamber, ciliary body or iris, massive infiltration (>3 mm) of the choroid, retrolaminar optic nerve infiltration, or focal choroidal disease in combination with any degree of nonretrolaminar optic nerve involvement.[80–88] Adjuvant chemotherapy is not indicated for patients with isolated prelaminar involvement[73,81] or isolated focal choroidal involvement.[73,82,83,86,89] Different chemotherapy regimens have been proposed. Six-month treatment with vincristine, doxorubicin, and cyclophosphamide; vincristine, carboplatin, and etoposide; or a hybrid option with alternating courses of both regimens, seems to be effective.

Bilateral Retinoblastoma

In the past, the treatment of patients with bilateral retinoblastoma has been enucleation of eyes with advanced intraocular disease and no visual potential, and the use of external beam radiation therapy for the remaining eyes. However, there are several complications associated with radiation therapy. Irradiation of the orbit during a period of rapid growth results in a major decrease in orbital volume, resulting in midfacial deformities. However, more important is the greatly increased risk for the development of a sarcoma within the radiation therapy field, greater than the already increased baseline underlying risk of secondary neoplasms in these predisposed individuals. This risk may be age related, and decreases as irradiation is delayed.[90] These concerns have resulted in the development of more conservative approaches. The treatment of patients with bilateral retinoblastoma now incorporates prior chemotherapy, which is intended to achieve maximum chemoreduction of the intraocular tumor burden early in the treatment, followed by aggressive focal therapies. This approach has resulted in an increase in the eye salvage rates and in a decrease (and delay) in the use of radiation therapy. Different chemotherapy combinations are used, although the best results are achieved with the combination of vincristine, carboplatin, and etoposide. For patients with early intraocular stages (R-E groups I–III, International Classification of Intraocular Retinoblastoma group B), a less intensive regimen with vincristine and carboplatin alone seems to be effective.[59] Salvage rates for group A and B eyes approaches 100% using these techniques. For patients with advanced intraocular tumors (groups C and D), chemotherapy intensification seems to correlate with outcome, and better results are obtained with protocols that include at least 6 courses of vincristine, etoposide, and carboplatin[91–93] Central retinal tumors usually respond better to chemotherapy than do tumors in the peripheral retina,[94] but large central tumors may be associated with subretinal seeds, which ultimately may cause treatment failure.[95] Despite the addition of aggressive sequential focal therapies, globe retention is still no better than 50% for group D eyes and most patients eventually require irradiation.[91] However, the use of radiation therapy is usually delayed for several months, which allows better orbital growth and a decrease in the risk of second malignancies. New agents with better intraocular penetration are being investigated. Topotecan, a topoisomerase-I inhibitor with well-documented efficacy against pediatric tumors, is a promising alternative. Studies performed in the animal model have shown that topotecan has excellent intraocular penetration and antitumor effect.[96] In a phase II study using an initial window of vincristine and topotecan in patients with advanced bilateral disease, responses were documented in 90% of the patients.[97]

INTRAVITREAL AND INTRA-ARTERIAL CHEMOTHERAPY FOR INTRAOCULAR RETINOBLASTOMA

Japanese investigators pioneered the administration of intravitreal and intra-arterial melphalan for patients with advanced or recurrent intraocular retinoblastoma.[98,99] Preclinical data suggest that retinoblastoma is very sensitive to melphalan, and that there is a synergistic effect with thermotherapy[100] and with other agents such as topotecan.[101] Direct delivery to the ocular vasculature has been limited in the past by the technical difficulties in the cannulation of the ophthalmic artery. Kaneko and Suzuki[98] initially reported the feasibility of injecting melphalan into the ipsilateral carotid artery, with documented efficacy. The technique was later perfected by Mohri[102] using a balloon catheter positioned within the internal carotid artery, distal to the origin of the ophthalmic artery, which allowed selective flow of the chemotherapy into the ophthalmic artery.[99,102] With recent technical advances in microcatheters and digital fluoroscopy, superselective direct catheterization of the ophthalmic artery by experienced practitioners is achievable in most cases, as pioneered and reported by Abramson and colleagues.[103] Successful catheterization and delivery of chemotherapy can be achieved in 98% of cases,[79,104] although in 16% of patients an alternative vascular route is required; often the orbital branch of the middle meningeal artery.[105] This approach has also been documented as feasible a tandem therapy in patients with bilateral disease.[106]

Although melphalan has remained the most commonly used and effective agent used intra-arterially, it is often combined with topotecan or with carboplatin when responses are suboptimal or the intraocular disease is very advanced.[79,104,107–110] The doses of the chemotherapeutic agents are determined by the age (and ocular volume) and by the angiographic anatomy; doses reported to result in a significant antitumor effect and limited toxicity are 2.7 to 7.5 mg for melphalan, 0.3 to 0.6 mg for topotecan, and 25 to 50 mg for carboplatin.[79,107,108,110,111]

Patients typically receive 1 to 6 (median 3) intra-arterial administrations of chemotherapy including melphalan alone or in combination, and responses are usually seen immediately after the first administration. For patients with treatment-naive eyes, the 2-year radiation-free ocular survival is 80% to 90%.[79,107,110] Similar outcomes are also being reported with single-agent carboplatin and in combination with topotecan.[108] Outcome correlates with the intraocular burden; patients with early intraocular disease (group B and C eyes) have excellent outcomes and may be treated with single-agent therapy.[108,109] Eyes with significant vitreous or subretinal seeding have worse outcomes, with radiation-free survival rates of 80% for eyes with subretinal seeding and 65% for eyes with vitreous seeding.[112] Ocular salvage rates when intra-arterial chemotherapy administration is used as salvage for patients with recurrent or progressive disease are consistently lower, with globe survival rates of 50% to 60%.[79,104,110,112] However, the use of a more intensive 3-drug regimen with melphalan, topotecan, and carboplatin in patients who have progressed after standard systemic and focal therapies has reported to result in radiation-free ocular salvage rates of 75% at 2 years.[111]

For neonates and very young infants in whom angiography and cannulation of the ophthalmic artery is associated with higher risk, a bridge treatment with single-agent systemic carboplatin until the baby is 3 months old or 6 kg, followed by consolidation with intra-arterial chemotherapy, has been shown to be very effective, with 1-year radiation-free ocular survival of 95%.[113]

Direct administration of high doses of chemotherapy to a sensitive organ such as the eye of a young child has complications. In a nonhuman primate model, treatment with 3 cycles of melphalan or carboplatin resulted in a significant inflammatory response, with leukostasis and central retinal arterial branch occlusion, with ultrastructural changes in the endothelial cells and surrounding pericytes. Eyes also showed nerve fiber infarcts and optic nerve hemorrhage and leukostasis, central retinal artery thrombosis, choroidal inflammation, and the presence of birefringent intravascular foreign bodies.[114] Similar histopathologic evidence of vasculopathy is seen in enucleated eyes of children with retinoblastoma after intra-arterial chemotherapy.[115] The impact of such intraocular vascular changes on vision has not been fully assessed because of the young age of the first cohorts of patients treated. Most patients do not have substantial electroretinographic changes,[116] and preservation of central vision has been reported.[117] However, in patients with heavily pretreated eyes, intensive intra-arterial chemotherapy may result in worsening of retinal function.[111] Major vascular complications are rare; no strokes or significant acute neurologic events have been reported by the most experienced groups.[79,99,104]

One additional risk associated with intra-arterial chemotherapy is the exposure to ionizing radiation during fluoroscopy. In experienced hands, the mean fluoroscopy time per procedure is 7 minutes.[118] Radiation doses per procedure can be as high as 191 mGy to the affected eye and 35 mGy to the contralateral eye,[119] although doses as low as 1 mGy per procedure have been reported by the most experienced center.[118] After multiple procedures, cumulative doses can reach 0.1 to 0.2 Gy, which can be cataractogenic and potentially carcinogenic in this susceptible population.[119] However, procedures for measuring target organ radiation exposure during fluoroscopy are not straightforward or standardized, and neither are angiographic techniques and equipment, resulting in the large disparities reported earlier. Long-term outcome data reported by Japanese investigators indicate that there is no increase in the incidence of second malignancies[99]; however, longer follow-up is required to fully ascertain the risks associated with the procedure.

In order to achieve the maximum concentrations of chemotherapy close to the tumor and in the vitreous, another technique explored by investigators has been direct intravitreal delivery. Clinical responses in patients with progressive retinoblastoma can be obtained using intravitreal melphalan followed by hyperthermia,[98] and more recent data indicate that intravitreal chemotherapy may have a role in the management of patients with progressive vitreous disease.[120,121]

The approach to the ocular salvage management for intraocular retinoblastoma is summarized in **Table 1**.

TREATMENT OF EXTRAOCULAR RETINOBLASTOMA

In Europe and the United States, fewer than 5% of patients present with extraocular disease, in contrast with up to 40% to 80% in less developed countries.[122,123] Three

Table 1
Recommended approach to the treatment of intraocular retinoblastoma

R-E Group	ICIR Group	Focal Tx	Intra-arterial Chemotherapy	Systemic Chemotherapy	Radiation
I–II	A	+	If PD	If PD	If PD
I–III	B	+	MEL 3–5 mg × 3–6 courses	VCR 0.05 mg/kg d 1 CBP 18.6 mg/kg d 1 For 2–6 courses	If PD
IV–V	C–D[a]	+	MEL 3–5 mg × 3–6 courses Consider addition of second agent (TOP, CBP)	VCR 0.05 mg/kg d 1 CBP 14 mg/kg d 1, 2 ETO 6 mg/kg d 1, 2 For 6 courses	If PD Consider early EBRT if massive vitreous seeding at completion of chemotherapy
V b	E	Enucleation			—

Abbreviations: CBP, carboplatin; EBRT, external beam radiation therapy; ETO, etoposide; ICIR, International Classification of Intraocular Retinoblastoma; MEL, melphalan; PD, progressive disease; TOP, topotecan; Tx, treatment; VCR, vincristine.
  [a] Consider prior enucleation if unilateral.

patterns of extraocular disease have been recognized: (1) locoregional dissemination, including orbital disease, tumor extending to the cut end of the optic nerve, and lymphatic spread to the preauricular lymph nodes; (2) CNS dissemination; and (3) metastatic retinoblastoma.

Orbital and Locoregional Retinoblastoma

Orbital retinoblastoma occurs as a result of progression of the tumor through the emissary vessels and sclera. For this reason, scleral disease is considered to be extraocular, and should be treated as such. Orbital retinoblastoma is isolated in 60% to 70% of cases; lymphatic, hematogenous, and CNS metastases occur in the remaining patients.[124] Treatment should include systemic chemotherapy and radiation therapy; with this approach, 60% to 85% of patients can be cured. Because most recurrences occur in the CNS, regimens using drugs with well-documented CNS penetration are recommended. Different chemotherapy regimens have proved to be effective, including vincristine, cyclophosphamide, and doxorubicin; platinum-based and epipodophyllotoxin-based regimens; or a combination of both.[59] For patients with macroscopic orbital disease, it is recommended that surgery be delayed until response to chemotherapy has been obtained (usually 2 or 3 courses of treatment). Enucleation should then be performed, and an additional 4 to 6 courses of chemotherapy administered. Local control should then be consolidated with orbital irradiation (40–45 Gy). Using this approach, orbital exenteration can be avoided.[125] Similar management is recommended for patients with scleral disease, including radiation therapy, although good outcomes without irradiation have also been reported.[122] Patients with isolated involvement of the optic nerve at the transection level should receive similar systemic treatment, and irradiation should include the entire orbit (36 Gy) with an 9-Gy to 10-Gy boost to the chiasm (total 45–46 Gy). The preauricular and cervical lymph nodes should be explored carefully, because 20% of patients with orbital retinoblastoma have lymphatic metastases.[124]

Central Nervous System Disease

Intracranial dissemination occurs by direct extension through the optic nerve, and its prognosis is dismal.[122,125] Treatment of these patients should include platinum-based intensive systemic chemotherapy and CNS-directed therapy. Although intrathecal chemotherapy has traditionally been used, there is no preclinical or clinical evidence to support its use. Although the use of irradiation in these patients is controversial, responses have been observed with craniospinal irradiation, using 23.4 to 36 Gy to the entire craniospinal axis, with a boost to achieve up to 45 Gy to sites of measurable disease. Therapeutic intensification with high-dose, marrow-ablative chemotherapy and autologous hematopoietic progenitor cell rescue has been explored, but its role is not yet clear.[126,127] Despite the intensity of the treatment and the documented responses of the intracranial disease, patients ultimately succumb to their disease, and reports of survivors are anecdotal.

(Extracranial) Metastatic Retinoblastoma

Hematogenous metastases may develop in the bones, bone marrow, and less frequently in the liver. Although long-term survivors have been reported with conventional chemotherapy, these reported cures should be considered anecdotal. However, in recent years it has been shown in small series of patients that metastatic retinoblastoma can be cured using high-dose, marrow-ablative chemotherapy and autologous hematopoietic progenitor cell rescue. The approach is similar to metastatic neuroblastoma; patients receive short and intensive induction regimens usually containing alkylating agents, anthracyclines, etoposide, and platinum compounds, and are then consolidated with marrow-ablative chemotherapy and autologous hematopoietic cell rescue. Using this approach, the outcome seems to be excellent.[127] Patients with distant (outside orbit and skull) bone metastases that show good response to induction chemotherapy may not require radiation therapy when treated with marrow-ablative chemotherapy.

LONG-TERM EFFECTS OF RETINOBLASTOMA AND ITS TREATMENT

The cumulative incidence of second cancers in patients with germline mutations of the *RB1* gene is greatly increased with the use of radiation therapy; this incidence is reported to increase steadily with age, reaching up to 40% to 60% at 40 to 50 years of age, although more recent studies estimate a considerably lower risk.[128–130] In contrast, patients with nonhereditary retinoblastoma are not inherently at an increased risk. Almost every neoplasm type has been reported in survivors of bilateral retinoblastoma, and 60% to 70% of the tumors occur in the head and neck areas.[128,129]

Most information on second malignancies in retinoblastoma survivors has derived from the prospective follow-up of a cohort of 1601 survivors of retinoblastoma who were diagnosed between 1914 and 1984 at institutions in Boston and New York.[128,131–133] In the most recent analysis, the median follow-up for patients with hereditary and nonhereditary retinoblastoma was 25.2 years and 29.5 years, respectively.[128] The standardized incidence ratio (SIR) in these studies was calculated as the ratio of the observed number of cancers to the expected number from the Connecticut Tumor Registry. The incidence of second cancers was significantly increased

Table 2
Risk and type of new cancers in 963 survivors of hereditary retinoblastoma

Cancer Site	N Observed (%)	SIR (95% CI)
All sites	260 (100)	19 (16–21)
Bone	75 (28.8)	360 (283–451)
Soft tissue	34 (13)	122 (84–170)
Nasal cavities	32 (12.3)	1111 (760–1569)
Melanoma	29 (11.1)	28 (18–40)
Eye and orbit	17 (6.5)	266 (155–426)
Brain	10 (3.8)	13.6 (6.5–25)
Breast	10 (3.8)	3.96 (1.9–7.3)
Corpus uteri	7 (2.7)	20 (8.0–41)
Buccal cavity	7 (2.7)	20 (8.2–42)
Lung	5 (1.9)	5.94 (1.9–14)
Pineoblastoma	5 (1.9)	90.8 (29–212)
Colon	3 (1.1)	6.28 (1.3–18)
Hodgkin lymphoma	3 (1.1)	3.4 (0.7–10)
Bladder	2 (0.7)	6.15 (0.7–22)
Thyroid	2 (0.7)	3.34 (0.4–12)
Leukemia	2 (0.7)	2.25 (0.3–8.1)

Abbreviation: CI, confidence interval.
Adapted from Kleinerman RA, Tucker MA, Tarone RE, et al. Risk of new cancers after radiotherapy in long-term survivors of retinoblastoma: an extended follow-up. J Clin Oncol 2005;23:2272–9.

in survivors of hereditary retinoblastoma (SIR, 19 vs 1.2 in patients with nonhereditary retinoblastoma)[128,134]; similar data have been reported using population-based registries (**Table 2**).[130]

Because their orbital growth is still in progress, children treated for retinoblastoma are at risk of functionally and cosmetically significant bony orbital abnormalities. These sequelae become evident by early adolescence, when orbital growth is largely complete, and results in the so-called hour-glass facial deformity. Both enucleation, which causes orbital contraction, and radiotherapy, which induces arrest of bone growth, adversely affect orbital growth. In children treated for bilateral retinoblastoma, the impact of enucleation in orbital development is not different from that of irradiation. However, final orbital volumes after enucleation correlate with the size of the prosthetic implant.

REFERENCES

1. Young JL, Smith MA, Roffers SD, et al. Retinoblastoma. SEER Monograph. 1999: 73–78.
2. Parkin DM, Stiller CA, Draper GJ, et al. The international incidence of childhood cancer. Int J Cancer 1988;42:511–20.
3. Stiller C, Parkin D. Geographic and ethnic variations in the incidence of childhood cancer. Br Med Bull 1996;52:682–703.
4. de Camargo B, de Oliveira Santos M, Rebelo M, et al. Cancer incidence among children and adolescents in Brazil: first report of 14 population-based cancer registries. Int J Cancer 2010;126:715–20.
5. Fajardo-Gutierrez A, Juarez-Ocana S, Gonzalez-Miranda G, et al. Incidence of cancer in children residing in ten jurisdictions of the Mexican Republic: importance of the cancer registry (a population-based study). BMC Cancer 2007;7:68.
6. Juarez-Ocana S, Palma-Padilla V, Gonzalez-Miranda G, et al. Epidemiological and some clinical characteristics of neuroblastoma in Mexican children (1996-2005). BMC Cancer 2009;9:266.
7. Bunin GR, Meadows AT, Emanuel BS, et al. Pre- and postconception factors associated with sporadic heritable and nonheritable retinoblastoma. Cancer Res 1989;49:5730–5.
8. Orjuela M, Titievsky L, Liu X, et al. Fruit and vegetable intake during pregnancy and risk for development of sporadic retinoblastoma. Cancer Epidemiol Biomarkers Prev 2005;14:1433–40.
9. Orjuela MA, Cabrera-Muñoz L, Paul L, et al. Risk of retinoblastoma is associated with a maternal polymorphism in dihydrofolatereductase (DHFR) and prenatal folic acid intake. Cancer 2012;118:5912–9.
10. Dryja TP, Mukai S, Petersen R, et al. Parental origin of mutations of the retinoblastoma gene. Nature 1989;339:556–8.
11. Moll AC, Imhof SM, Kuik J, et al. High parental age is associated with sporadic hereditary retinoblastoma: The Dutch Retinoblastoma Register 1862-1994. Hum Genet 1996;98:109–12.
12. Heck J, Lombardi C, Meyers T, et al. Perinatal characteristics and retinoblastoma. Cancer Causes Control 2012;23:1567–75.
13. Bunin GR, Petrakova A, Meadows AT, et al. Occupations of parents of children with retinoblastoma: a report from the Children's Cancer Study Group. Cancer Res 1990;50:7129–33.
14. Jemal A, Devesa SS, Fears TR, et al. Retinoblastoma incidence and sunlight exposure. Br J Cancer 2000;82:1875–8.

15. Hooper ML. Is sunlight an aetiological agent in the genesis of retinoblastoma? Br J Cancer 1999;79:1273–6.
16. Heck JE, Park AS, Qiu J, et al. Retinoblastoma and ambient exposure to air toxics in the perinatal period. J Expo Sci Environ Epidemiol 2013. [Epub ahead of print].
17. Niemitz EL, Feinberg AP. Epigenetics and assisted reproductive technology: a call for investigation. Am J Hum Genet 2004;74:599–609.
18. Moll A, Imhof S, Cruysberg JR, et al. Incidence of retinoblastoma in children born after in-vitro fertilisation. Lancet 2003;361:309–10.
19. Marees T, Dommering CJ, Imhof SM, et al. Incidence of retinoblastoma in Dutch children conceived by IVF: an expanded study. Hum Reprod 2009;24:3220–4.
20. Bunin GR, Felice MA, Davidson W, et al. Medical radiation exposure and risk of retinoblastoma resulting from new germline RB1 mutation. Int J Cancer 2011; 128:2393–404.
21. Knudson AG. Mutation and childhood cancer: a probabilistic model for the incidence of retinoblastoma. Proc Natl Acad Sci U S A 1971;72:820–3.
22. Lee WH, Bookstein R, Hong F, et al. Human retinoblastoma susceptibility gene: cloning, identification, and sequence. Science 1987;235:1394–9.
23. Friend SH, Bernards R, Rogelj S, et al. A human DNA segment with properties of the gene that predisposes to retinoblastoma and osteosarcoma. Nature 1986; 323:643–6.
24. Laurie NA, Donovan SL, Shih CS, et al. Inactivation of the p53 pathway in retinoblastoma. Nature 2006;444:61–6.
25. Dimaras H, Khetan V, Halliday W, et al. Loss of RB1 induces non-proliferative retinoma: increasing genomic instability correlates with progression to retinoblastoma. Hum Mol Genet 2008;17:1363–72.
26. Hernando E, Nahle Z, Juan G, et al. Rb inactivation promotes genomic instability by uncoupling cell cycle progression from mitotic control. Nature 2004;430:797–802.
27. Manning AL, Longworth MS, Dyson NJ. Loss of pRB causes centromere dysfunction and chromosomal instability. Genes Dev 2010;24:1364–76.
28. Zhang J, Benavente CA, McEvoy J, et al. A novel retinoblastoma therapy from genomic and epigenetic analyses. Nature 2012;481:329–34.
29. Rushlow DE, Mol BM, Kennett JY, et al. Characterisation of retinoblastomas without RB1 mutations: genomic, gene expression, and clinical studies. Lancet Oncol 2013;14:327–34.
30. McEvoy J, Nagahawatte P, Finkelstein D, et al. RB1 inactivation by chromothripsis in human retinoblastoma. Oncotarget 2014;5(2):438–50.
31. Goddard AG, Kingston JE, Hungerford JL. Delay in diagnosis of retinoblastoma: risk factors and treatment outcome. Br J Ophthalmol 1999;83:1320–3.
32. Chantada GL, Qaddoumi I, Canturk S, et al. Strategies to manage retinoblastoma in developing countries. Pediatr Blood Cancer 2011;56:341–8.
33. Committee on Practice and Ambulatory Medicine, Section on Ophthalmology, American Association of Certified Orthoptists, American Association for Pediatric Ophthalmology and Strabismus, American Academy of Ophthalmology. Eye examination in infants, children, and young adults by pediatricians. Pediatrics 2003;111:902–7.
34. Draper GJ, Sanders BM, Brownhill PA, et al. Patterns of risk of hereditary retinoblastoma and applications to genetic counselling. Br J Cancer 1992;66:211–9.
35. Richter S, Vandezande K, Chen N, et al. Sensitive and efficient detection of RB1 gene mutations enhances care for families with retinoblastoma. Am J Hum Genet 2003;72:253–69.

36. Houdayer C, Gauthier-Villars M, Laug A, et al. Comprehensive screening for constitutional RB1 mutations by DHPLC and QMPSF. Hum Mutat 2004;23: 193–202.

37. Abramson DH, Frank CM, Susman M, et al. Presenting signs of retinoblastoma. J Pediatr 1998;132:505–8.

38. Baud O, Cormier-Daire V, Lyonnet S, et al. Dysmorphic phenotype and neurological impairment in 22 retinoblastoma patients with constitutional cytogenetic 13q deletion. Clin Genet 1999;55:478–82.

39. Holladay DA, Holladay A, Montebello JF, et al. Clinical presentation, treatment, and outcome of trilateral retinoblastoma. Cancer 1991;67:710–5.

40. Wright KD, Qaddoumi I, Patay Z, et al. Successful treatment of early detected trilateral retinoblastoma using standard infant brain tumor therapy. Pediatr Blood Cancer 2010;55:570–2.

41. Kivel T. Trilateral retinoblastoma: a meta-analysis of hereditary retinoblastoma associated with primary ectopic intracranial retinoblastoma. J Clin Oncol 1999;17:1829–37.

42. Beck-Popovic M, Balmer A, Maeder P, et al. Benign pineal cysts in children with bilateral retinoblastoma: a new variant of trilateral retinoblastoma? Pediatr Blood Cancer 2006;46:755–61.

43. Ramasubramanian A, Kytasty C, Meadows AT, et al. Incidence of pineal gland cyst and pineoblastoma in children with retinoblastoma during the chemoreduction era. Am J Ophthalmol 2013;156:825–9.

44. Beets-Tan RG, Hendriks MJ, Ramos LM, et al. Retinoblastoma: CT and MRI. Neuroradiology 1994;36:59–62.

45. Wilson MW, Rodriguez-Galindo C, Billups C, et al. Lack of correlation between the histologic and magnetic resonance imaging results of optic nerve involvement in eyes primarily enucleated for retinoblastoma. Ophthalmology 2009; 116:1558–63.

46. Khurana A, Eisenhut C, Wan W, et al. Comparison of the diagnostic value of MR imaging and ophthalmoscopy for the staging of retinoblastoma. Eur Radiol 2013;23:1271–80.

47. Song KD, Eo H, Kim JH, et al. Can preoperative MR imaging predict optic nerve invasion of retinoblastoma? Eur J Radiol 2012;81:4041–5.

48. Laurent VE, Sampor C, Solernou V, et al. Detection of minimally disseminated disease in the cerebrospinal fluid of children with high-risk retinoblastoma by reverse transcriptase-polymerase chain reaction for GD2 synthase mRNA. Eur J Cancer 2013;49:2892–9.

49. Chantada GL, Rossi J, Casco F, et al. An aggressive bone marrow evaluation including immunocytology with GD2 for advanced retinoblastoma. J Pediatr Hematol Oncol 2006;28:369–73.

50. Terry J, Calicchio ML, Rodriguez-Galindo C, et al. Immunohistochemical expression of CRX in extracranial malignant small round cell tumors. Am J Surg Pathol 2012;36:1165–9. http://dx.doi.org/10.097/PAS.0b013e3182601d84.

51. Reese AB, Ellsworth RM. The evaluation and current concept of retinoblastoma therapy. Trans Am Acad Ophthalmol Otolaryngol 1963;67:164–72.

52. Shields CL, Mashayekhi A, Au AK, et al. The International Classification of Retinoblastoma predicts chemoreduction success. Ophthalmology 2006;113:2276–80.

53. Murphree AL. Intraocular retinoblastoma: the case for a new group classification. Ophthalmol Clin North Am 2005;18:41–53.

54. Grabowski EF, Abramson DH. Intraocular and extraocular retinoblastoma. Hematol Oncol Clin North Am 1987;1:721–35.

55. Pratt CB, Fontanesi J, Lu X, et al. Proposal for a new staging scheme for intraocular and extraocular retinoblastoma based on an analysis of 103 globes. Oncologist 1997;2:1–5.
56. AJCC. Retinoblastoma. In: Edge SB, Byrd DR, Compton CC, et al, editors. AJCC cancer staging manual. 7th edition. New York: Springer; 2010. p. 562–3.
57. Chantada G, Doz F, Antonelli CBG, et al. A proposal for an international retinoblastoma staging system. Pediatr Blood Cancer 2006;47:801–5.
58. Chantada GL, Sampor C, Bosaleh A, et al. Comparison of staging systems for extraocular retinoblastoma: analysis of 533 patients. JAMA Ophthalmol 2013; 131:1127–34.
59. Rodriguez-Galindo C, Chantada GL, Haik B, et al. Retinoblastoma: current treatment and future perspectives. Curr Treat Options Neurol 2007;9:294–307.
60. Shields CL, Shields JA. Recent developments in the management of retinoblastoma. J Pediatr Ophthalmol Strabismus 1999;36:8–18.
61. Wilson M. Treatment of intraocular retinoblastoma. In: Rodriguez-Galindo C, Wilson MW, editors. Retinoblastoma. New York (NY): Springer; 2010. p. 91–9.
62. Shields JA, Shields CL, DePotter P. Photocoagulation of retinoblastoma. Int Ophthalmol Clin 1993;33:95–9.
63. Shields JA, Parsons H, Shields CL, et al. The role of cryotherapy in the management of retinoblastoma. Am J Ophthalmol 1989;108:260–4.
64. Shields CL, Santos MC, Diniz W, et al. Thermotherapy for retinoblastoma. Arch Ophthalmol 1999;117:885–93.
65. Scott IU, Murray TG, Feuer WJ, et al. External beam radiotherapy in retinoblastoma: tumor control and comparison of 2 techniques. Arch Ophthalmol 1999; 117:766–70.
66. Hungerford JL, Toma NM, Plowman PN, et al. External beam radiotherapy for retinoblastoma: I. Whole eye technique. Br J Ophthalmol 1995;79:109–11.
67. Toma NM, Hungerford JL, Plowman PN, et al. External beam radiotherapy for retinoblastoma: II. Lens sparing technique. Br J Ophthalmol 1995;79:112–7.
68. Merchant TE. Radiation therapy in the management of retinoblastoma retinoblastoma. In: Rodriguez-Galindo, Wilson MW, editors. Retinoblastoma. New York (NY): Springer; 2010. p. 55–64.
69. Fass D, McCormick B, Abramson D, et al. Cobalt60 plaques in recurrent retinoblastoma. Int J Radiat Oncol Biol Phys 1991;21:625–7.
70. Freire JE, De Potter P, Brady LW, et al. Brachytherapy in primary ocular tumors. Semin Surg Oncol 1997;13:167–76.
71. Al-Haj AN, Lobriguito AM, Lagarde CS. Radiation dose profile in 125I brachytherapy: an 8-year review. Radiat Prot Dosimetry 2004;111:115–9.
72. Abouzeid H, Moeckli R, Gaillard MC, et al. (106)Ruthenium brachytherapy for retinoblastoma. Int J Radiat Oncol Biol Phys 2008;71:821–8.
73. Chantada GL, Davila MT, Fandiño A, et al. Retinoblastoma with low risk for extraocular relapse. Ophthalmic Genet 1999;20:133–40.
74. Merchant TE, Gould CJ, Hilton NE, et al. Ocular preservation after 36 Gy external beam radiation therapy for retinoblastoma. J Pediatr Hematol Oncol 2002;24:246–9.
75. Berry JL, Jubran R, Kim JW, et al. Long-term outcomes of Group D eyes in bilateral retinoblastoma patients treated with chemoreduction and low-dose IMRT salvage. Pediatr Blood Cancer 2013;60:688–93.
76. Shields CL, Ramasubramanian A, Thangappan A, et al. Chemoreduction for group E retinoblastoma: comparison of chemoreduction alone versus

chemoreduction plus low-dose external radiotherapy in 76 eyes. Ophthalmology 2009;116:544–51.e1.

77. Sethi RV, Shih HA, Yeap BY, et al. Second nonocular tumors among survivors of retinoblastoma treated with contemporary photon and proton radiotherapy. Cancer 2014;120:126–33.

78. Ross G, Lipper EG, Abramson D, et al. The development of young children with retinoblastoma. Arch Pediatr Adolesc Med 2001;155:80–3.

79. Gobin Y, Dunkel IJ, Marr BP, et al. Intra-arterial chemotherapy for the management of retinoblastoma: four-year experience. Arch Ophthalmol 2011;129:732–7.

80. Honavar SG, Singh AD, Shields CL, et al. Postenucleation adjuvant therapy in high-risk retinoblastoma. Arch Ophthalmol 2002;120:923–31.

81. Uusitalo MS, Van Quill KR, Scott IU, et al. Evaluation of chemoprophylaxis in patients with unilateral retinoblastoma with high-risk features on histopathologic examination. Arch Ophthalmol 2001;119:41–8.

82. Khelfaoui F, Validire P, Auperin A, et al. Histopathologic risk factors in retinoblastoma. A retrospective study of 172 patients treated in a single institution. Cancer 1996;77:1206–13.

83. Chantada G, Fandiño A, Davila MT, et al. Results of a prospective study for the treatment of retinoblastoma. Cancer 2004;100:834–42.

84. Chantada GL, Casco F, Fandiño AC, et al. Outcome of patients with retinoblastoma and postlaminar optic nerve invasion. Ophthalmology 2007;114:2083–9.

85. Cuenca A, Giron F, Castro D, et al. Microscopic scleral invasion in retinoblastoma: clinicopathological features and outcome. Arch Ophthalmol 2009;127: 1006–10.

86. Bosaleh A, Sampor C, Solernou V, et al. Outcome of children with retinoblastoma and isolated choroidal invasion. Arch Ophthalmol 2012;130:724–9.

87. Kaliki S, Shields CL, Shah SU, et al. Postenucleation adjuvant chemotherapy with vincristine, etoposide, and carboplatin for the treatment of high-risk retinoblastoma. Arch Ophthalmol 2011;129:1422–7.

88. Kaliki S, Shields CL, Rojanaporn D, et al. High-risk retinoblastoma based on International Classification of Retinoblastoma: analysis of 519 enucleated eyes. Ophthalmology 2013;120:997–1003.

89. Schvartzman E, Chantada G, Fandiño A, et al. Results of a stage-based protocol for the treatment of retinoblastoma. J Clin Oncol 1996;14:1532–6.

90. Abramson DH, Frank CM. Second nonocular tumors in survivors of bilateral retinoblastoma. A possible age effect on radiation-related risk. Ophthalmology 1998;105:573–80.

91. Shields CL, Honavar SG, Meadows AT, et al. Chemoreduction plus focal therapy for retinoblastoma: factors predictive of need for treatment with external beam radiotherapy or enucleation. Am J Ophthalmol 2002;133:657–64.

92. Gündüz K, Shields CL, Shields JA, et al. The outcome of chemoreduction treatment in patients with Reese-Ellsworth group V retinoblastoma. Arch Ophthalmol 1998;116:1613–7.

93. Shields CL, Shields JA, Needle M, et al. Combined chemoreduction and adjuvant treatment for intraocular retinoblastoma. Ophthalmology 1997;104:2101–11.

94. Gombos DS, Kelly A, Coen PG, et al. Retinoblastoma treated with primary chemotherapy alone: the significance of tumor size, location, and age. Br J Ophthalmol 2002;86:80–3.

95. Shields CL, Honavar SG, Shields JA, et al. Factors predictive of recurrence of retinal tumors, vitreous seeds, and subretinal seeds following chemoreduction for retinoblastoma. Arch Ophthalmol 2002;120:460–4.

96. Laurie NA, Gray JK, Zhang J, et al. Topotecan combination chemotherapy in two new rodent models of retinoblastoma. Clin Cancer Res 2005;11:7569–78.

97. Qaddoumi I, Billups CA, Tagen M, et al. Topotecan and vincristine combination is effective against advanced bilateral intraocular retinoblastoma and has manageable toxicity. Cancer 2012;118:5663–70.

98. Kaneko A, Suzuki S. Eye-preservation treatment of retinoblastoma with vitreous seeding. Jpn J Clin Oncol 2003;33:601–7.

99. Suzuki S, Yamane T, Mohri M, et al. Selective ophthalmic arterial injection therapy for intraocular retinoblastoma: the long-term prognosis. Ophthalmology 2011;118:2081–7.

100. Inomata M, Kaneko A. Chemosensitivity profiles of primary and cultured human retinoblastoma cells in a human tumor clonogenic assay. Jpn J Cancer Res 1987;78:858–68.

101. Schaiquevich P, Buitrago E, Taich P, et al. Pharmacokinetic analysis of melphalan after superselective ophthalmic artery infusion in preclinical models and retinoblastoma patients. Invest Ophthalmol Vis Sci 2012;53:4205–12.

102. Mohri M. The technique of selective ophthalmic arterial infusion for conservative treatment of recurrent intraocular retinoblastoma (in Japanese). Keio Igaku 1993;70:679–87.

103. Abramson DH, Dunkel IJ, Brodie SE, et al. A phase I/II study of direct intraarterial (ophthalmic artery) chemotherapy with melphalan for intraocular retinoblastoma: initial results. Ophthalmology 2008;115:1398–404.

104. Shields CL, Bianciotto CG, Jabbour P, et al. Intra-arterial chemotherapy for retinoblastoma: Report no. 1, control of retinal tumors, subretinal seeds, and vitreous seeds. Arch Ophthalmol 2011;129:1399–406.

105. Klufas MA, Gobin YP, Marr B, et al. Intra-arterial chemotherapy as a treatment for intraocular retinoblastoma: alternatives to direct ophthalmic artery catheterization. AJNR Am J Neuroradiol 2012;33:1608–14.

106. Abramson DD, Dunkel IJ, Brodie SE, et al. Bilateral superselective ophthalmic artery chemotherapy for bilateral retinoblastoma: tandem therapy. Arch Ophthalmol 2010;128:370–2.

107. Abramson DH, Dunkel IJ, Brodie SE, et al. Superselective ophthalmic artery chemotherapy as primary treatment for retinoblastoma (chemosurgery). Ophthalmology 2010;117:1623–9.

108. Francis J, Gobin Y, Dunkel I, et al. Carboplatin +/- topotecan ophthalmic artery chemosurgery for intraocular retinoblastoma. PLoS One 2013;8:e72441.

109. Abramson DH, Marr BP, Brodie SE, et al. Ophthalmic artery chemosurgery for less advanced intraocular retinoblastoma: five year review. PLoS One 2012;7:e34120.

110. Schaiquevich P, Ceciliano A, Millan N, et al. Intra-arterial chemotherapy is more effective than sequential periocular and intravenous chemotherapy as salvage treatment for relapsed retinoblastoma. Pediatr Blood Cancer 2013;60:766–70.

111. Marr BP, Brodie SE, Dunkel IJ, et al. Three-drug intra-arterial chemotherapy using simultaneous carboplatin, topotecan and melphalan for intraocular retinoblastoma: preliminary results. Br J Ophthalmol 2012;96:1300–3.

112. Abramson DH, Marr BP, Dunkel IJ, et al. Intra-arterial chemotherapy for retinoblastoma in eyes with vitreous and/or subretinal seeding: 2-year results. Br J Ophthalmol 2012;96:499–502.

113. Gobin Y, Dunkel I, Marr BP, et al. Combined, sequential intravenous and intra-arterial chemotherapy (bridge chemotherapy) for young infants with retinoblastoma. PLoS One 2012;7:e44322.

114. Tse BC, Steinle JJ, Johnson D, et al. Superselective intraophthalmic artery chemotherapy in a nonhuman primate model: Histopathologic findings. JAMA Ophthalmol 2013;131:903–11.
115. Eagle RC, Shields CL, Bianciotto C, et al. Histopathologic observations after intra-arterial chemotherapy for retinoblastoma. Arch Ophthalmol 2011;129:1416–21.
116. Abramson DH. Chemosurgery for retinoblastoma: what we know after 5 years. Arch Ophthalmol 2011;129:1492–4.
117. Brodie S, Munier F, Francis J, et al. Persistence of retinal function after intravitreal melphalan injection for retinoblastoma. Doc Ophthalmol 2013;126:79–84.
118. Gobin Y, Rosenstein LM, Marr BP, et al. Radiation exposure during intra-arterial chemotherapy for retinoblastoma. Arch Ophthalmol 2012;130:403–5.
119. Vijayakrishnan R, Shields CL, Ramasubramanian A, et al. Irradiation toxic effects during intra-arterial chemotherapy for retinoblastoma: should we be concerned? Arch Ophthalmol 2010;128:1427–31.
120. Munier FL, Gaillard MC, Balmer A, et al. Intravitreal chemotherapy for vitreous disease in retinoblastoma revisited: from prohibition to conditional indications. Br J Ophthalmol 2012;96:1078–83.
121. Shields CL, Manjandavida FP, Arepalli S, et al. Intravitreal melphalan for persistent or recurrent retinoblastoma vitreous seeds: preliminary results. JAMA Ophthalmol 2014;132:319–25.
122. Antonelli CB, Steinhorst F, Ribeiro KC, et al. Extraocular retinoblastoma: a 13-year experience. Cancer 2003;98:1292–8.
123. Menon BS, Reddy SC, Maziah W, et al. Extraocular retinoblastoma. Med Pediatr Oncol 2000;35:75–6.
124. Doz F, Khelfaoui F, Mosseri V, et al. The role of chemotherapy in orbital involvement of retinoblastoma. Cancer 1994;74:722–32.
125. Chantada G, Fandiño A, Casak S, et al. Treatment of overt extraocular retinoblastoma. Med Pediatr Oncol 2003;40:158–61.
126. Namouni F, Doz F, Tanguy ML, et al. High-dose chemotherapy with carboplatin, etoposide and cyclophosphamide followed by a haematopoietic stem cell rescue in patients with high-risk retinoblastoma: a SFOP and SFGM study. Eur J Cancer 1997;33:2368–75.
127. Dunkel IJ, Khakoo Y, Kernan NA, et al. Intensive multimodality therapy for patients with stage 4a metastatic retinoblastoma. Pediatr Blood Cancer 2010;55:55–9.
128. Kleinerman RA, Tucker MA, Tarone RE, et al. Risk of new cancers after radiotherapy in long-term survivors of retinoblastoma: an extended follow-up. J Clin Oncol 2005;23:2272–9.
129. Kleinerman RA, Tucker MA, Abramson DH, et al. Risk of soft tissue sarcomas by individual subtype in survivors of hereditary retinoblastoma. J Natl Cancer Inst 2007;99:24–31.
130. Shinohara ET, DeWees T, Perkins SM. Subsequent malignancies and their effect on survival in patients with retinoblastoma. Pediatr Blood Cancer 2014;61:116–9.
131. Kleinerman RA, Tarone RE, Abramson DH, et al. Hereditary retinoblastoma and risk of lung cancer. J Natl Cancer Inst 2000;92:2037–9.
132. Yu CL, Tucker MA, Abramson DH, et al. Cause-specific mortality in long-term survivors of retinoblastoma. J Natl Cancer Inst 2009;101:581–91.
133. Kleinerman RA, Yu CL, Little MP, et al. Variation of second cancer risk by family history of retinoblastoma among long-term survivors. J Clin Oncol 2012;30:950–7.
134. Fletcher O, Easton D, Anderson K, et al. Lifetime risks of common cancers among retinoblastoma survivors. J Natl Cancer Inst 2004;96:357–63.

Neuroblastoma

Paradigm for Precision Medicine

Meredith S. Irwin, MD[a], Julie R. Park, MD[b],*

KEYWORDS

- Neuroblastoma • Risk stratification • MYCN
- Segmental chromosome aberrations (SCA) • ALK (anaplastic lymphoma kinase)
- Phox2B • Myeloablative therapy (MAT) • Immunotherapy

KEY POINTS

- Neuroblastoma (NB) is the most common extracranial pediatric tumor, most frequently diagnosed cancer in infancy, and has a heterogeneous presentation and prognosis.
- Clinical and biological prognostic factors are used to risk stratify patients into groups with low, intermediate, and high risk for recurrence; most protocols now use the International Neuroblastoma Risk Group classification system.
- Age, stage, histology, and amplification of the MYCN oncogene are currently the most robust prognostic factors.
- Outcomes for low- and intermediate-risk NB are excellent, but survival for high-risk NB is less than 50%.
- High-risk NB tumors contain many segmental chromosome aberrations (eg, loss of heterozygosity 1p, 11q); but recurrent somatic mutations are rare, with anaplastic lymphoma kinase (ALK) being the most commonly altered gene in approximately 10% of NB.
- Survival after relapse of metastatic NB is uncommon; current and upcoming trials will rely on incorporation of novel immunotherapies, inhibitors of aberrant pathways (eg MYC, ALK), and radioisotope-containing regimens, such as high-dose iodine-131-metaiodobenzylguanidine.

INTRODUCTION

Neuroblastoma (NB), the most common extracranial tumor of childhood, is a cancer of primordial neural crest cells that give rise to sympathetic neural ganglia and adrenal medulla. NB has a diverse pattern of clinical presentation and prognosis that ranges

a Division of Hematology-Oncology, Hospital for Sick Children, University of Toronto, 555 University Ave, Toronto, ON M5G1X8, Canada; b Division of Hematology-Oncology, Seattle Children's Hospital, University of Washington School of Medicine, Fred Hutchinson Cancer Research Center, 4800 Sandpoint Way NE, Seattle, WA 98105, USA
* Corresponding author.
E-mail address: julie.park@seattlechildrens.org

Pediatr Clin N Am 62 (2015) 225–256
http://dx.doi.org/10.1016/j.pcl.2014.09.015
0031-3955/15/$ – see front matter © 2015 Elsevier Inc. All rights reserved.
pediatric.theclinics.com

from spontaneous regression to aggressive metastatic tumors. For more than 2 decades, NB treatment has served as a paradigm for the incorporation of clinical and biological factors to stratify patients and tailor therapies. Using clinical, pathologic, and increasingly genetic factors, patients can be categorized as low, intermediate (IR), and high risk (HR) for recurrence. The overall survival (OS) for patients with low and IR NB is excellent at greater than 90% with relatively minimal surgical or medical interventions (**Fig. 1**). The goal of recent trials for non-HR patients has been to decrease treatments further and minimize chemotherapy-related toxicities. In contrast, long-term survival for HR patients remains 40% to 50% despite intensification of treatments and incorporation of immunotherapies. Current protocols are aimed at identifying better predictors of response and outcome as well as discovering genetic aberrations that may represent tractable therapeutic targets. This article summarizes the clinical presentations and current understanding of NB biology and prognostic features, their roles in risk stratification–based treatments, and novel therapies for patients with recurrent disease.

EPIDEMIOLOGY AND GENETIC PREDISPOSITION

The incidence of NB in North America and Europe is 10.5 per million children between 0 and 14 years of age, with a slight male predominance (1.2:1.0).[1–4] NB is the most common cancer diagnosed in infancy, with most patients diagnosed between 0 and 4 years of age (median age 19 months[5]), and less than 5% at greater than 10 years. NB accounts for 8% to 10% of all pediatric cancers and 12% to 15% of cancer-related deaths in children. Although there are no significant geographic variations in incidence, there are ethnic disparities in outcome. African American and Native American patients are more likely to have HR features and poor outcomes, in part because of genetic differences.[6–8] Environmental factors, including parental exposures, have not been clearly linked with NB development.[9,10]

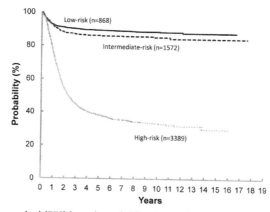

Fig. 1. Event-free survival (EFS) based on children's oncology group (COG) risk stratification. EFS Kaplan-Meier survival curves calculated from the time of diagnosis for children enrolled onto COG (since 2001); Children's Cancer Group and Pediatric Oncology Group Neuroblastoma Biology trials and were classified as low risk, IR, or HR at the time of diagnosis based on clinical and biological factors (current COG classification is summarized in **Table 2**). (*From* Park JR, Bagatell R, London WB, et al. Children's Oncology Group 2013 blueprint for research: neuroblastoma. Pediatr Blood Cancer 2013;60(6):986, with permission. © 2012 Wiley Periodicals, Inc.)

NB is the only solid tumor of childhood for which there have been large screening initiatives, pioneered largely in Japan. Universal screening of 6-month-old asymptomatic infants by detection of elevated urinary catecholamines resulted in a 2-fold increase in NB incidence to 20.1 per million children; however, most of the detected tumors had favorable clinical and biological characteristics.[11–13] Studies in Germany and Quebec also demonstrated an increased incidence and detection of tumors with favorable biology and pathology.[14,15] In general, universal screening has not detected poor prognosis disease, which usually presents at an older age and, thus, has not affected mortality rates.[16] In contrast, in selected populations with an inherited genetic predisposition to NB, screening may be indicated.

Genetic Predisposition

The incidence of familial NB is estimated at 1% to 2%.[17] Cases often involve multifocal and/or bilateral adrenal primary tumors with a median age of onset of 9 months. The pattern of inheritance is autosomal dominant with incomplete penetrance. NB can occur in patients with other neural crest disorders, such as Hirschsprung disease (HSCR), congenital central hypoventilation syndrome (CCHS), and neurofibromatosis type 1 (NF1). Mutations in the *Phox2b* homeobox gene have been detected in subsets of patients with familial NB and usually are associated with other neurocristopathies, such as HSCR and CCHS.[18–20] *Phox2b* mutations have also been detected in approximately 2% of sporadic NB. There are many reports of NB in patients with NF; however, there are conflicting data as to whether germline *NF1* mutations are associated with an increased risk to develop NB.[21,22]

Linkage studies in familial NB pedigrees identified candidate chromosomal predisposition regions including 16p, 12p, and 2p[23–26] and led to the identification of germline mutations in the tyrosine kinase domain of the anaplastic lymphoma kinase (*ALK*) oncogene.[27,28] ALK is involved in nervous system development,[29] and central nervous system (CNS) anomalies have been reported in some patients with germline *ALK* mutations.[29] Sporadic NB tumors also harbor *ALK* abnormalities, including genomic amplification (2%–3%) and missense mutations (8%–12%)[27,28,30–33] (see "Somatic Gene Mutations"), that can be targeted by pharmacologic inhibitors.[34–36] Studies of ALK inhibitors in NB and other tumors with *ALK* aberrations (eg, anaplastic large cell lymphoma) have shown promising results.[37] NB cases are also detected in other familial cancer syndromes, including Beckwith-Wiedemann syndrome,[38] Li-Fraumeni,[39,40] Noonan (*PTPN11*), some subtypes of Fanconi anemia, and some chromosomal breakage syndromes.[41,42]

Recent genome-wide association studies using peripheral blood from thousands of patients with NB have also identified germline genetic variants that may predispose to the development of sporadic NB. These variants include single nucleotide polymorphisms (SNPs) in *LINC00340, BARD1, LMO1, DUSP12, DDX4, LIN28B, HACE1*, and *TP53*.[43–48] Unlike the rare germline mutations in *ALK* and *Phox2B* described earlier, these SNPs are more frequent but individually have less dramatic impacts on the NB risk.[49] The interplay between multiple germline variants and somatic alterations, discussed later, may influence the initiation and progression of NB.

PRESENTATION, DIAGNOSIS, AND STAGING
Symptoms

NB presentations vary based on the disease extent and tumor location, which may occur anywhere along the sympathetic chain resulting in local effects on organs, vessels, or nerves (**Fig. 2, Table 1**). Most of them (65%) arise in the abdomen, most

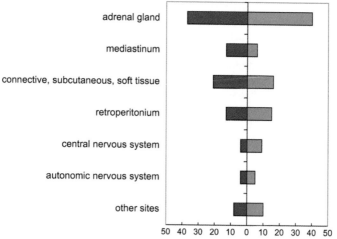

Fig. 2. Percent distribution of NBs by primary site and age; Surveillance, Epidemiology and End Results Program (1975 to 1995). (*Adapted from* Ries L, Smith M, Gurney J, et al. Cancer incidence and survival among children and adolescents: United States SEER Program 1975–1995, National Cancer Institute, SEER Program. Bethesda (MD): NIH Pub; 1999. p. 99–4649. NIH Publication No. 99–4649.)

commonly the adrenal gland, and may be asymptomatic or associated with hypertension, abdominal pain, distension, and constipation. Other sites include the neck, chest, and pelvis. The primary site location is associated with age and outcome.[50] Cervical and thoracic tumors are more common in infants and may present with Horner syndrome (unilateral ptosis, anhidrosis, and myosis) and respiratory

Table 1 Clinical presentation and symptoms of NB	
Location	**Signs and Symptoms**
Abdomen/pelvis	Pain, constipation, distension, urinary retention, hypertension
Thorax	Respiratory distress, Horner syndrome
Presacral and paraspinal (includes abdominal and thoracic masses)	Symptoms of cord compression (urinary retention, paraplegia/paraparesis, clonus)
Neck	Mass/swelling
Metastases	Irritability, bone pain, cytopenias (petechiae, ecchymoses, pallor), periorbital ecchymoses, fever, weight loss, lymphadenopathy
4S/4M metastases	Hepatomegaly, coagulopathy, hyperbilirubinemia, respiratory distress (from abdominal enlargement), skin nodules
Paraneoplastic syndromes	• OMS: myoclonic jerking and random eye movement, with or without cerebellar ataxia • VIP secreting tumors: intractable secretory diarrhea caused by tumor secretion of VIP

Patients may be asymptomatic or may have one or more of the listed symptoms or findings on exam.

Abbreviations: OMS, opsoclonus myoclonus ataxia syndrome; VIP, vasoactive intestinal peptide.

symptoms. Epidural or intradural tumor extension occurs in 5% to 15% of patients and may result in spinal cord compression and paraplegia.[51] Two rare paraneoplastic syndromes associated with NB include secretory diarrhea caused by tumor production of vasoactive intestinal peptide[52,53] and opsoclonus myoclonus ataxia syndrome (OMS). OMS is reported in 2% to 3% of patients and is commonly associated with favorable well-differentiated tumors.[54,55] OMS is characterized by myoclonic jerks and random eye movements with or without ataxia, is attributed to immune-mediated effects, and often persists after resection, resulting in significant neurodevelopmental sequelae.

Approximately half of patients present with localized or regional disease, and 35% have regional lymph node spread at the time of diagnosis. Distant metastases are detected in 50% of patients at diagnosis and occur through both lymphatic and hematogenous routes. The most common sites include bone, bone marrow, and liver. NB has a particular predilection to spread to metaphyseal, skull, and orbital bone sites, resulting in a classic presentation characterized by periorbital ecchymoses (raccoon eyes), proptosis, and potentially visual impairment. In contrast to the frequent lack of symptoms for locoregional tumors, patients with widespread disease are often ill appearing with fever, pain, irritability, and weight loss. Less common sites of metastases at diagnosis include the lung[56] and brain; however, CNS disease at relapse is increasingly common.[57,58] In infants there is an unusual pattern of metastases, stage 4S or MS (see "Staging" later), characterized by skin nodules and/or diffuse liver involvement and hepatomegaly often associated with respiratory compromise.[59]

Diagnosis is confirmed either by (1) tumor tissue biopsy and histopathology (**Fig. 3**) or (2) a combination of NB tumor cells detected in bone marrow together with elevated urine or serum catecholamine or catecholamine metabolites (dopamine, vanillylmandelic acid, and homovanillic acid). Evaluation includes cross-sectional imaging with computed tomography or MRI to determine size, regional extent (including intraspinal invasion), distant spread to neck, thorax, abdomen and pelvis (see **Fig. 4**).[60,61] Bilateral iliac crest bone marrow aspirates and biopsies are required to determine tumor involvement by histology. Radioiodine-labeled metaiodobenzylguanidine (MIBG), a norepinephrine analogue that selectively concentrates in sympathetic nervous tissue, is used to detect primary tumors and metastatic sites.[62] Approximately 90% of patients have MIBG-avid disease, and semiquantitative scoring systems are being integrated into NB response criteria.[63,64] [(18)F-fluorodeoxyglucose positron emission tomography (FDG-PET) scans are recommended for detecting metastatic disease in patients whose tumors are not MIBG avid.[65–67] Technetium bone scans can be used to detect cortical bone disease if MIBG and PET scan are not available.

Staging

Until recently, the criteria for diagnosis and staging were based on the surgical-pathologic International Neuroblastoma Staging System (INSS) (**Box 1**).[68,69] INSS stages 1 to 3 are localized tumors that are classified based on the amount of resection, local invasion, and node involvement. Stage 4 is defined as distant metastases; 4S (4Special) is characterized by metastases to the liver, skin, and/or marrow in infants, which is usually associated with favorable biological features and can undergo spontaneous regression. In 2009, the International Neuroblastoma Risk Group's (INRG) stratification system was developed by representatives from a major consortium in North America (Children's Oncology Group [COG]) Europe (SIOPEN, International Society of Pediatric Oncology European Neuroblastoma), and Germany, Japan, and Australia. The INRG staging system (INRGSS) uses surgical risk factors (SRFs), which are preoperative radiological features to distinguish locoregional tumors that do not

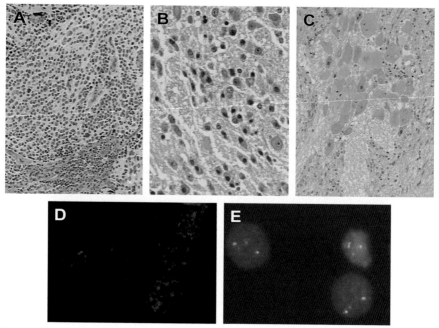

Fig. 3. Histopathology and fluorescence in situ hybridization (FISH) assays (*A–C*). Shown are representative images (hematoxylin-eosin, original magnification ×200 [*A* and *C*] ×400) from 3 different histologic appearances of NB: (*A*) poorly differentiated NB, (*B*) differentiating NB, and (*C*) ganglioneuroblastoma (stroma-rich NB). The fluffy pink material separating the cells is neuropil (categorized as stroma-poor). (*A*) The poorly differentiated NB cells have minimal cytoplasm, discernible only as purple-stained nuclei. (*B*) The neuroblasts are differentiating as reflected by defined pink cytoplasm and larger nuclei. (*C*) The neuroblasts have the features of fully differentiated ganglion cells, and the spindle cell areas in the 4 corners are composed of Schwann cells (categorized as stroma-rich). (*D*) FISH showing MYCN amplification (MYCNA). The presence of multiple copies of MYCN is detected in tumor cells using a labeled probe (*red*) for the chromosomal location 2p region that includes the *MYCN* gene. MYCNA is defined as greater than 10 copies. (*E*) FISH showing 1p loss of heterozygosity (LOH). Cells show 2 signals from the control 1q probe (*green*) and 1 signal for the 1p 36 probe (*red*) indicating that there is loss of one copy of 1p36 loci (LOH) and 2 normal copies of 1q. (*Courtesy of* Dr Paul Thorner, Pathology Department, and Dr Mary Shago, Cytogenetics Laboratory, Hospital for Sick Children, Toronto.)

involve local structures (INRGS L1) from locally invasive tumors with imaging-defined risk factors (IDRFs) (INRGS L2) (**Boxes 2** and **3**).[70,71] INRGS M and MS refer to tumors with distant metastases and have the INSS 4 or 4S pattern of spread, respectively.

CLINICAL AND BIOLOGICAL RISK FACTORS, PROGNOSIS, AND RISK STRATIFICATION

NB is classified into low risk, IR, and HR based on clinical and biological factors that have been shown to predict prognosis and risk of recurrence, including age, stage, histopathology, DNA index (ploidy), and *MYCN* amplification (*MYCNA*) and are used to assign treatment (**Table 2**). In comparison, the recently developed INRG classification system defines similar cohorts using the INRG database (8800 patients treated between 1990–2002) to facilitate comparisons across international clinical trials (**Box 4**).[70]

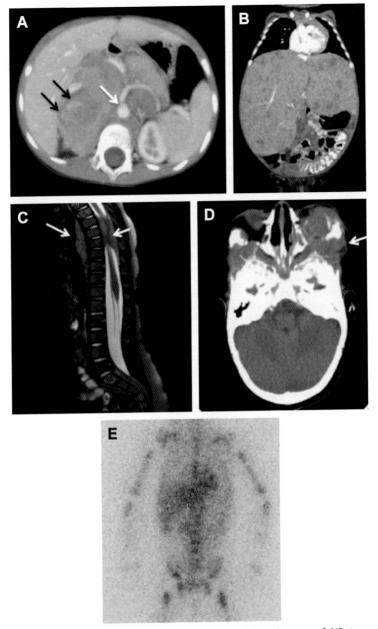

Fig. 4. Diagnostic imaging of NB. Shown are representative images of NB tumors from different primary locations from diagnostic evaluations. (*A*) Computed tomography (CT) scan (axial view) shows a typical retroperitoneal mass arising from the adrenal with calcifications (white speckles in tumor mass, *black arrows*) and tumor encasement of vessels (aorta, *white arrow*). The left kidney demonstrates mild pelviectasis, which is commonly seen secondary to the mass effect. (*B*) CT scan (coronal view) of very large liver with multiple NB tumor nodules (darker than surrounding liver parenchyma), which is typically seen in infants with International Neuroblastoma Staging System stage 4S/INRG MS. (*C*) MRI scan (sagittal view) shows a paraspinal thoracic mass (*arrows*) with intraspinal extension and spinal cord compression. (*D*) Brain and orbital CT (axial) with large metastases involving the orbits, with more extensive involvement on the left (*arrow*). (*E*) I-123 metaiodobenzylguanidine scan demonstrates widespread bony metastases in the extremities, vertebrae, and pelvis (darker lesions). Note the normal physiologic uptake in the heart, liver, and bladder.

Box 1
International Neuroblastoma Staging System (INSS)

Stage[c,d]	Description
1	Localized tumor with complete gross excision, with or without microscopic residual disease representative ipsilateral lymph nodes negative for tumor microscopically (nodes attached to and removed with the primary tumor may be positive)
2A	Localized tumor with incomplete gross resection; representative ipsilateral nonadherent lymph nodes negative for tumor microscopically
2B	Localized tumor with or without complete gross excision, with ipsilateral nonadherent lymph nodes positive for tumor; enlarged contralateral lymph nodes must be negative microscopically.
3	Unresectable unilateral tumor infiltrating across the midline[a], with or without regional lymph node involvement; or localized unilateral tumor with contralateral regional lymph node involvement; or midline tumor with bilateral extension by infiltration (unresectable) or by lymph node involvement
4	Any primary tumor with dissemination to distant lymph nodes, bone, bone marrow, liver, skin, and/or other organs (except as defined for stage 4S)
4S	Localized primary tumor (as defined for stage 1, 2A or 2B) with dissemination limited to skin, liver, and/or bone marrow[b] (limited to infants <1 y of age)

[a] The midline is defined as the vertebral column. Tumors originating on one side and crossing the midline must infiltrate to or beyond the opposite side of the vertebral column.
[b] Marrow involvement in stage 4S should be minimal (ie, less than 10% of total nucleated cells identified as malignant on bone marrow biopsy or marrow aspirate). More extensive marrow involvement would be considered to be stage 4.
[c] Multifocal primary tumors (eg, bilateral adrenal primary tumors) should be staged according to the greatest extent of disease, as defined earlier, and followed by a subscript M (eg, 3_M).
[d] Proven malignant effusion within the thoracic cavity if it is bilateral or the abdominal cavity upstages patients to INSS 3.

Data from Brodeur GM, Pritchard J, Berthold F, et al. Revisions of the international criteria for neuroblastoma diagnosis, staging, and response to treatment. J Clin Oncol 1993;11(8):1466–77; and Brodeur GM, Seeger RC, Barrett A, et al. International criteria for diagnosis, staging, and response to treatment in patients with neuroblastoma. J Clin Oncol 1988;6(12):1874–81.

Stage and Age

Many studies have consistently demonstrated the independent prognostic value of the INSS stage, including an INRG database analysis that reported superior event-free survival (EFS) and OS for patients with nonmetastatic NB (INSS stages 1, 2, and 3) and INSS stage 4S ($83 \pm 1\%$ and $91 \pm 1\%$) compared with only 35 ± 1 and $42 \pm 1\%$, for patients with INSS stage 4 disease.[70] With the exception of stage 4S, specific metastatic sites have not been incorporated into staging systems. However, retrospective studies suggest that spread confined to distant lymph nodes may predict improved outcomes,[72] whereas there is a trend toward inferior outcomes for patients with metastases to the lung[56] or bone marrow.[73] Although retrospective studies have demonstrated the prognostic significance of the INRGSS, which incorporates SRFs,[60,61,71] this will be prospectively validated across North America and Europe.[64]

Age was one of the first prognostic indicators identified. In comparison to infants, patients older than 1 to 2 years at diagnosis have an inferior outcome; this effect is more prominent for patients with metastatic disease. Historically, a cutoff of 365 days had been used as a surrogate for tumor behavior; however, London and

---

Box 2
International Risk Group Staging System (INRGSS)

Stage[a]	Description
L1	Localized tumor not involving vital structures as defined by the list of image-defined risk factors and confined to one body compartment
L2	Locoregional tumor with presence of one or more IDRFs (see **Box 1**)
M	Distant metastatic disease (except stage MS)
MS	Metastatic disease in children younger than 18 mo with metastases confined to skin, liver, and/or bone marrow

[a] Patients with multifocal primary tumors should be staged according to the greatest extent of disease as defined in the table.

Data from Monclair T, Brodeur GM, Ambros PF, et al. The International Neuroblastoma Risk Group (INRG) staging system: an INRG task force report. J Clin Oncol 2009;27(2):298–303.

---

colleagues[5] studied the continuous nature of age for 3666 patients and concluded that the most prognostic cutoff was 460 days (15.1 months). Several retrospective studies specifically examined whether 18 months might represent a more clinically relevant cutoff and demonstrated that EFS and OS for patients with INSS stage 4 disease aged 12 to 18 months (with favorable tumor biology) was similar to that of patients aged less than 12 months.[74,75] Similarly, patients with INSS stage 3 disease aged 12 to 18 months had a superior outcome to those older than 18 months.[76] Prospective COG trials will determine whether reduction of therapy for toddlers aged 12 to 18 months with biologically favorable tumors, traditionally treated with more intensive regimens, will still provide superior outcomes.[77] Older children, adolescents, and young adults with NB have a more indolent course and worse overall outcome despite infrequent *MYCN* oncogene amplification (*MYCNA*); however, no specific prognostic age cutoffs greater than 18 months have been identified.[78]

Histopathology

Pathologic characteristics have been used to further classify tumors into favorable and unfavorable categories, initially using a system developed by Shimada and colleagues[79] that provided the basis for the more recently revised International Neuroblastoma Pathology Committee (INPC) criteria. The prognostic value of INPC classification, based on age, presence of Schwannian stroma, grade of neuroblastic differentiation, and Mitosis-karyorrhexis index, has been validated in large cooperative group studies[80,81] to identify specific patient risk groups that may benefit from modified therapy. In the COG P9641, patients with INSS stage 1 and 2 disease with favorable histology had a significantly better outcome than those with unfavorable histology (UH) (EFS $90 \pm 3\%$ and $72 \pm 7\%$, OS $99 \pm 1\%$ and $86 \pm 5\%$).[82]

Tumor Genetics

NB genetic features have been used for risk stratification for more than 20 years. Two broad categories of genetic aberration patterns include (1) tumors with whole chromosome gains, lack of structural changes, and hyperdiploid karyotype and (2) tumors with segmental chromosomal aberrations (SCAs) and diploid DNA content, which are often associated with poor outcomes. SCAs often include partial gains and losses of chromosomal regions predicted to encode oncogenes and tumor suppressors, respectively.

Box 3
Image Defined Risk Factors (IDRFs)

Ipsilateral tumor extension within 2 body compartments

Neck-chest, chest-abdomen, abdomen-pelvis

Neck

Encases carotid and/or vertebral artery and/or internal jugular vein; extends to skull base; compresses trachea

Cervicothoracic junction

Encases brachial plexus roots or subclavian vessels and/or vertebral or carotid artery; compresses trachea

Thorax

Encases the aorta and/or major branches; compresses trachea and/or principal bronchi; lower mediastinal tumor infiltrating costovertebral junction between T9 and 12

Thoracoabdominal

Encases the aorta and/or vena cava

Abdomen/pelvis

Infiltrates the porta hepatis and/or the hepatoduodenal ligament; encases branches of the superior mesenteric artery at the mesenteric root or origin of celiac axis and/or superior mesenteric artery; invades one or both renal pedicles; encases aorta and/or vena cava or iliac vessels, crossing sciatic notch

Intraspinal tumor extension whatever the location provided that

More than one-third of the spinal canal in the axial plane invaded and/or the perimedullary leptomeningeal spaces not visible and/or the spinal cord signal abnormal

Infiltration of adjacent organs/structures

Pericardium, diaphragm, kidney, liver, duodeno-pancreatic block, and mesentery

Conditions to be recorded but not considered IDRFs

Multifocal primary tumors

Pleural effusion, with or without malignant cells

Ascites, with or without malignant cells

IDRFs are used to determine the ability to completely resect locoregional tumors at diagnosis based on surgical risk factors that can be defined by IDRFs detected on cross-sectional imaging with CT and/or MRI.
    Data from Monclair T, Brodeur GM, Ambros PF, et al. The International Neuroblastoma Risk Group (INRG) staging system: an INRG task force report. J Clin Oncol 2009;27(2):298–303.

Allelic Gains, Amplifications, and Oncogenes

MYCNA defined as greater than 10 copies[83] is detected in approximately 20% of NB tumors, with a higher incidence in INSS stages 3 and 4 (40%) but only 5% of stages 1, 2, and 4s.[70] Many studies have demonstrated that in comparison to patients with non-*MYCNA* tumors, patients with *MYCNA* have a significantly worse outcome[84,85] (reviewed in Refs.[49,86,87]). All patients with *MYCNA* stage 3, 4 and 4S tumors are classified as HR, including infants; however, the prognostic significance of *MYCNA* in rare cases of localized resected NB remains controversial.[88,89] Importantly, most laboratory animal models for NB rely on overexpression of MYCN in neural crest cells[36,90]; recent studies have identified drugs that target MYCN to inhibit NB growth.[91]

Table 2
Children's Oncology Group Neuroblastoma Risk Stratification

Risk Group	Stage	Age	MYCN	Ploidy	Shimada
Low risk	1	Any	Any	Any	Any
Low risk	2a/2b	Any	Not amp	Any	Any
HR	2a/2b	Any	Amp	Any	Any
IR	3	<547 d	Not amp	Any	Any
IR	3	≥547 d	Not amp	Any	FH
HR	3	Any	Amp	Any	Any
HR	3	≥547 d	Not amp	Any	UH
HR	4	<365 d	Amp	Any	Any
IR	4	<365 d	Not amp	Any	Any
HR	4	365–<547 d	Amp	Any	Any
HR	4	365–<547 d	Any	DI = 1	Any
HR	4	365–<547 d	Any	Any	UH
IR	4	365–<547 d	Not amp	DI>1	FH
HR	4	≥547 d	Any	Any	Any
Low risk	4s	<365 d	Not amp	DI>1	FH
IR	4s	<365 d	Not amp	DI = 1	Any
IR	4s	<365 d	Not amp	Any	UH
HR	4s	<365 d	Amp	Any	Any

COG currently uses the International Neuroblastoma Staging System's stage, age, MYCN status, DNA index or ploidy, and INPC histology to determine patient's risk category as high, intermediate or low.[64]

Abbreviations: amp, amplification; DI, DNA index; FH, favorable histology; UH, unfavorable histology.

From Park JR, Bagatell R, London WB, et al. Children's Oncology Group's 2013 blueprint for research: neuroblastoma. Pediatr Blood Cancer 2013;60(6):985–93.

Amplification of *ALK*, located at 2p23 in close proximity to *MYCN* at 2p24, is detected in 2% to 3% of NB and is more common, though not exclusively, observed in tumors with *MYCN* amplification.[92] A 17q gain detected in greater than 60% of tumors is often associated with other poor prognostic markers (eg, *MYCNA*, older age).[93,94] Although the specific genes that may have oncogenic roles on 17q have not been identified, candidates include *BIRC5* (survivin), *PPMID* (WIP1), and *NME1/2*.

Allelic Losses and Tumor Suppressor Genes

The most frequently deleted chromosomal regions in NB include 1p, 4p, 11q, and 14q. Chromosome 1p loss of heterozygosity (LOH), detected in 23%–30% of tumors, predicts poor outcome.[95,96] 1p36 LOH correlates with *MYCNA* and other HR features (eg, metastasis, age >1, UH), and thus, 1pLOH may be most relevant as an independent prognostic factor in infants and patients without *MYCNA*.[97] The 1p candidate tumor suppressor genes include the chromatin remodeling protein CHD5[98] and transcription factor CASZ1.[99] Chromosome 11qLOH is detected in approximately 30% to 40% of patients.[95,100] Like 17q gain and 1pLOH, 11qLOH is more common in patients with stage 4 disease and predicts poor prognosis; however, 11qLOH is rarely associated with *MYCNA* and, therefore, may predict additional HR subsets within the non-*MYCNA* tumors. One 11q candidate gene, *CADM1*, has been implicated in NB growth and proliferation.[101] Although INRG currently includes 11qLOH as criteria to upstate to

Box 4
INRG consensus pretreatment classification schema

INRG Stage	Age (mo)	Histologic Category	Grade of Tumor Differentiation	MYCN	11q Aberration	Ploidy	Pretreatment Risk Group
L1/L2	—	GN maturing; GNB intermixed	—	—	—	—	A. Very low
L1	—	Any, except GN maturing or GNB intermixed	—	NA	—	—	B. Very low
				Amp	—	—	K. High
L2	<18	Any, except GN maturing or GNB intermixed	—	NA	No	—	D. Low
				NA	Yes	—	G. Intermediate
	≥18	GNB nodular; neuroblastoma	Differentiating	NA	No	—	E. Low
					Yes	—	—
			Poorly differentiated or undifferentiated	NA	—	—	H. Intermediate
				Amp	—	—	N. High
M	<18	—	—	NA	—	Hyperdiploid	F. Low
	<12	—	—	NA	—	Diploid	I. Intermediate
	12–<18	—	—	NA	—	Diploid	J. Intermediate
	<18	—	—	Amp	—	—	O. High
	≥18	—	—	—	—	—	P. High
MS	<18	—	—	NA	No	—	C. Very low
			—	NA	Yes	—	Q. High
			—	Amp	—	—	R. High

Classification schema is based on analysis of 8800 patients in the INRG database (1990–2002). Risk groups are very low risk (5-year event-free survival [EFS] >85%); low risk (5-year EFS >75% to ≤85%); IR (5-year EFS ≥50% to ≤75%); HR (5-year EFS <50%). Staging of L1, L2, M, and MS described in **Fig. 2B**.

Abbreviations: Amp, amplified; EFS, event-free survival; GN, ganglioneuroma; GNB, ganglioneuroblastoma; NA, not amplified.

Adapted from Cohn SL, Pearson AD, London WB, et al. The International Neuroblastoma Risk Group [INRG] classification system: an INRG task force report. J Clin Oncol 2009;27(2):295.

HR classification, prospective trials are ongoing to determine whether 11qLOH predicts poor outcomes for non-HR patients.

Segmental Chromosome Aberrations

Historically, individual chromosomal loci were analyzed using polymerase chain reaction or fluorescent in situ hybridization–based assays. Recent studies using techniques that assess the whole genome, such as comparative genome hybridization and SNP arrays, demonstrate that it is the genomic pattern and not individual losses/gains that is most prognostic. Tumors with numerical chromosomal abnormalities (NCAs) characterized by whole chromosome gains and losses have an excellent outcome, even in patients greater than 18 mo. In contrast, patients with segmental chromosome aberrations (SCA), characterized by gains and losses of smaller fragments, have an inferior outcome.[102,103] SCAs may be a particularly strong predictor of poor outcome in infants with locally unresectable or metastatic non-*MYCN* amplified tumors.[104] Prospective trials in North America and Europe will determine whether the presence of SCAs ($\geq$1 of the following: segmental loss at 1p, 3p, 4p, 11q or gain at 1q, 2p, or 17q) can distinguish less favorable subsets of patients within the non-HR groups of patients and potentially replace tests that detect single gene losses/gains.

DNA Content

Ploidy or tumor DNA content (chromosome number) is a powerful predictor of survival. Hyperdiploid tumors (DNA index >1) with an increased amount of DNA in comparison with diploid tumors (DNA index = 1) are associated with a more favorable prognosis.[105,106] Ploidy is most prognostic in infants and patients with localized disease[74,107] and has been used prospectively to inform risk assignment and tailor therapy for patients with non-HR NB.[108]

Somatic Gene Mutations

Recently, next-generation sequencing approaches have revealed that, in contrast to adult carcinomas, there is a striking lack of recurrent NB tumor (somatic) mutations.[109–112] The most commonly mutated gene is *ALK* (8%–10%), with an additional 3% harboring *ALK* amplification.[10] *ALK* genomic aberrations are detected in all risk groups and are associated with an adverse outcome,[33] and high levels of ALK protein or amplification may correlate with poor outcomes independent of mutation status.[32,113,114] Mutations in *ATRX* (alpha thalassemia/mental retardation syndrome X linked), which is involved in telomere maintenance, are detected more frequently in older patients with NB.[112] Deletions and point mutations of the chromatin remodeling proteins AT-rich interactive domain 1A and B (*ARID1a/1b*) were detected in 11% of tumors.[111] Other mutations detected in less than 5% of tumors include *MYCN, TP53, PTPN11*, and genes involved in Ras/MAPK signaling. Current studies are exploring whether mutations may be more common at recurrence[115] and whether epigenetic regulation of transcription and genomic organization, which has recently been reported to be involved in the medulloblastoma,[116] may be playing similar roles in NB.

Molecular Factors and Expression Signatures

Because recurrent mutations are not frequent in NB, the identification of genes and signaling pathways with altered expression have also been used to discover additional prognostic factors and therapeutic targets involved in NB differentiation, apoptosis, drug resistance, angiogenesis, metastasis, and inflammation. Extensive reviews of these molecular factors have been the subject of several recent reviews,[49,117,118] and a subset of the most well studied are included later.

Neurotrophin signaling has central roles in normal neuronal cell development, and the clinical and biological roles of TRK receptors (NTRK1, 2, 3 encoding TrkA, B, C) and their ligands (NGF, BDNF, and NT-3) have been extensively studied in NB (reviewed in Ref.[119]). TrkA expression is highest in tumors with favorable biological characteristics and outcomes, and TrkA induces apoptosis and/or differentiation in vitro. TrkA signaling has been implicated in mediating spontaneous regression that is often observed in infants with localized or stage 4S disease.[120] In contrast, TrkB has pro-proliferative and migratory properties, enhances chemoresistance, and is highly expressed in biologically unfavorable *MYCNA* NB. Although the TrkB inhibitor lestaurtinib did not show efficacy in a phase 1 trial,[121] trks and proteins involved in neural crest development and differentiation pathways may still represent potential therapeutic targets.

Disruption of proteins involved in apoptotic pathways, including multidrug-resistance proteins, such as MDR-1, bcl-2 family proteins, caspase-8, mTOR/PI3 kinase, and TP53/HDM2, have also been shown to play important roles in NB initiation and progression. There are many ongoing pre-clinical studies to determine the ability to pharmacologically target these pathways.[122–126] Many genes involved in NB, including *caspase 8* and the *RASSF1A* tumor suppressor, are inactivated by the promoter hypermethylation,[126–128] which contributes to resistance to apoptosis induced by many therapies. Demethylating agents, such as decitabine, have been tested in phase I studies.[129] Enhanced angiogenesis and high expression of proangiogenic factors, such as vascular endothelial growth factor and basic fibroblast growth factor are associated with more aggressive NB tumors; early phase clinical trials of drugs that block these pathways have been completed.[130–132]

Rather than focusing on specific candidate genes, several investigators have identified multigene expression profiles that predict outcome and may lead to further refinement of risk categories. One large study demonstrated that the expression of 59 genes was an independent predictor of outcome, even after controlling for currently used risk factors, with an odds ratio of 19.3 for OS and 3.96 for progression-free survival.[133] Additional retrospective studies have identified other multigene classifiers (ranging from 3 to >50 genes).[134–138] Although most of these signatures have not been studied in specific NB risk groups, Asgharzadah and colleagues[139,140] recently demonstrated that a 14-gene classifier can be used to specifically identify subsets of HR patients with the worst prognosis. Many of these signatures include genes implicated in NB pathogenesis, neural development, and inflammation/immune response. Recent reports also demonstrate prognostic profiles of microRNAs, small 22 to 25 nucleotide RNAs that inhibit protein translation or target mRNA degradation[141–143] (reviewed in Ref.[144]).

MANAGEMENT GOALS

Diagnosis and therapy requires a multidisciplinary approach. Surgical biopsy is usually required to assess tumor genetic and histologic features and is most critical for patients less than 18 months of age with metastatic disease and those with localized unresectable tumors. The improved understanding of NB biology and its impact on prognosis has resulted in successful tailoring based on risk stratification (low risk, IR, and HR) using many of the pretreatment clinical and biological risk factors discussed earlier (see **Box 4**, **Table 2**). The requirements for further surgical resection, chemotherapy, radiotherapy and/or immunotherapy is based on the patients' specific risk category (**Table 3**) and, in part, response as outlined in the International Neuroblastoma Response Criteria, which is currently under revision. When possible, exposure to chemotherapy is limited for patients with regional disease, whereas radiotherapy is limited to those with advanced disease with unfavorable characteristics.

Low Risk

Survival rates for patients with INSS stage 1 disease, regardless of biological factors, are excellent with surgery alone and rare recurrences can often be cured with salvage chemotherapy.[145,146] Similarly, chemotherapy can be omitted for most patients with biologically favorable but incompletely resected localized tumors (INSS 2A, 2B), with survival rates greater than 95%.[82,146–148] In general, for patients with INSS stage 1, 2A, and 2B (mostly INRG stage L1), chemotherapy is reserved for patients with localized NB who have life- or organ-threatening symptoms or the minority of patients who experience recurrence or progressive disease.

Because previous infant screening studies[15,16,149–151] and European trials[152,153] have suggested that subsets of biologically favorable NB can spontaneously differentiate and regress, a recent COG trial (ANBL00P2) studied whether infants less than 6 months of age with small localized adrenal masses (including those detected by prenatal ultrasound) could be observed without biopsy, surgery, or chemotherapy.[154] Eighty-one percent of patients demonstrated spontaneous regression without surgical intervention; the 3-year EFS and OS were 97% and 100%, respectively.

Like many localized tumors in infants, most of stage 4S NB without MYCNA undergo spontaneous regression.[59,155] Chemotherapy or low-dose radiotherapy is reserved for symptoms of large tumors or massive hepatomegaly causing mechanical obstruction, respiratory distress, and/or liver dysfunction and should be initiated as soon as possible to prevent the morbidity and mortality frequently associated with this form of the disease, especially in very young infants.[105,156,157]

Overall, these data support continued reduction of chemotherapy exposure and surgery for most low risk asymptomatic patients, while strategies to improve survival for the rare subsets of non-HR patients with unfavorable pathology or biology (eg,

Table 3
Treatment strategies based on risk group (COG)

	Low (40%)	IR (20%)	HR (40%)
Survival (EFS)	>95	80–95	40–50
Patient/tumor characteristics	• Localized, resectable tumors	• Localized unresectable • Infants with metastases (no MYCNA)	• Metastases >18 mo • Unresectable with unfavorable biology (eg, MYCNA)
Treatment	Observation OR surgery (chemotherapy only for symptoms (eg, stage 4S or cord compression))	Chemotherapy (2–8 cycles based on biology), surgery	Chemotherapy, surgery, radiation, myeloablative therapy with autologous stem cell rescue, immunotherapy and biological agents (isotretinoin)

Summarized are general treatment strategies and characteristics for each risk group based on recent COG trials. This chart includes the most common characteristics for each group and overall treatment strategies. These treatments may vary across different cooperative groups internationally and change based on ongoing and future clinical trials. The approximate relative proportion of patients in each risk group is based on data from the COG ANBL00B1 Biology Study (since 2001).[64]

diploid tumors with SCAs)[82,158] are being examined in prospective SIOPEN and COG trials.[64]

Intermediate Risk

IR classification encompasses a wide spectrum of disease for which surgical resection and moderate-dose multiagent chemotherapy are the backbone of most regimens. IR includes subsets of patients with INSS stage 3 (mostly INRG L2) disease and infants with stage 4/M disease with favorable biological features. Survival following surgical resection and moderate-dose chemotherapy, including carboplatin or cisplatin, doxorubicin, etoposide, and cyclophosphamide, is greater than 90% for children whose tumors exhibit favorable characteristics, including infants with stage 4/M who lack *MYCNA*.[159–161] These high survival rates were maintained in 2 prospective COG IR trials in which therapy was reduced further based on histology, ploidy, and 1p and 11qLOH status.[108,157] Small series have suggested that IR patients with localized NB with favorable biology can be observed without chemotherapy.[153,162] Ongoing prospective international trials will determine whether SCA status can be used to refine treatment assignment to further reduce, and in some cases eliminate, therapy for most IR patients with favorable histology and genomics.

High Risk

Outcome of HR patients (mainly stage 4 > 18 months of age and stage 3 *MYCNA* or stage 3 > 18 months with unfavorable histology tumors) remains poor despite improvements in survival (**Fig. 5**).[163–168] Standard HR therapy involves 3 components: (1) induction chemotherapy and local control, (2) consolidation, and (3) postconsolidation/maintenance. These regimens have evolved significantly over the past 20 years based on work by several international cooperative groups and smaller cohort studies summarized later.

Induction therapy

There is a correlation between survival and end-of-induction response[63,169]; despite chemotherapy dose intensification, approximately 20% of patient will progress or have inadequate response to induction therapy. Standard North American (COG) induction regimens include combinations of anthracyclines, alkylators, platinum compounds, and topoisomerase II inhibitors delivered every 21 days for 5 to 7 cycles. SIOPEN uses a rapid regimen whereby cycles are delivered every 10 days based on results that demonstrated superior 5-year EFS of 30%, compared with 18% for standard interval chemotherapy.[165] The topoisomerase I inhibitor topotecan, which has demonstrated efficacy in recurrent NB,[170] has recently been incorporated into COG induction regimens.[64,171]

Local control

Optimal local control is achieved with a combination of aggressive surgical resection and external beam radiotherapy to the primary tumor. Surgery of the primary and bulky metastatic disease is usually delayed until after 4 to 6 cycles of chemotherapy to improve resectability and minimize complications[172]; however, there are conflicting reports as to whether complete primary tumor resection impacts patient outcomes in HR NB.[173–176]

NB is one of the most radiosensitive pediatric solid tumors, and doses of 2160 cGy in daily 180 cGY fractions to the primary sites decrease local recurrence rates for HR patients.[177,178] A recently completed prospective COG trial will determine whether higher radiation doses delivered to incompletely resected tumors improves local control rates. Radiation is also often delivered to residual MIBG-avid metastatic sites, and

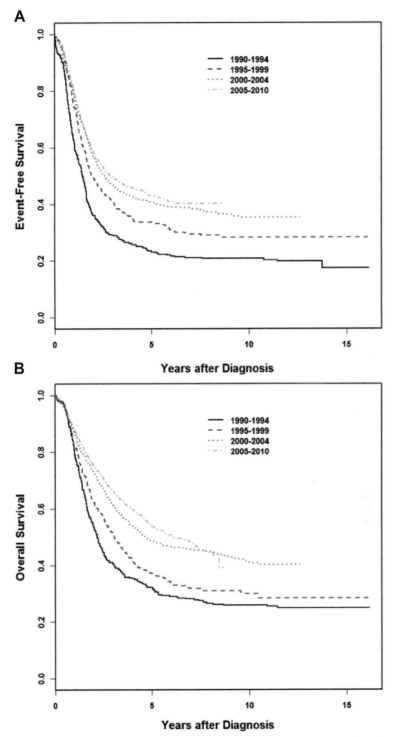

Fig. 5. Survival for HR patients with NB based on treatment era. The EFS (*A*) and OS (*B*) Kaplan-Meier survival curves calculated from the time of diagnosis for children enrolled onto COG (since 2001) and Children's Cancer Group and Pediatric Oncology Group Neuro-blastoma Biology trials between 1990 and 2010 (N = 3389) shown in 5-year intervals, beginning in 1990. (*With permission from* Children's Oncology Group Statistical Data Center.)

a recent report suggests that nonirradiated lesions have a higher likelihood of involvement at the time of first relapse.[179]

Myeloablative consolidation therapy

Over the past 2 decades, several clinical trials performed in Germany, Europe, and North America demonstrated improved outcomes following myeloablative therapy (MAT) with autologous bone marrow or, more recently, autologous peripheral blood stem cell rescue as compared with maintenance chemotherapy or observation.[167,169,180,181] These data together with a recent Cochrane systems meta-analysis suggest that MAT has resulted in improvements in EFS.[182] Recent and ongoing trials are aimed at identifying the optimal intensity and chemotherapy combinations for MAT regimens. Preliminary SIOPEN results suggest that patients randomized to a Busulfan-Melphalan (Bu-Mel) regimen had outcomes superior to those who received carboplatin-etoposide-melphalan.[175] Before adoption of Bu-Mel, the COG and other groups are examining the efficacy and toxicities of Bu-Mel MAT in combination with different induction regimens and postconsolidation immunotherapy.[64] In addition, data will soon be available from COG study ANBL0532, which randomized patients to single and tandem MAT and was based on a limited institution tandem MAT study with 3- and 5-year EFS rates of 55% and 47%.[183] Future trials will also aim to identify those at highest risk for recurrence and assess whether additional therapies during induction or consolidation improve their outcome.[64]

Postconsolidation biologic and immunotherapies

Initial results from CCG-3891 demonstrated efficacy for the synthetic retinoid isotretinoin [cis-retinoic acid (cis-RA)] in treating minimal residual NB after MAT and established a standard for the use of noncytotoxic differentiation therapy for minimal residual disease.[164] A recent randomized-controlled trial led by Yu and colleagues[166] demonstrated that the addition of the anti-GD2 chimeric monoclonal antibody (mAb) in conjunction with cytokines (granulocyte-macrophage colony-stimulation factor and interleukin 2) improved survival, establishing a role for immunotherapy in the standard treatment of HR patients. Additional studies have shown efficacy for different anti-GD2 regimens at diagnosis and recurrence.[184,185] Future immunotherapy regimens are aimed at determining the importance of cytokines and mAb and examining biomarkers that may predict which patients are most likely to respond favorably to this regimen, which has many side effects, including allergic reactions, fever, hypotension, capillary leak syndrome, and pain (caused by cross-reactivity with GD2 expressed on peripheral nerve cells). Early phase trials are also examining different antibodies and addition of immunomodulators (see "Recurrence" section).

LATE EFFECTS

There are few comprehensive reports of the prevalence of long-term effects in NB survivors, in part because of the poor prognosis for HR NB. Late effects are generally related to chemotherapy/radiation dose intensities, with the highest toxicities in patients who underwent MAT.[186–190] Recent pharmacogenomic studies have begun to identify germline variants or SNPs that may predict which patients are most susceptible to specific chemotherapy toxicities.[191] Ototoxicity, renal dysfunction, and endocrine late effects, including hypothyroidism, ovarian dysfunction and infertility, have been detected in most HR patients with NB.[186] Secondary cancers, most commonly myelodysplastic syndrome and acute myelogenous leukemia, have been reported in 1% to 8% of patients enrolled on trials and small series of NB survivors[187,192,193] and have been attributed to etoposide exposure, radiation, high-dose MIBG, and other agents. In addition to hematopoietic malignancies, solid tumors of the thyroid, bone, and kidney have been reported. Patients may also have effects related to tumor location, such as visual impairment caused by orbital metastases and neurologic complications or scoliosis following spinal cord compression.[194,195]

RECURRENCE

Despite recent advances, greater than 50% of patients with HR NB experience tumor recurrence. Although there are no proven curative therapies, some patients achieve prolonged survival even after multiple relapses. In the INRG database, low/IR patients with NB who relapsed had an OS of 65% 5 years after recurrence, whereas for those with metastatic disease, 5-year OS was 8%.[96] Thus, research into novel therapies is a high priority and has been the subject of several recent reviews.[117,196,197]

Relapse strategies can be divided into chemotherapies, MIBG/radioisotopes, immunotherapies, and targeted therapies. Current phase I and II trials often involve combinations of these approaches. Cytotoxic chemotherapies commonly used for relapse include topotecan or irinotecan-based regimens[170,198–200] as well as ifosfamide, carboplatin, etoposide[201] and often result in transient responses or stable disease but poor long-term survival. Iodide-131- MIBG, which targets high doses of radiation to NB cells, is the most effective single agent for relapsed NB, with response rates greater than 30%.[202–205] Current MIBG trials will determine the efficacy of concurrent radiosensitizing chemotherapies and feasibility of delivering MIBG followed by MAT to potentially incorporate MIBG into upfront therapy for HR NB.[64]

Building on the success of anti-GD2 mAbs, novel approaches to enhance mAb efficacy, such as the addition of lenolidomide,[206] which activates natural killer cells, and active immunization with anti-idiotype antibodies, are being studied in relapsed patients.[207] Among the most promising phase I trials are those that use a patient's own cytotoxic T cells (CTLs) that can be redirected against tumor-associated antigens (eg, GD2, L1CAM). Autologous CTLs engineered to overexpress chimeric antigen receptors are infused and have been shown to persist and demonstrate antitumor activity in patients with NB.[208–211]

There are several potential targets, and respective inhibitors, for recurrent NB based on preclinical and, in certain cases, phase I trials. A subset of ALK aberrant tumors can be targeted with crizotinib, and trials with second-generation ALK inhibitors and combinations with chemotherapy are underway.[37,92,212] For patients with *MYCNA*, preclinical studies suggest that bromodomain and extraterminal domain (BET) inhibitors can induce cell death by interfering with *MYCN* transcription.[91] Other drugs that have effects on MYCN stability (aurora kinase A and mTOR inhibitors)[213] as well as those that target MYC-dependent metabolic changes[214] are being studied. There is significant interest in drugs, such as histone deacetylase inhibitors, that are less targeted and instead modulate the expression of many genes to induce death, differentiation, and enhance the response to chemotherapies in NB cells.[215] Other drugs targeting cell cycle (eg, Chk1, Wee-1, CDK4/6), angiogenesis, and differentiation are also under investigation.[196]

Current trial designs for patients with relapsed NB have incorporated novel approaches, such as *pick the winner* whereby patients are randomized to receive different novel agents in combination with a common chemotherapy backbone regimens. In addition, many early phase NB trials will incorporate precision medicine by tailoring treatment based on individual patient tumor aberrations. These studies will increasingly depend on genomic and molecular studies of tumors, particularly at the time of relapse, when mutations may be more common.[216]

FUTURE DIRECTIONS

NB is a heterogeneous tumor for which molecular and genetic determinants affect clinical behavior. Further advances in the understanding of aberrantly expressed genes and pathways will continue to inform and refine risk stratification and treatment and identify novel therapeutic targets. For patients with low risk and IR NB, these genetic factors will help to identify rare patients who still require treatment as we continue to reduce exposures to chemotherapy and surgery for most non-HR patients. In contrast, for HR patients, we need to better predict those at greatest risk of treatment failure or recurrence, either at diagnosis (eg, genetic signatures) or based on their response to treatment (eg, persistent MIBG positive metastases). Furthermore, molecular and genetic studies of tumors at the time of recurrence will be required to specifically identify targets in this chemoresistant population. International collaborations, including INRG databases, are critical for the development of risk stratification and response classifications as well as advances in basic and translational studies, especially for rare populations (eg 4S, OMS). Future studies will move toward more refined risk classifications and treatments based on individual tumor aberrations as well as more attention to survivors to better understand the extent and individual susceptibility to long-term side effects of our treatments.

REFERENCES

1. Ries L, Smith M, Gurney J, et al. Cancer incidence and survival among children and adolescents: United States SEER Program 1975–1995, National Cancer Institute, SEER Program. Bethesda (MD): NIH Pub; 1999. p. 99–4649.
2. Stiller CA, Parkin DM. International variations in the incidence of neuroblastoma. Int J Cancer 1992;52(4):538–43.
3. Heck JE, Ritz B, Hung RJ, et al. The epidemiology of neuroblastoma: a review. Paediatr Perinat Epidemiol 2009;23(2):125–43.
4. Spix C, Pastore G, Sankila R, et al. Neuroblastoma incidence and survival in European children (1978–1997): report from the automated childhood cancer information system project. Eur J Cancer 2006;42(13):2081–91.
5. London WB, Castleberry RP, Matthay KK, et al. Evidence for an age cutoff greater than 365 days for neuroblastoma risk group stratification in the Children's Oncology Group. J Clin Oncol 2005;23(27):6459–65.
6. Johnson KA, Aplenc R, Bagatell R. Survival by race among children with extracranial solid tumors in the United States between 1985 and 2005. Pediatr Blood Cancer 2011;56(3):425–31.
7. Henderson TO, Bhatia S, Pinto N, et al. Racial and ethnic disparities in risk and survival in children with neuroblastoma: a Children's Oncology Group study. J Clin Oncol 2011;29(1):76–82.
8. Pinto N, Cipkala DA, Ladd PE, et al. Treatment of two cases with refractory, metastatic intermediate-risk neuroblastoma with isotretinoin alone or observation. Pediatr Blood Cancer 2014;61(6):1104–6.
9. Zahm SH, Devesa SS. Childhood cancer: overview of incidence trends and environmental carcinogens. Environ Health Perspect 1995;103(Suppl 6): 177–84.
10. Connelly JM, Malkin MG. Environmental risk factors for brain tumors. Curr Neurol Neurosci Rep 2007;7(3):208–14.
11. Yamamoto K, Hayashi Y, Hanada R, et al. Mass screening and age-specific incidence of neuroblastoma in Saitama Prefecture, Japan. J Clin Oncol 1995;13(8): 2033–8.

12. Yamamoto K, Ohta S, Ito E, et al. Marginal decrease in mortality and marked increase in incidence as a result of neuroblastoma screening at 6 months of age: cohort study in seven prefectures in Japan. J Clin Oncol 2002;20(5):1209–14.

13. Hiyama E, Iehara T, Sugimoto T, et al. Effectiveness of screening for neuroblastoma at 6 months of age: a retrospective population-based cohort study. Lancet 2008;371(9619):1173–80.

14. Schilling FH, Spix C, Berthold F, et al. Neuroblastoma screening at one year of age. N Engl J Med 2002;346(14):1047–53.

15. Woods WG, Gao RN, Shuster JJ, et al. Screening of infants and mortality due to neuroblastoma. N Engl J Med 2002;346(14):1041–6.

16. Maris JM, Woods WG. Screening for neuroblastoma: a resurrected idea? Lancet 2008;371(9619):1142–3.

17. Shojaei-Brosseau T, Chompret A, Abel A, et al. Genetic epidemiology of neuroblastoma: a study of 426 cases at the Institut Gustave-Roussy in France. Pediatr Blood Cancer 2004;42(1):99–105.

18. Trochet D, Bourdeaut F, Janoueix-Lerosey I, et al. Germline mutations of the paired-like homeobox 2B (PHOX2B) gene in neuroblastoma. Am J Hum Genet 2004;74(4):761–4.

19. Rohrer T, Trachsel D, Engelcke G, et al. Congenital central hypoventilation syndrome associated with Hirschsprung's disease and neuroblastoma: case of multiple neurocristopathies. Pediatr Pulmonol 2002;33(1):71–6.

20. Mosse YP, Laudenslager M, Khazi D, et al. Germline PHOX2B mutation in hereditary neuroblastoma. Am J Hum Genet 2004;75(4):727–30.

21. Brems H, Beert E, de Ravel T, et al. Mechanisms in the pathogenesis of malignant tumours in neurofibromatosis type 1. Lancet Oncol 2009;10(5):508–15.

22. Clausen N, Andersson P, Tommerup N. Familial occurrence of neuroblastoma, von Recklinghausen's neurofibromatosis, Hirschsprung's agangliosis and jaw-winking syndrome. Acta Paediatr Scand 1989;78(5):736–41.

23. Longo L, Panza E, Schena F, et al. Genetic predisposition to familial neuroblastoma: identification of two novel genomic regions at 2p and 12p. Hum Hered 2007;63(3–4):205–11.

24. Tonini GP, McConville C, Cusano R, et al. Exclusion of candidate genes and chromosomal regions in familial neuroblastoma. Int J Mol Med 2001;7(1):85–9.

25. Maris JM, Kyemba SM, Rebbeck TR, et al. Familial predisposition to neuroblastoma does not map to chromosome band 1p36. Cancer Res 1996;56(15):3421–5.

26. Maris JM, Weiss MJ, Mosse Y, et al. Evidence for a hereditary neuroblastoma predisposition locus at chromosome 16p12-13. Cancer Res 2002;62(22):6651–8.

27. Mosse YP, Laudenslager M, Longo L, et al. Identification of ALK as a major familial neuroblastoma predisposition gene. Nature 2008;455(7215):930–5.

28. Janoueix-Lerosey I, Lequin D, Brugieres L, et al. Somatic and germline activating mutations of the ALK kinase receptor in neuroblastoma. Nature 2008;455(7215):967–70.

29. de Pontual L, Kettaneh D, Gordon CT, et al. Germline gain-of-function mutations of ALK disrupt central nervous system development. Hum Mutat 2011;32(3):272–6.

30. George RE, Sanda T, Hanna M, et al. Activating mutations in ALK provide a therapeutic target in neuroblastoma. Nature 2008;455(7215):975–8.

31. Chen Y, Takita J, Choi YL, et al. Oncogenic mutations of ALK kinase in neuroblastoma. Nature 2008;455(7215):971–4.

32. Schulte JH, Bachmann HS, Brockmeyer B, et al. High ALK receptor tyrosine kinase expression supersedes ALK mutation as a determining factor of an unfavorable phenotype in primary neuroblastoma. Clin Cancer Res 2011;17(15):5082–92.

33. Weiser DA, Bresler SC, Laudenslager M, et al. Stratification of patients with neuroblastoma for targeted ALK inhibitor therapy. J Clin Oncol 2011;29 [abstract: 9514].

34. Berry T, Luther W, Bhatnagar N, et al. The ALK (F1174L) mutation potentiates the oncogenic activity of MYCN in neuroblastoma. Cancer Cell 2012;22(1):117–30.

35. Heukamp LC, Thor T, Schramm A, et al. Targeted expression of mutated ALK induces neuroblastoma in transgenic mice. Sci Transl Med 2012;4(141):141ra191.

36. Zhu S, Lee JS, Guo F, et al. Activated ALK collaborates with MYCN in neuroblastoma pathogenesis. Cancer Cell 2012;21(3):362–73.

37. Mosse YP, Lim MS, Voss SD, et al. Safety and activity of crizotinib for paediatric patients with refractory solid tumours or anaplastic large-cell lymphoma: a children's oncology group phase 1 consortium study. Lancet Oncol 2013;14(6): 472–80.

38. DeBaun MR, Tucker MA. Risk of cancer during the first four years of life in children from The Beckwith-Wiedemann Syndrome Registry. J Pediatr 1998; 132(3 Pt 1):398–400.

39. Birch JM, Alston RD, McNally RJ, et al. Relative frequency and morphology of cancers in carriers of germline TP53 mutations. Oncogene 2001;20(34):4621–8.

40. Rossbach HC, Baschinsky D, Wynn T, et al. Composite adrenal anaplastic neuroblastoma and virilizing adrenocortical tumor with germline TP53 R248W mutation. Pediatr Blood Cancer 2008;50(3):681–3.

41. Bissig H, Staehelin F, Tolnay M, et al. Co-occurrence of neuroblastoma and nephroblastoma in an infant with Fanconi's anemia. Hum Pathol 2002;33(10): 1047–51.

42. Reid S, Schindler D, Hanenberg H, et al. Biallelic mutations in PALB2 cause Fanconi anemia subtype FA-N and predispose to childhood cancer. Nat Genet 2007;39(2):162–4.

43. Maris JM, Mosse YP, Bradfield JP, et al. Chromosome 6p22 locus associated with clinically aggressive neuroblastoma. N Engl J Med 2008;358(24):2585–93.

44. Diskin SJ, Capasso M, Schnepp RW, et al. Common variation at 6q16 within HACE1 and LIN28B influences susceptibility to neuroblastoma. Nat Genet 2012;44(10):1126–30.

45. Capasso M, Devoto M, Hou C, et al. Common variations in BARD1 influence susceptibility to high-risk neuroblastoma. Nat Genet 2009;41(6):718–23.

46. Diskin SJ, Hou C, Glessner JT, et al. Copy number variation at 1q21.1 associated with neuroblastoma. Nature 2009;459(7249):987–91.

47. Wang K, Diskin SJ, Zhang H, et al. Integrative genomics identifies LMO1 as a neuroblastoma oncogene. Nature 2011;469(7329):216–20.

48. Diskin SJ, Capasso M, Diamond M, et al. Rare variants in TP53 and susceptibility to neuroblastoma. J Natl Cancer Inst 2014;106(4):dju047.

49. Maris JM. Recent advances in neuroblastoma. N Engl J Med 2010;362(23): 2202–11.

50. Vo KT, Matthay KK, Neuhaus J, et al. Clinical, biological and prognostic differences based on primary tumor site in neuroblastoma: a report from the International Neuroblastoma Risk Group (INRG) project. J Clin Oncol 2014;32(28):3169–76.

51. De Bernardi B, Pianca C, Pistamiglio P, et al. Neuroblastoma with symptomatic spinal cord compression at diagnosis: treatment and results with 76 cases. J Clin Oncol 2001;19(1):183–90.

52. El Shafie M, Samuel D, Klippel CH, et al. Intractable diarrhea in children with VIP-secreting ganglioneuroblastomas. J Pediatr Surg 1983;18(1):34–6.
53. Scheibel E, Rechnitzer C, Fahrenkrug J, et al. Vasoactive intestinal polypeptide (VIP) in children with neural crest tumours. Acta Paediatr Scand 1982;71(5):721–5.
54. Matthay KK, Blaes F, Hero B, et al. Opsoclonus myoclonus syndrome in neuroblastoma a report from a workshop on the dancing eyes syndrome at the advances in neuroblastoma meeting in Genoa, Italy, 2004. Cancer Lett 2005;228(1–2):275–82.
55. Gorman MP. Update on diagnosis, treatment, and prognosis in opsoclonus-myoclonus-ataxia syndrome. Curr Opin Pediatr 2010;22(6):745–50.
56. Dubois SG, London WB, Zhang Y, et al. Lung metastases in neuroblastoma at initial diagnosis: a report from the International Neuroblastoma Risk Group (INRG) project. Pediatr Blood Cancer 2008;51(5):589–92.
57. Kramer K, Kushner B, Heller G, et al. Neuroblastoma metastatic to the central nervous system. The Memorial Sloan-Kettering Cancer Center experience and a literature review. Cancer 2001;91(8):1510–9.
58. Matthay KK, Brisse H, Couanet D, et al. Central nervous system metastases in neuroblastoma: radiologic, clinical, and biologic features in 23 patients. Cancer 2003;98(1):155–65.
59. Evans AE, Chatten J, D'Angio GJ, et al. A review of 17 IV-S neuroblastoma patients at the Children's Hospital of Philadelphia. Cancer 1980;45(5):833–9.
60. Simon T, Hero B, Benz-Bohm G, et al. Review of image defined risk factors in localized neuroblastoma patients: results of the GPOH NB97 trial. Pediatr Blood Cancer 2008;50(5):965–9.
61. Cecchetto G, Mosseri V, De Bernardi B, et al. Surgical risk factors in primary surgery for localized neuroblastoma: the LNESG1 study of the European International Society of Pediatric Oncology Neuroblastoma Group. J Clin Oncol 2005;23(33):8483–9.
62. Messina JA, Cheng SC, Franc BL, et al. Evaluation of semi-quantitative scoring system for metaiodobenzylguanidine (mIBG) scans in patients with relapsed neuroblastoma. Pediatr Blood Cancer 2006;47(7):865–74.
63. Yanik GA, Parisi MT, Shulkin BL, et al. Semiquantitative mIBG scoring as a prognostic indicator in patients with stage 4 neuroblastoma: a report from the children's oncology group. J Nucl Med 2013;54(4):541–8.
64. Park JR, Bagatell R, London WB, et al. Children's Oncology Group's 2013 blueprint for research: neuroblastoma. Pediatr Blood Cancer 2013;60(6):985–93.
65. Sharp SE, Shulkin BL, Gelfand MJ, et al. 123I-MIBG scintigraphy and 18F-FDG PET in neuroblastoma. J Nucl Med 2009;50(8):1237–43.
66. Zhang H, Huang R, Cheung NK, et al. Imaging the norepinephrine transporter in neuroblastoma: a comparison of [18F]-MFBG and 123I-MIBG. Clin Cancer Res 2014;20(8):2182–91.
67. Taggart DR, Han MM, Quach A, et al. Comparison of iodine-123 metaiodobenzylguanidine (MIBG) scan and [18F]fluorodeoxyglucose positron emission tomography to evaluate response after iodine-131 MIBG therapy for relapsed neuroblastoma. J Clin Oncol 2009;27(32):5343–9.
68. Brodeur GM, Pritchard J, Berthold F, et al. Revisions of the international criteria for neuroblastoma diagnosis, staging, and response to treatment. J Clin Oncol 1993;11(8):1466–77.

69. Brodeur GM, Seeger RC, Barrett A, et al. International criteria for diagnosis, staging, and response to treatment in patients with neuroblastoma. J Clin Oncol 1988;6(12):1874–81.
70. Cohn SL, Pearson AD, London WB, et al. The International Neuroblastoma Risk Group (INRG) classification system: an INRG task force report. J Clin Oncol 2009;27(2):289–97.
71. Monclair T, Brodeur GM, Ambros PF, et al. The International Neuroblastoma Risk Group (INRG) staging system: an INRG task force report. J Clin Oncol 2009; 27(2):298–303.
72. Morgenstern DA, London WB, Stephens D, et al. Metastatic neuroblastoma confined to distant lymph nodes (stage 4N) predicts outcome in patients with stage 4 disease: a study from the International Neuroblastoma Risk Group Database. J Clin Oncol 2014;32(12):1228–35.
73. Hartmann O, Valteau-Couanet D, Vassal G, et al. Prognostic factors in metastatic neuroblastoma in patients over 1 year of age treated with high-dose chemotherapy and stem cell transplantation: a multivariate analysis in 218 patients treated in a single institution. Bone Marrow Transplant 1999;23(8): 789–95.
74. George RE, London WB, Cohn SL, et al. Hyperdiploidy plus nonamplified MYCN confers a favorable prognosis in children 12 to 18 months old with disseminated neuroblastoma: a pediatric oncology group study. J Clin Oncol 2005;23(27): 6466–73.
75. Schmidt ML, Lal A, Seeger RC, et al. Favorable prognosis for patients 12 to 18 months of age with stage 4 nonamplified MYCN neuroblastoma: a Children's Cancer Group study. J Clin Oncol 2005;23(27):6474–80.
76. Park JR, Villablanca JG, London WB, et al. Outcome of high-risk stage 3 neuroblastoma with myeloablative therapy and 13-cis-retinoic acid: a report from the children's oncology group. Pediatr Blood Cancer 2009;52(1):44–50.
77. Park JR, Eggert A, Caron H. Neuroblastoma: biology, prognosis, and treatment. Hematol Oncol Clin North Am 2010;24(1):65–86.
78. Mosse YP, Deyell RJ, Berthold F, et al. Neuroblastoma in older children, adolescents and young adults: a report from the International Neuroblastoma Risk Group project. Pediatr Blood Cancer 2014;61(4):627–35.
79. Shimada H, Chatten J, Newton WA Jr, et al. Histopathologic prognostic factors in neuroblastic tumors: definition of subtypes of ganglioneuroblastoma and an age-linked classification of neuroblastomas. J Natl Cancer Inst 1984;73(2):405–16.
80. Shimada H, Stram DO, Chatten J, et al. Identification of subsets of neuroblastomas by combined histopathologic and N-myc analysis. J Natl Cancer Inst 1995;87(19):1470–6.
81. Shimada H, Ambros IM, Dehner LP, et al. The International Neuroblastoma Pathology Classification (the Shimada system). Cancer 1999;86(2):364–72.
82. Strother DR, London WB, Schmidt ML, et al. Outcome after surgery alone or with restricted use of chemotherapy for patients with low-risk neuroblastoma: results of children's oncology group study P9641. J Clin Oncol 2012;30(15): 1842–8.
83. Ambros PF, Ambros IM, Brodeur GM, et al. International consensus for neuroblastoma molecular diagnostics: report from the International Neuroblastoma Risk Group (INRG) Biology Committee. Br J Cancer 2009;100(9):1471–82.
84. Seeger RC, Brodeur GM, Sather H, et al. Association of multiple copies of the N-myc oncogene with rapid progression of neuroblastomas. N Engl J Med 1985;313(18):1111–6.

85. Brodeur GM, Seeger RC, Schwab M, et al. Amplification of N-myc in untreated human neuroblastomas correlates with advanced disease stage. Science 1984; 224(4653):1121–4.
86. Huang M, Weiss WA. Neuroblastoma and MYCN. Cold Spring Harb Perspect Med 2013;3(10):a014415.
87. Maris JM, Hogarty MD, Bagatell R, et al. Neuroblastoma. Lancet 2007; 369(9579):2106–20.
88. Cohn SL, Look AT, Joshi VV, et al. Lack of correlation of N-myc gene amplification with prognosis in localized neuroblastoma: a Pediatric Oncology Group study. Cancer Res 1995;55(4):721–6.
89. Bagatell R, Beck-Popovic M, London WB, et al. Significance of MYCN amplification in international neuroblastoma staging system stage 1 and 2 neuroblastoma: a report from the International Neuroblastoma Risk Group database. J Clin Oncol 2009;27(3):365–70.
90. Weiss WA, Aldape K, Mohapatra G, et al. Targeted expression of MYCN causes neuroblastoma in transgenic mice. EMBO J 1997;16(11):2985–95.
91. Puissant A, Frumm SM, Alexe G, et al. Targeting MYCN in neuroblastoma by BET bromodomain inhibition. Cancer Discov 2013;3(3):308–23.
92. Carpenter EL, Mosse YP. Targeting ALK in neuroblastoma–preclinical and clinical advancements. Nat Rev Clin Oncol 2012;9(7):391–9.
93. Bown N, Cotterill S, Lastowska M, et al. Gain of chromosome arm 17q and adverse outcome in patients with neuroblastoma. N Engl J Med 1999;340(25): 1954–61.
94. Meddeb M, Danglot G, Chudoba I, et al. Additional copies of a 25 Mb chromosomal region originating from 17q23.1-17qter are present in 90% of high-grade neuroblastomas. Genes Chromosomes Cancer 1996;17(3):156–65.
95. Attiyeh EF, London WB, Mosse YP, et al. Chromosome 1p and 11q deletions and outcome in neuroblastoma. N Engl J Med 2005;353(21):2243–53.
96. Caron H, van Sluis P, de Kraker J, et al. Allelic loss of chromosome 1p as a predictor of unfavorable outcome in patients with neuroblastoma. N Engl J Med 1996;334(4):225–30.
97. Riley RD, Heney D, Jones DR, et al. A systematic review of molecular and biological tumor markers in neuroblastoma. Clin Cancer Res 2004;10(1 Pt 1):4–12.
98. Fujita T, Igarashi J, Okawa ER, et al. CHD5, a tumor suppressor gene deleted from 1p36.31 in neuroblastomas. J Natl Cancer Inst 2008;100(13):940–9.
99. Liu Z, Yang X, Li Z, et al. CASZ1, a candidate tumor-suppressor gene, suppresses neuroblastoma tumor growth through reprogramming gene expression. Cell Death Differ 2011;18(7):1174–83.
100. Guo C, White PS, Weiss MJ, et al. Allelic deletion at 11q23 is common in MYCN single copy neuroblastomas. Oncogene 1999;18(35):4948–57.
101. Nowacki S, Skowron M, Oberthuer A, et al. Expression of the tumour suppressor gene CADM1 is associated with favourable outcome and inhibits cell survival in neuroblastoma. Oncogene 2008;27(23):3329–38.
102. Janoueix-Lerosey I, Schleiermacher G, Michels E, et al. Overall genomic pattern is a predictor of outcome in neuroblastoma. J Clin Oncol 2009;27(7):1026–33.
103. Schleiermacher G, Mosseri V, London WB, et al. Segmental chromosomal alterations have prognostic impact in neuroblastoma: a report from the INRG project. Br J Cancer 2012;107(8):1418–22.
104. Schleiermacher G, Michon J, Huon I, et al. Chromosomal CGH identifies patients with a higher risk of relapse in neuroblastoma without MYCN amplification. Br J Cancer 2007;97(2):238–46.

105. Katzenstein HM, Bowman LC, Brodeur GM, et al. Prognostic significance of age, MYCN oncogene amplification, tumor cell ploidy, and histology in 110 infants with stage D(S) neuroblastoma: the Pediatric Oncology Group experience–a pediatric oncology group study. J Clin Oncol 1998;16(6):2007–17.

106. Look AT, Hayes FA, Shuster JJ, et al. Clinical relevance of tumor cell ploidy and N-myc gene amplification in childhood neuroblastoma: a Pediatric Oncology Group study. J Clin Oncol 1991;9(4):581–91.

107. Bowman LC, Castleberry RP, Cantor A, et al. Genetic staging of unresectable or metastatic neuroblastoma in infants: a Pediatric Oncology Group study. J Natl Cancer Inst 1997;89(5):373–80.

108. Baker DL, Schmidt ML, Cohn SL, et al. Outcome after reduced chemotherapy for intermediate-risk neuroblastoma. N Engl J Med 2010;363(14):1313–23.

109. Molenaar JJ, Koster J, Zwijnenburg DA, et al. Sequencing of neuroblastoma identifies chromothripsis and defects in neuritogenesis genes. Nature 2012; 483(7391):589–93.

110. Pugh TJ, Morozova O, Attiyeh EF, et al. The genetic landscape of high-risk neuroblastoma. Nat Genet 2013;45:279–84.

111. Sausen M, Leary RJ, Jones S, et al. Integrated genomic analyses identify ARID1A and ARID1B alterations in the childhood cancer neuroblastoma. Nat Genet 2013;45(1):12–7.

112. Cheung NK, Zhang J, Lu C, et al. Association of age at diagnosis and genetic mutations in patients with neuroblastoma. JAMA 2012;307(10):1062–71.

113. De Brouwer S, De Preter K, Kumps C, et al. Meta-analysis of neuroblastomas reveals a skewed ALK mutation spectrum in tumors with MYCN amplification. Clin Cancer Res 2010;16(17):4353–62.

114. Passoni L, Longo L, Collini P, et al. Mutation-independent anaplastic lymphoma kinase overexpression in poor prognosis neuroblastoma patients. Cancer Res 2009;69(18):7338–46.

115. Schleiermacher G, Javanmardi N, Bernard V, et al. Emergence of new ALK mutations at relapse of neuroblastoma. J Clin Oncol 2014;32:2727–34.

116. Hovestadt V, Jones DT, Picelli S, et al. Decoding the regulatory landscape of medulloblastoma using DNA methylation sequencing. Nature 2014;510(7506): 537–41.

117. Cole KA, Maris JM. New strategies in refractory and recurrent neuroblastoma: translational opportunities to impact patient outcome. Clin Cancer Res 2012; 18(9):2423–8.

118. Cheung NK, Dyer MA. Neuroblastoma: developmental biology, cancer genomics and immunotherapy. Nat Rev Cancer 2013;13(6):397–411.

119. Brodeur GM, Minturn JE, Ho R, et al. Trk receptor expression and inhibition in neuroblastomas. Clin Cancer Res 2009;15(10):3244–50.

120. Diede SJ. Spontaneous regression of metastatic cancer: learning from neuroblastoma. Nat Rev Cancer 2014;14(2):71–2.

121. Minturn JE, Evans AE, Villablanca JG, et al. Phase I trial of lestaurtinib for children with refractory neuroblastoma: a new approaches to neuroblastoma therapy consortium study. Cancer Chemother Pharmacol 2011;68(4):1057–65.

122. Pastorino F, Di Paolo D, Loi M, et al. Recent advances in targeted anti-vasculature therapy: the neuroblastoma model. Curr Drug Targets 2009; 10(10):1021–7.

123. Barone G, Tweddle DA, Shohet JM, et al. MDM2-p53 interaction in paediatric solid tumours: preclinical rationale, biomarkers and resistance. Curr Drug Targets 2014;15(1):114–23.

124. Goldsmith KC, Lestini BJ, Gross M, et al. BH3 response profiles from neuroblastoma mitochondria predict activity of small molecule Bcl-2 family antagonists. Cell Death Differ 2010;17(5):872–82.

125. Henderson MJ, Haber M, Porro A, et al. ABCC multidrug transporters in childhood neuroblastoma: clinical and biological effects independent of cytotoxic drug efflux. J Natl Cancer Inst 2011;103(16):1236–51.

126. Teitz T, Wei T, Valentine MB, et al. Caspase 8 is deleted or silenced preferentially in childhood neuroblastomas with amplification of MYCN. Nat Med 2000;6(5): 529–35.

127. Yang Q, Zage P, Kagan D, et al. Association of epigenetic inactivation of RASSF1A with poor outcome in human neuroblastoma. Clin Cancer Res 2004; 10(24):8493–500.

128. Astuti D, Agathanggelou A, Honorio S, et al. RASSF1A promoter region CpG island hypermethylation in phaeochromocytomas and neuroblastoma tumours. Oncogene 2001;20(51):7573–7.

129. George RE, Lahti JM, Adamson PC, et al. Phase I study of decitabine with doxorubicin and cyclophosphamide in children with neuroblastoma and other solid tumors: a children's oncology group study. Pediatr Blood Cancer 2010;55(4): 629–38.

130. Rossler J, Taylor M, Geoerger B, et al. Angiogenesis as a target in neuroblastoma. Eur J Cancer 2008;44(12):1645–56.

131. Glade Bender J, Yamashiro DJ, Fox E. Clinical development of VEGF signaling pathway inhibitors in childhood solid tumors. Oncologist 2011;16(11):1614–25.

132. Glade Bender J, Blaney SM, Borinstein S, et al. A phase I trial and pharmacokinetic study of aflibercept (VEGF Trap) in children with refractory solid tumors: a children's oncology group phase I consortium report. Clin Cancer Res 2012; 18(18):5081–9.

133. Vermeulen J, De Preter K, Naranjo A, et al. Predicting outcomes for children with neuroblastoma using a multigene-expression signature: a retrospective SIOPEN/COG/GPOH study. Lancet Oncol 2009;10(7):663–71.

134. De Preter K, Vermeulen J, Brors B, et al. Accurate outcome prediction in neuroblastoma across independent data sets using a multigene signature. Clin Cancer Res 2010;16(5):1532–41.

135. Oberthuer A, Berthold F, Warnat P, et al. Customized oligonucleotide microarray gene expression-based classification of neuroblastoma patients outperforms current clinical risk stratification. J Clin Oncol 2006;24(31):5070–8.

136. Oberthuer A, Hero B, Berthold F, et al. Prognostic impact of gene expression-based classification for neuroblastoma. J Clin Oncol 2010;28(21):3506–15.

137. Garcia I, Mayol G, Rios J, et al. A three-gene expression signature model for risk stratification of patients with neuroblastoma. Clin Cancer Res 2012;18(7):2012–23.

138. Stricker TP, Morales La Madrid A, Chlenski A, et al. Validation of a prognostic multi-gene signature in high-risk neuroblastoma using the high throughput digital NanoString nCounter system. Mol Oncol 2014;8(3):669–78.

139. Asgharzadeh S, Pique-Regi R, Sposto R, et al. Prognostic significance of gene expression profiles of metastatic neuroblastomas lacking MYCN gene amplification. J Natl Cancer Inst 2006;98(17):1193–203.

140. Asgharzadeh S, Salo JA, Ji L, et al. Clinical significance of tumor-associated inflammatory cells in metastatic neuroblastoma. J Clin Oncol 2012;30(28):3525–32.

141. Buckley PG, Alcock L, Bryan K, et al. Chromosomal and microRNA expression patterns reveal biologically distinct subgroups of 11q- neuroblastoma. Clin Cancer Res 2010;16(11):2971–8.

142. Chen Y, Stallings RL. Differential patterns of microRNA expression in neuroblastoma are correlated with prognosis, differentiation, and apoptosis. Cancer Res 2007;67(3):976–83.
143. De Preter K, Mestdagh P, Vermeulen J, et al. miRNA expression profiling enables risk stratification in archived and fresh neuroblastoma tumor samples. Clin Cancer Res 2011;17(24):7684–92.
144. Buechner J, Einvik C. N-myc and noncoding RNAs in neuroblastoma. Mol Cancer Res 2012;10(10):1243–53.
145. Alvarado CS, London WB, Look AT, et al. Natural history and biology of stage A neuroblastoma: a Pediatric Oncology Group study. J Pediatr Hematol Oncol 2000;22(3):197–205.
146. Perez CA, Matthay KK, Atkinson JB, et al. Biologic variables in the outcome of stages I and II neuroblastoma treated with surgery as primary therapy: a Children's Cancer Group study. J Clin Oncol 2000;18(1):18–26.
147. Simon T, Spitz R, Faldum A, et al. New definition of low-risk neuroblastoma using stage, age, and 1p and MYCN status. J Pediatr Hematol Oncol 2004;26(12): 791–6.
148. Simon T, Spitz R, Hero B, et al. Risk estimation in localized unresectable single copy MYCN neuroblastoma by the status of chromosomes 1p and 11q. Cancer Lett 2006;237(2):215–22.
149. Yamamoto K, Hanada R, Kikuchi A, et al. Spontaneous regression of localized neuroblastoma detected by mass screening. J Clin Oncol 1998; 16(4):1265–9.
150. Woods WG, Tuchman M, Robison LL, et al. A population-based study of the usefulness of screening for neuroblastoma. Lancet 1996;348(9043): 1682–7.
151. Oue T, Inoue M, Yoneda A, et al. Profile of neuroblastoma detected by mass screening, resected after observation without treatment: results of the wait and see pilot study. J Pediatr Surg 2005;40(2):359–63.
152. Rubie H, De Bernardi B, Gerrard M, et al. Excellent outcome with reduced treatment in infants with nonmetastatic and unresectable neuroblastoma without MYCN amplification: results of the prospective INES 99.1. J Clin Oncol 2011; 29(4):449–55.
153. Hero B, Simon T, Spitz R, et al. Localized infant neuroblastomas often show spontaneous regression: results of the prospective trials NB95-S and NB97. J Clin Oncol 2008;26(9):1504–10.
154. Nuchtern JG, London WB, Barnewolt CE, et al. A prospective study of expectant observation as primary therapy for neuroblastoma in young infants: a children's oncology group study. Ann Surg 2012;256(4):573–80.
155. D'Angio GJ, Evans AE, Koop CE. Special pattern of widespread neuroblastoma with a favourable prognosis. Lancet 1971;1(7708):1046–9.
156. Nickerson HJ, Matthay KK, Seeger RC, et al. Favorable biology and outcome of stage IV-S neuroblastoma with supportive care or minimal therapy: a Children's Cancer Group study. J Clin Oncol 2000;18(3):477–86.
157. Twist C, London WB, Naranjo AN, et al. Maintaining outstanding outcomes using response- and biology-based therapy for intermediate-risk neuroblastoma: a report from the Children's Oncology Group study ANBL0531. J Clin Oncol 2014;32:5s [suppl; abstract: 10006].
158. De Bernardi B, Mosseri V, Rubie H, et al. Treatment of localised resectable neuroblastoma. Results of the LNESG1 study by the SIOP Europe Neuroblastoma Group. Br J Cancer 2008;99(7):1027–33.

159. Matthay KK, Perez C, Seeger RC, et al. Successful treatment of stage III neuro-blastoma based on prospective biologic staging: a Children's Cancer Group study. J Clin Oncol 1998;16(4):1256–64.

160. Schmidt ML, Lukens JN, Seeger RC, et al. Biologic factors determine prognosis in infants with stage IV neuroblastoma: a prospective Children's Cancer Group study. J Clin Oncol 2000;18(6):1260–8.

161. Meany HJ, London WB, Ambros PF, et al. Significance of clinical and biologic features in Stage 3 neuroblastoma: a report from the International Neuroblas-toma Risk Group Project. Pediatr Blood Cancer 2014;61:1932–9.

162. Kushner BH, Cheung NK, LaQuaglia MP, et al. Survival from locally invasive or widespread neuroblastoma without cytotoxic therapy. J Clin Oncol 1996;14(2): 373–81.

163. Ladernstein RL, Poetschger U, Luksch R, et al. Busulfan-melphalan as a mye-loablative therapy (MAT) for high risk neuroblastoma: results from the HR-NBL1/SIOPEN trial. ASCO Annual Meeting Proceedings. J Clin Oncol 2011;29 [abstract: 2].

164. Matthay KK, Reynolds CP, Seeger RC, et al. Long-term results for children with high-risk neuroblastoma treated on a randomized trial of myeloablative therapy followed by 13-cis-retinoic acid: a Children's Oncology Group study. J Clin Oncol 2009;27(7):1007–13 [Erratum appears in J Clin Oncol 2014;32:1862–3].

165. Pearson AD, Pinkerton CR, Lewis IJ, et al. High-dose rapid and standard induc-tion chemotherapy for patients aged over 1 year with stage 4 neuroblastoma: a randomised trial. Lancet Oncol 2008;9(3):247–56.

166. Yu AL, Gilman AL, Ozkaynak MF, et al. Anti-GD2 antibody with GM-CSF, inter-leukin-2, and isotretinoin for neuroblastoma. N Engl J Med 2010;363(14): 1324–34.

167. Berthold F, Boos J, Burdach S, et al. Myeloablative megatherapy with autolo-gous stem-cell rescue versus oral maintenance chemotherapy as consolidation treatment in patients with high-risk neuroblastoma: a randomised controlled trial. Lancet Oncol 2005;6(9):649–58.

168. Kreissman SG, Seeger RC, Matthay KK, et al. Purged versus non-purged peripheral blood stem-cell transplantation for high-risk neuroblastoma (COG A3973): a randomised phase 3 trial. Lancet Oncol 2013;14(10):999–1008.

169. Matthay KK, Villablanca JG, Seeger RC, et al. Treatment of high-risk neuroblas-toma with intensive chemotherapy, radiotherapy, autologous bone marrow trans-plantation, and 13-cis-retinoic acid. Children's Cancer Group. N Engl J Med 1999;341(16):1165–73.

170. London WB, Frantz CN, Campbell LA, et al. Phase II randomized comparison of topotecan plus cyclophosphamide versus topotecan alone in children with recurrent or refractory neuroblastoma: a Children's Oncology Group study. J Clin Oncol 2010;28(24):3808–15.

171. Park JR, Scott JR, Stewart CF, et al. Pilot induction regimen incorporating phar-macokinetically guided topotecan for treatment of newly diagnosed high-risk neuroblastoma: a Children's Oncology Group study. J Clin Oncol 2011;29(33): 4351–7.

172. Adkins ES, Sawin R, Gerbing RB, et al. Efficacy of complete resection for high-risk neuroblastoma: a Children's Cancer Group study. J Pediatr Surg 2004; 39(6):931–6.

173. Zwaveling S, Tytgat GA, van der Zee DC, et al. Is complete surgical resection of stage 4 neuroblastoma a prerequisite for optimal survival or may >95 % tumour resection suffice? Pediatr Surg Int 2012;28(10):953–9.

174. Simon T, Haberle B, Hero B, et al. Role of surgery in the treatment of patients with stage 4 neuroblastoma age 18 months or older at diagnosis. J Clin Oncol 2013;31(6):752–8.

175. Holmes K, ASarnacki S, Poetschger U, et al. Influence of surgical excision on survival of patients with high risk neuroblastoma: report from Study 1 of SIOPEN. Advances in Neuroblastoma Research Meeting, May 15, 2014. Cologne, 2014; PL-012.

176. Von Allmen D, Davidoff A, London WB, et al. Influence of extent of resection on survival in high risk neuroblasotma: report from COG A3793 Study. Advances in Neuroblastoma Research Meeting, May 15, 2014. Cologne, 2014. 2014; OR-067.

177. Haas-Kogan DA, Swift PS, Selch M, et al. Impact of radiotherapy for high-risk neuroblastoma: a Children's Cancer Group study. Int J Radiat Oncol Biol Phys 2003;56(1):28–39.

178. Kushner BH, Wolden S, LaQuaglia MP, et al. Hyperfractionated low-dose radiotherapy for high-risk neuroblastoma after intensive chemotherapy and surgery. J Clin Oncol 2001;19(11):2821–8.

179. Polishchuk AL, Li R, Hill-Kayser C, et al. Likelihood of bone recurrence in prior sites of metastasis in patients with high-risk neuroblastoma. Int J Radiat Oncol Biol Phys 2014;89(4):839–45.

180. Ladenstein R, Potschger U, Hartman O, et al. 28 years of high-dose therapy and SCT for neuroblastoma in Europe: lessons from more than 4000 procedures. Bone Marrow Transplant 2008;41(Suppl 2):S118–27.

181. Pritchard J, Cotterill SJ, Germond SM, et al. High dose melphalan in the treatment of advanced neuroblastoma: results of a randomised trial (ENSG-1) by the European Neuroblastoma Study Group. Pediatr Blood Cancer 2005;44(4):348–57.

182. Yalcin B, Kremer LC, Caron HN, et al. High-dose chemotherapy and autologous haematopoietic stem cell rescue for children with high-risk neuroblastoma. Cochrane Database Syst Rev 2013;(8):CD006301.

183. George RE, Li S, Medeiros-Nancarrow C, et al. High-risk neuroblastoma treated with tandem autologous peripheral-blood stem cell-supported transplantation: long-term survival update. J Clin Oncol 2006;24(18):2891–6.

184. Simon T, Hero B, Faldum A, et al. Long term outcome of high-risk neuroblastoma patients after immunotherapy with antibody ch14.18 or oral metronomic chemotherapy. BMC Cancer 2011;11:21.

185. Cheung NK, Cheung IY, Kushner BH, et al. Murine anti-GD2 monoclonal antibody 3F8 combined with granulocyte-macrophage colony-stimulating factor and 13-cis-retinoic acid in high-risk patients with stage 4 neuroblastoma in first remission. J Clin Oncol 2012;30(26):3264–70.

186. Cohen LE, Gordon JH, Popovsky EY, et al. Late effects in children treated with intensive multimodal therapy for high-risk neuroblastoma: high incidence of endocrine and growth problems. Bone Marrow Transplant 2014;49(4):502–8.

187. Laverdiere C, Liu Q, Yasui Y, et al. Long-term outcomes in survivors of neuroblastoma: a report from the Childhood Cancer Survivor Study. J Natl Cancer Inst 2009;101(16):1131–40.

188. Moreno L, Vaidya SJ, Pinkerton CR, et al. Long-term follow-up of children with high-risk neuroblastoma: the ENSG5 trial experience. Pediatr Blood Cancer 2013;60(7):1135–40.

189. Perwein T, Lackner H, Sovinz P, et al. Survival and late effects in children with stage 4 neuroblastoma. Pediatr Blood Cancer 2011;57(4):629–35.

190. Trahair TN, Vowels MR, Johnston K, et al. Long-term outcomes in children with high-risk neuroblastoma treated with autologous stem cell transplantation. Bone Marrow Transplant 2007;40(8):741–6.

191. Ross CJ, Katzov-Eckert H, Dube MP, et al. Genetic variants in TPMT and COMT are associated with hearing loss in children receiving cisplatin chemotherapy. Nat Genet 2009;41(12):1345–9.
192. Martin A, Schneiderman J, Helenowski IB, et al. Secondary malignant neoplasms after high-dose chemotherapy and autologous stem cell rescue for high-risk neuroblastoma. Pediatr Blood Cancer 2014;61(8):1350–6.
193. Kushner BH, Kramer K, Modak S, et al. Reduced risk of secondary leukemia with fewer cycles of dose-intensive induction chemotherapy in patients with neuroblastoma. Pediatr Blood Cancer 2009;53(1):17–22.
194. De Bernardi B, Quaglietta L, Haupt R, et al. Neuroblastoma with symptomatic epidural compression in the infant: the AIEOP experience. Pediatr Blood Cancer 2014;61(8):1369–75.
195. London WB, Castel V, Monclair T, et al. Clinical and biologic features predictive of survival after relapse of neuroblastoma: a report from the International Neuroblastoma Risk Group project. J Clin Oncol 2011;29(24):3286–92.
196. Morgenstern DA, Baruchel S, Irwin MS. Current and future strategies for relapsed neuroblastoma: challenges on the road to precision therapy. J Pediatr Hematol Oncol 2013;35(5):337–47.
197. Modak S, Cheung NK. Neuroblastoma: therapeutic strategies for a clinical enigma. Cancer Treat Rev 2010;36(4):307–17.
198. Di Giannatale A, Dias-Gastellier N, Devos A, et al. Phase II study of temozolomide in combination with topotecan (TOTEM) in relapsed or refractory neuroblastoma: a European Innovative Therapies for Children with Cancer-SIOP-European Neuroblastoma study. Eur J Cancer 2014;50(1):170–7.
199. Kushner BH, Kramer K, Modak S, et al. Differential impact of high-dose cyclophosphamide, topotecan, and vincristine in clinical subsets of patients with chemoresistant neuroblastoma. Cancer 2010;116(12):3054–60.
200. Garaventa A, Luksch R, Biasotti S, et al. A phase II study of topotecan with vincristine and doxorubicin in children with recurrent/refractory neuroblastoma. Cancer 2003;98(11):2488–94.
201. Kushner BH, Modak S, Kramer K, et al. Ifosfamide, carboplatin, and etoposide for neuroblastoma: a high-dose salvage regimen and review of the literature. Cancer 2013;119(3):665–71.
202. Lashford LS, Lewis IJ, Fielding SL, et al. Phase I/II study of iodine 131 metaiodobenzylguanidine in chemoresistant neuroblastoma: a United Kingdom Children's Cancer Study Group investigation. J Clin Oncol 1992;10(12):1889–96.
203. Matthay KK, Tan JC, Villablanca JG, et al. Phase I dose escalation of iodine-131-metaiodobenzylguanidine with myeloablative chemotherapy and autologous stem-cell transplantation in refractory neuroblastoma: a new approaches to Neuroblastoma Therapy Consortium Study. J Clin Oncol 2006;24(3):500–6.
204. Matthay KK, DeSantes K, Hasegawa B, et al. Phase I dose escalation of 131I-metaiodobenzylguanidine with autologous bone marrow support in refractory neuroblastoma. J Clin Oncol 1998;16(1):229–36.
205. Matthay KK, Yanik G, Messina J, et al. Phase II study on the effect of disease sites, age, and prior therapy on response to iodine-131-metaiodobenzylguanidine therapy in refractory neuroblastoma. J Clin Oncol 2007;25(9):1054–60.
206. Xu Y, Sun J, Sheard MA, et al. Lenalidomide overcomes suppression of human natural killer cell anti-tumor functions by neuroblastoma microenvironment-associated IL-6 and TGFbeta1. Cancer Immunol Immunother 2013;62(10):1637–48.
207. Koehn TA, Trimble LL, Alderson KL, et al. Increasing the clinical efficacy of NK and antibody-mediated cancer immunotherapy: potential predictors of

successful clinical outcome based on observations in high-risk neuroblastoma. Front Pharmacol 2012;3:91.

208. Heczey A, Louis CU. Advances in chimeric antigen receptor immunotherapy for neuroblastoma. Discov Med 2013;16(90):287–94.

209. Louis CU, Savoldo B, Dotti G, et al. Antitumor activity and long-term fate of chimeric antigen receptor-positive T cells in patients with neuroblastoma. Blood 2011;118(23):6050–6.

210. Pule MA, Savoldo B, Myers GD, et al. Virus-specific T cells engineered to coexpress tumor-specific receptors: persistence and antitumor activity in individuals with neuroblastoma. Nat Med 2008;14(11):1264–70.

211. Park JR, Digiusto, DL, Slovak M, et al. Adoptive transfer of chimeric antigen receptor re-directed cytolytic T lymphocyte clones in patients with neuroblastoma. Mol Ther 2007;15(4):825–33.

212. Bresler SC, Wood AC, Haglund EA, et al. Differential inhibitor sensitivity of anaplastic lymphoma kinase variants found in neuroblastoma. Sci Transl Med 2011;3(108):108ra114.

213. Barone G, Anderson J, Pearson AD, et al. New strategies in neuroblastoma: therapeutic targeting of MYCN and ALK. Clin Cancer Res 2013;19(21):5814–21.

214. Hogarty MD, Norris MD, Davis K, et al. ODC1 is a critical determinant of MYCN oncogenesis and a therapeutic target in neuroblastoma. Cancer Res 2008; 68(23):9735–45.

215. Witt O, Deubzer HE, Lodrini M, et al. Targeting histone deacetylases in neuroblastoma. Curr Pharm Des 2009;15(4):436–47.

216. Schleirmacher G, Javanmardi N, Bernard V, et al. Emergence of new ALK mutations at relapse in neuroblastoma. J Clin Oncol 2014;32(25):2727–34.

Hematopoietic Cell Transplantation and Cellular Therapeutics in the Treatment of Childhood Malignancies

Kanwaldeep Mallhi, MD[a], Lawrence G. Lum, MD, DSc[b],
Kirk R. Schultz, MD[a],*, Maxim Yankelevich, MD[c]

KEYWORDS

- Hematopoietic cell transplantation • Cellular therapy • Children • Adolescents
- Cancer

KEY POINTS

- Hematopoietic cell transplantation continues to be the only established immune therapy for childhood cancer.
- Cellular therapy shows great promise to either replace HCT and act as an adjuvant to standard chemotherapy for childhood cancer.
- Survival after HCT has improved primarily due to new approaches to decrease it's toxicity.
- Better understanding of the immune mechanisms of the graft-versus-leukemia/tumor effect are needed to improve the efficacy of HCT.

INTRODUCTION

Hematopoietic cell transplantation (HCT) represents the most common and effective form of immunotherapy for childhood malignancies. The role of the graft-versus-leukemia (GVL) effect in allogeneic HCT has been well established in childhood malignancies, but is also associated with short-term and long-term morbidity. HCT may be ineffective in some settings at obtaining control of the malignancy, and as such cannot

[a] Department of Pediatrics, BC Children's Hospital, 4480 Oak Street, Vancouver, British Columbia V6H 3V4, Canada; [b] Department of Oncology, Barbara Ann Karmanos Cancer Institute, Wayne State University, 3901 Beaubien, Detroit, MI 48201, USA; [c] Division of Hematology/Oncology, Children's Hospital of Michigan, Wayne State University, 3901 Beaubien, Detroit, MI 48201, USA
* Corresponding author. Division of Hematology/Oncology/Bone Marrow Transplantation, Department of Pediatrics, BC Children's Hospital, University of British Columbia, 4480 Oak Street, Vancouver, British Columbia V6H 3V4, Canada.
E-mail address: kschultz@mail.ubc.ca

Pediatr Clin N Am 62 (2015) 257–273
http://dx.doi.org/10.1016/j.pcl.2014.10.001   **pediatric.theclinics.com**
0031-3955/15/$ – see front matter © 2015 Elsevier Inc. All rights reserved.

be used as a universal cancer immunotherapy. Novel therapies using dendritic cell vaccinations, tumor-infiltrating lymphocytes, and chimeric antigen receptor T cells are being evaluated as potential adjuvants to HCT.

Hematopoietic Cell Transplantation

Allogeneic HCT refers to the transfer of hematopoietic stem cells from one individual to another with the intent to obtain lifelong engraftment of the administered cells. The use of allogeneic HCT as a cellular immune therapy for acute leukemia first became feasible in the early 1960s after the identification and typing of major histocompatibility complexes (human leukocyte antigen [HLA] system). In the 1970s Thomas and colleagues[1] cured several patients with end-stage leukemia by using HLA-identical siblings after ablating the recipient marrow with total-body irradiation combined with cyclophosphamide. It was evident that the occurrence of graft-versus-host disease (GVHD) reduced the incidence of leukemic relapse, suggesting that donor lymphocytes can eradicate tumor cells that survive preparative regimens.[2]

FACTORS THAT AFFECT THE OUTCOME OF HEMATOPOIETIC CELL TRANSPLANTATION

The outcome and efficacy of HCT in malignancies is influenced by several factors, including the underlying disorder, the level of residual tumor, donor source, HLA matching, the degree of graft-versus-leukemia/tumor (GVL/T) effect, and the toxicities associated with the preparative chemotherapy regimens.

Donor Source

Various allogeneic graft sources have the potential to produce a potent antineoplastic GVL/T effect to sustain complete remission of malignant disease. Donor sources for HCT in children include cells from bone marrow (BM), umbilical cord blood (UCB), or mobilized peripheral blood (PBSC) from related or unrelated donors. In addition to the type of the allogeneic graft, secondary non-HLA selection factors such as age of the donor, sex of the donor, total cell count, cytomegalovirus status, and ABO blood groups may contribute to the selection of a donor. However, the most important selection criterion for a donor source is HLA matching. At present, the role of high-resolution matching at HLA-A, HLA-B, and HLA-DRB1 is clearly established. However, the significance of the other loci, including HLA-C, HLA-DQ, HLA-DRB3 and DRB5, and HLA-DPB1, is less clear and is currently under investigation.[3]

HLA-identical sibling donors are considered the preferred stem cell source for allogeneic HCT; they have less transplantation-related mortality, acute GVHD (aGVHD), and chronic GVHD (cGVHD), along with better disease-free and overall survival (OS) than the unrelated donors.[4] Past studies have shown that use of a PBSC source produces a more rapid hematopoietic reconstitution; however, they are associated with a significant increase in cGVHD.[5] Not only is cGVHD significantly higher for patients receiving PBSC in comparison with BM (33% vs 19%, respectively; $P<.001$) but in the pediatric population treatment-related mortality, treatment failure, and overall mortality are also higher in the PBSC group.[6] The use of antithymocyte globulin (ATG) in the preparative regimen lowers the incidence of cGVHD.[7] A distinct advantage of unrelated donor UCB or haploidentical related donors is their rapid availability, and transplantation with cord blood requires less stringent HLA matching than transplant with bone marrow or peripheral stem cells. In general, mismatched cord blood cells are less likely than BM to cause both aGVHD and cGVHD, without losing the GVL effect.[8,9] Hematologic and immunologic reconstitution is slower in UCB transplants than in BM recipients, which is associated with an increase in infection-related morbidity. A limiting factor of UCB transplants is the cell dose. Blood from the umbilical cord and placenta is rich in hematopoietic stem cells but is often limited in volume. Data from pediatric studies reveal a lower survival in patients who receive a cell dose of less than 3×10^7/kg when compared with patients who received greater than 3×10^7 cells/kg.[10] This limitation can be partially overcome by using double UCB over single cord. Thus current practice supports the use of UCB donors, which provide a cell dose of greater than 3×10^7 cells/kg. Because of the limitation in cell number presented by UCB, newer ex vivo expansion approaches are being used to target molecular pathways involved in stem cell self-renewal, such as the Notch signaling system.[11] The use of T-cell depleted haploidentical donors (usually parents) is another option that has been explored to overcome the limitation of obtaining matched unrelated donors or UCB. However, the overall rate of chronic GVHD was significantly higher in patients who underwent haploidentical transplants while the relapse-free survival and disease-free survival (DFS) rates did not differ significantly between the groups.[12] Alloreactive natural killer (NK) cells, which express combinations of activation and inhibitory killer-cell immunoglobulin-like receptors, seem to be the primary mechanism for the GVL effect.

Preparative Chemotherapy Regimen

Several factors contribute to the outcome of HCT. In particular, the preparative chemotherapy regimens play a key part. The goal of preparative or conditioning regimens in patients undergoing HCT for malignant diseases includes providing significant immune ablation to prevent graft rejection and reduce the tumor burden. Traditionally myeloablative conditioning (MAC) regimens were thought to be the only means of achieving these goals. However, in recent years the reduced-intensity conditioning (RIC) regimens have been shown to be effective in HCT. Selecting the intensity of the conditioning regimen depends on the disease type, remission status, age of the patient, donor availability, and comorbid conditions. Myeloablative regimens often consist of alkylating agents with or without total-body irradiation (TBI) and are expected to ablate marrow hematopoiesis, preventing autologous hematologic recovery. High-dose TBI has been widely used as part of myeloablative regimens, especially in patients with acute lymphoblastic leukemia (ALL). Data from a large retrospective study and a randomized controlled trial in pediatric ALL patients with TBI as part of the preparative regimen demonstrated better event-free survival (EFS) outcomes when compared with myeloablative preparative regimens containing high-dose chemotherapy alone.[13,14] Although TBI reduces the risk of relapse, TBI-based regimens have significant late effects in children, and is often associated with an increased risk of gastrointestinal, hepatic, and pulmonary toxicities, cataracts, endocrinopathies, second malignancies, impaired growth and development, and cognitive delay.[15]

In recent years, use of a RIC for allogeneic HCT has demonstrated efficacy with an acceptable rate of donor engraftment and lower transplant-related morbidity and mortality relative to MAC regimens. Results of a phase 2 trial of RIC transplantation in children ineligible for MAC conditioning found that favorable outcomes could be achieved using a RIC regimen of busulfan, fludarabine, and antithymocyte globulin.[16,17] A retrospective comparison of RIC and MAC regimens in pediatric patients with acute myeloid leukemia (AML) showed that relapse rates were similar for both RIC and MAC regimens, and interestingly the transplant-related mortality (TRM) was also similar for both regimen groups.[18] These data indicate that long-term DFS can be achieved using reduced-intensity conditioning regimens, and may be considered in patients who are ineligible for MAC regimens.

The addition of antibodies targeting T cells, such as ATG and alemtuzumab (Campath 1H), to conditioning regimens is a commonly used approach to decrease the incidence of graft rejection and prevent GVHD. Several studies have shown that the administration of horse or rabbit ATG results in a significant reduction in the risk of aGVHD grades III and IV.[19] Alemtuzumab has been shown to be effective in decreasing the incidence of GVHD without increasing the risk of relapse and, with a significant delay in immune reconstitution, there was no increase in infectious complications or relapse in recipients of alemtuzumab.[20]

Recipient Characteristics

In children with a malignancy, sometimes the underlying nonmalignant disorder requires consideration when planning conditioning regimens. For example, patients with inherited DNA repair disorders such as Fanconi anemia are very sensitive to conventional conditioning protocols because of high chromosome fragility, and MAC regimens involving alkylating agents and ionizing radiation have been associated with a high incidence of transplantation-related toxicity and mortality.[21] RIC regimens are often used in patients with nonmalignant disorders and have been shown to be associated with a low TRM; however, these patients have been shown to have a significantly higher incidence of primary graft failure.[22]

EFFICACY OF ALLOGENEIC STEM CELL TRANSPLANTATION IN THE TREATMENT OF CHILDHOOD MALIGNANCIES
Acute Lymphoblastic Leukemia

Relapsed ALL is the most common malignant childhood disease for which an HCT is offered, particularly in those who experience marrow relapse on treatment or within 18 months of stopping therapy. The role of HCT in treating isolated central nervous system (CNS) disease is uncertain, with most opting to use intensive chemotherapy and delayed CNS radiation as the first option.[23] Another group in which HCT is being explored is that with a high risk of relapse. A prospective study in 7 countries investigated the outcome of patients with very high-risk ALL in first complete remission (CR1) found that the 5-year DFS was 40.6% in children allocated to chemotherapy alone, compared with 56.7% in those assigned to HCT ($P = .2$).[24] The Children's Cancer Study group (CCG-1921) investigated the role of HCT from HLA-matched family donors in ALL patients with ultrahigh-risk features, and reported the 5-year EFS for all patients to be 58.6%; patients without cytogenetic abnormalities had a 5-year EFS of 77.8%.[25]

Acute Myeloid Leukemia

The use of HCT for patients with AML has evolved significantly in the last 3 decades. In the 1980s a common practice in North America was to offer matched family donor stem cell transplantation in CR1, whereas the European groups favored a more conservative approach with HCT in second complete remission (CR2).[5] In the Children's Cancer Group (CCG) and Pediatric Oncology Group (POG) studies, the outcome was better for those allocated to matched related HCT in CR1, and the OS and DFS was superior for allogeneic HCT in comparison with chemotherapy alone or autologous purged HCT.[26–28] In the POG study, there was no advantage for autologous bone marrow transplantation (BMT) in CR1 over chemotherapy alone.[28] A more recent analysis of combined CCG and POG AML studies, however, demonstrated that the superior survival advantage of allogeneic BMT for AML in CR1 may be limited to the intermediate-risk group of patients, with no significant benefit over chemotherapy for low-risk and high-risk patients.[29] At present, AML-CR1 allogeneic BMT is not recommended to low-risk patients (those with RUNX1-ETO, inv16, t[16;16], and NPM1 mutations; Down syndrome AML; acute promyelocytic leukemia).[30] By contrast, allogeneic BMT remains the only curative treatment option after relapse regardless of the initial risk factors.

Chronic Myeloid Leukemia

Chronic myeloid leukemia (CML) is a relatively rare hematopoietic malignancy in the pediatric and adolescent population. In CML, allogeneic HCT offers a long-term DFS in patients in chronic phase and is the only proven curative approach. In the European Group for Blood and Marrow Transplantation (EBMT) study the OS ranged from 60% to 80%, with better results in matched sibling donors (87%) than in matched unrelated donors (59%).[31] Over recent years, the increased use of tyrosine kinase inhibitors (TKIs), such as imatinib, and clinical efficacy in CML have been well established, resulting in only a minority of pediatric patients undergoing upfront HCT.[32] Achieving a major cytogenetic remission by prior imatinib treatment at the time of HCT has been found to predict a 5-year OS of 81% to 89% in unrelated matched HCT in adults.[33] The exact role of HCT for children and adolescents with CML is controversial, with studies to establish its role being considered in the International BFM Study Group and the Children's Oncology Group (COG).

Myelodysplastic Syndrome

Myelodysplastic syndrome (MDS) is a clonal disorder of hematopoiesis with variable BM dysplasia and cellularity, progressive cytopenias, and susceptibility for transformation to AML. Current World Health Organization criteria classify MDS into the following subdivisions: refractory cytopenia (RC), refractory anemia with excess blasts (RAEB), and RAEB in transformation (RAEB-T). MDS in children has a poor prognosis and, despite attempts to use various treatment modalities, currently the curative treatment choice is allogeneic HCT. Smith and colleagues[34] reviewed 37 pediatric MDS cases at a single institution and revealed factors associated with improved 3-years DFS, including not having received pre-HCT chemotherapy and a shorter interval (<140 days) from time of diagnosis to transplant. The 3-year DFS in patients who did not receive pre-HCT chemotherapy and those who had a shorter interval to transplant was 80%. Therefore, children with MDS should be referred for allogeneic HCT soon after diagnosis, and pre-HCT chemotherapy does not appear to improve outcome.

Juvenile Myelomonocytic Leukemia

Juvenile myelomonocytic leukemia (JMML) is an uncommon disease occurring exclusively in young children that includes among its symptoms fevers, infections, massive hepatosplenomegaly, pulmonary infiltrates, and rash. Intensive chemotherapy is mostly unsuccessful in JMML because of an increased risk of treatment-related death. The European Working Group on Childhood Myelodysplastic Syndromes and Bone Marrow Transplant Working Group (EWOG-MDS/EBMT) reported the largest cohort to date (N = 100) in which the 5-year EFS was 52%, and used a myeloablative preparative regimen with high doses of busulfan/cyclophosphamide/melphalan (BU-CY-MEL).[35] The OS was 64%, without significant differences in the EFS between matched related or matched unrelated donors. Both acute and chronic GVHD are associated with a lower risk of relapse.[36] At present the COG is conducting a randomized phase II study comparing a busulfan/fludarabine (BU-FLU) conditioning regimen with a BU-CY-MEL conditioning regimen, hypothesizing less TRM and comparable EFS with the BU-FLU regimen.

Lymphoma

The OS of children and adolescents with newly diagnosed Hodgkin lymphoma and non-Hodgkin lymphoma (NHL) disease approaches 90%, with the use of combination chemotherapy with either autologous or allogeneic HCT considered for refractory patients. Unfortunately, greater than 60% of patients with Hodgkin lymphoma who undergo autologous HCT fail to achieve complete remission.[37] Evidence suggests that allogeneic HCT have been associated with a significantly lower incidence of relapse of Hodgkin lymphoma compared with autologous HCT, but with no impact on OS and a high incidence of TRM. Gross and colleagues[38] examined the role of allogeneic and autologous HCT in children with refractory or recurrent Burkitt, lymphoblastic, diffuse large B-cell (DLBCL), and anaplastic large cell lymphomas. The 5-year EFS was similar after allogeneic and autologous HCT for DLBCL (50% vs 52%), Burkitt (31% vs 27%), and anaplastic large cell lymphoma (46% vs 35%). However, it was higher for lymphoblastic lymphoma after allogeneic HCT (40% vs 4%; $P<.01$).

Limitations to Hematopoietic Cell Transplantation

For most patients undergoing allogeneic HCT the major causes of morbidity and mortality are related to disease relapse, aGVHD and cGVHD, infection, regimen-related toxicity, and graft failure. Other serious acute adverse effects include idiopathic pneumonia syndrome (IPS), engraftment syndrome, and sinusoidal obstruction syndrome (SOS). IPS is defined as the presence of widespread alveolar injury in the absence of active lower respiratory tract infection that occurs following allogeneic HCT.[39] The lung injury generally occurs within 4 months of transplant and is associated with a high mortality rate exceeding 60%. Immunologic cell-mediated injury and inflammatory cytokines contributes to the lung injury.[40] Prompt treatment with corticosteroids and etanercept may reduce the injury.[41]

Engraftment syndrome occurs usually before neutrophil recovery, especially after UCB HCT, and is characterized by fever, rash, weight gain, pulmonary edema, liver and renal dysfunction, and/or encephalopathy. Engraftment syndrome is due to a cytokine storm with capillary leak and is associated with interstitial pneumonitis.[42] Engraftment syndrome has a higher progression to aGVHD and has a lower OS at 2 years (38% vs 54%, $P<.001$). Prompt treatment of engraftment syndrome with corticosteroid therapy should be initiated on diagnosis.

Another severe complication is the potentially fatal hepatic SOS, previously known as veno-occlusive disease, characterized by the presence of painful hepatomegaly, jaundice, and fluid retention. The mechanism of action involves damaged sinusoidal endothelium that sloughs out and obstructs the hepatic circulation, leading to centrilobular hepatocyte injury.[43] Several risk factors increase the incidence of sinusoidal obstruction syndrome, including chronic liver disease, the presence of the C282Y allele of the HFE hemochromatosis gene, and common variants of the glutathione S-transferase gene that alters the metabolism of busulfan and cyclophosphamide.[44,45]

Acute Graft-Versus-Host Disease

aGVHD is an immune response stimulated and accentuated by injury resulting from the preparative regimen used before transplantation.[46] A postulated mechanism of aGVHD involves the activation of toll-like receptors on various cells, which then leads to the release of inflammatory cytokines. Activation of toll-like receptors blocks the suppressive effects of regulatory T cells, thus permitting the activated alloreactive cytotoxic T cells to enter the circulation and damage organs such as the gut, liver, and skin, resulting in aGVHD.[47,48]

The reported incidence of aGVHD in children varies widely from 20% to 80%, depending on the major risk factors of HLA matching and donor type (matched or mismatched, sibling) and stem cell source.[49] The National Institutes of Health (NIH) Consensus Development Project defines classic aGVHD as occurring before 100 days after transplant with the presence of aGVHD symptoms and the absence of cGVHD symptoms. Persistent or late-onset aGVHD is defined as occurring after day 100 with the presence of aGVHD symptoms (such as intestinal aGVHD) and the absence of cGVHD symptoms.[36,50] This situation is not uncommon after unrelated UCB HCT.

Standard aGVHD prophylaxis regimens usually combine a calcineurin inhibitor (tacrolimus or cyclosporine) with short-course methotrexate. The initial treatment of aGVHD involves optimizing the present GVHD prophylaxis and initiation of corticosteroids. Only 50% to 70% of aGVHD cases will have a complete response to steroid treatment. Steroid-refractory aGVHD has been treated with equivalent success with anti–tumor necrosis factor α antibodies (infliximab, etanercept), mycophenolate mofetil (MMF), mTOR inhibitors (sirolimus), interleukin-2 receptor antibodies (daclizumab), ATG, or extracorporeal photopheresis as second-line treatments.[51,52]

Chronic Graft-Versus-Host Disease

cGVHD is believed to involve autoimmune and alloimmune dysregulation, leading to disordered immunologic reactivity against autologous (self) and allogeneic (donor) antigens.[53–57] Based on the NIH Consensus Development Project, classic cGVHD is defined as occurring after day 100 post-HCT with the presence of cGVHD symptoms and the absence of aGVHD symptoms. Overlap syndrome is then defined as occurring 100 days post-HCT with the presence of both aGVHD and cGVHD symptoms. cGVHD can potentially affect any organ of the body, although the skin, eyes, oral cavity, gastrointestinal tract, genitourinary system, liver, and lungs are most commonly affected. Other organ systems such as the kidneys or heart can also be affected, although far less frequently. cGVHD of the skin can present as sclerosis (lichen sclerosus–like or lichen planus–like), hypopigmentation or hyperpigmentation, alopecia, keratosis pilaris, and ichthyosis. Musculoskeletal involvement of cGVHD can result in myositis, fasciitis, muscle weakness, cramping, edema, and pain and joint contracture. Ocular cGVHD affects up to 80% of patients and typically presents with dry or gritty eyes (sicca syndrome), photophobia, keratoconjunctivitis, punctate keratopathy, and blepharitis. Pulmonary cGVHD is classified as either obstructive lung disease or restrictive lung disease, and the incidence of lung toxicity ranges from 30% to 60% in children. Bronchiolitis obliterans (BO) is a serious life-threatening manifestation of cGVHD characterized by an inflammatory process resulting in bronchiolar obliteration, fibrosis, and progressive obstructive lung disease. Pulmonary function tests should be routinely checked at 3 and 12 months after transplantation and at the onset of cGVHD, to determine whether obstructive lung mechanics are present and whether therapy for BO should be initiated. Initial therapy for BO includes a trial of enhanced systemic immunosuppression, with inhaled corticosteroids and pulmonary rehabilitation. Hyposplenism leading to increased susceptibility to encapsulated organism should be considered, with active cGVHD and penicillin prophylaxis initiated. First-line therapy for cGVHD continues to be corticosteroids. Second-line immunosuppressive agents such as MMF, sirolimus, imatinib, rituximab, and extracorporeal photopheresis may be considered. Imatinib may improve sclerodermatous cGVHD, and rituximab may benefit skin and musculoskeletal cGVHD.

Long-Term Effects Not Associated with Graft-Versus-Host Disease

Advances in allogeneic HCT have led to improved patient survival, and long-term complications have increased in importance. Long-term effects may involve the cardiovascular system, lungs, kidneys, CNS, endocrine system, second malignancies, and the psychosocial implications of survivorship.[54,55] Factors that increase cardiovascular mortality include high cumulative doses of anthracyclines and exposure to radiation therapy that may have included the heart or mediastinum. The metabolic syndrome (central obesity, insulin resistance, glucose intolerance, dyslipidemia, and hypertension), associated with development of type 2 diabetes mellitus and atherosclerotic cardiovascular disease is also increased, and needs to be monitored for at follow-up visits. Both busulfan and TBI preparative regimens can lead to impaired pulmonary function tests, either obstructive or restrictive, not related to cGVHD up to 10 years after transplant, necessitating close follow-up. Renal function should also be monitored long term at all follow-up visits, as chronic renal insufficiency can be caused by radiation-induced renal injury and cGVHD.

There is a high prevalence of endocrine dysfunction in long-term survivors, resulting in disturbances in thyroid function, onset of puberty, fertility, bone health, and growth and development. The long-term use of corticosteroids to treat cGVHD can result in a variety of complications including, but not limited to, aseptic necrosis of the bone and osteoporosis, adrenal suppression, and metabolic syndrome. Craniospinal radiation has been implicated as the primary cause of growth failure after HCT as a result of damage to the hypothalamic-pituitary axis, leading to decreased production of growth hormone. Preparative regimens that include TBI and busulfan can lead to premature ovarian failure in some survivors, resulting in absence of or delayed puberty and amenorrhea. As they enter their reproductive years, many women will fail to ovulate after undergoing transplantation, while men potentially become infertile. In addition, the frequency of secondary cancers such as cancers of the skin, oral mucosa, brain, thyroid, bone, and posttransplant lymphoproliferative disease are increased.[58] Any female patient who has had TBI should have monitoring for breast cancer by MRI, initiated in her early 20s. As the number of long-term pediatric HCT survivors increases, more attention is being focused on neurocognitive and psychosocial outcomes. Studies have shown that there is a small but significant decline in IQ in children transplanted for malignant disorders when compared with control subjects, and especially in children who received TBI or craniospinal radiation and those who developed aGVHD. Socioeconomic status continues to be an important determinant of cognitive and academic function. Recognizing the nature and complexity of long-term side effects in children after HCT, it is necessary to maintain frequent and thorough follow-up evaluations to detect issues that may arise as early as possible. Early diagnosis can lead to early intervention and may improve the manifestations of many late effects.

Graft-Versus-Leukemia/Tumor

Allogeneic HCT represents the most common and effective form of immunotherapy in childhood leukemia. Over the past several decades, clinical studies have revealed that the effectiveness of GVL/T in eradicating malignant disease is linked closely to the activity of immunoreactive cells in the graft, particularly the T cells and NK cells from allogeneic BM, PBSC, or UBC. In haploidentical or multiple HLA antigen–mismatched donors, the donor NK cells carry receptors for peptide–major histocompatibility complex molecules on recipient target and are the primary mediators of GVHD.[56] Donor T cells seem to primarily respond to minor histocompatibility antigens expressed on both hematopoietic and nonhematopoietic cells, causing both GVL/T and GVHD.[53] Comparison of relapse rates seen in patients who develop no GVHD, aGVHD, cGVHD, or both aGVHD and cGVHD continue to reveal that the GVL effect is strongly associated with the development of GVHD. This claim is further supported by the fact that there are increased rates of leukemia relapse after T-cell–depleted and identical twin allogeneic HCT.[57]

The GVL effect is affected by several factors, the primary one being minimal residual disease status before transplant, resulting in a higher risk of relapse after HCT in ALL.[59,60] In haploidentical HCT, it is clear that alloreactive NK cells that kill recipient cells through the recognition of mismatches in the NK cell killer immunoglobulin-like receptor (KIR) play a large role in GVL.[61,62] Current trials are under way to evaluate the impact of KIR mismatches in the setting of matched unrelated donor HCT in high-risk AML (COG study). An additional advantage of this approach is that activated NK cells can directly lyse GVHD-inducing T cells and host antigen-presenting cells, potentially controlling GVHD.[63,64]

Novel Cellular Therapies in the Treatment of Childhood Malignancies

Despite the effectiveness of allogeneic HCT and GVL/T in the treatment of hematopoietic malignancies, the leading cause of treatment failure remains relapse of disease. Attempts to generate and enhance cellular cytotoxic responses in vivo have been made using monoclonal antibodies. Although monoclonal antibodies may be directly cytotoxic, most induce antitumor responses via antibody-dependent effector mechanisms, including complement-mediated lysis and antibody-dependent cellular cytotoxicity (ADCC). Monoclonal antibody therapy has resulted in clinical improvements in several malignancies; however, monoclonal antibody therapy has not been curative in most patients. Recently, application of anti-GD2 antibodies in high-risk neuroblastoma with minimal residual disease resulted in significant improvement of survival, but the disease still progressed in at least 40% of the patients.[65] Several cellular-based therapies to create a GVL effect are currently under investigation, including dendritic cell (DC) immunotherapy, bispecific antibodies, chimeric antibody receptor T cells, NK cells, and adjuvant immune therapies.

Dendritic Cell Immunotherapy

DCs can capture and present tumor antigens to T cells, resulting in the development of tumor-specific cytotoxic T cells that can mediate protective antitumor responses.[66,67] Since the first published DC vaccine trial,[68] numerous clinical studies have established the feasibility and safety of DC vaccinations; however, clinical and immunologic responses have been infrequent and unpredictable, as in a case of pediatric high-grade gliomas (**Fig. 1**). Several DC vaccines have been used in pediatric tumors, fibrosarcoma, and malignant brain tumors, some with significant responses.[69,70] Combining DC vaccines with the demethylating agent decitabine to upregulate TAA expression for a child with advanced neuroblastoma[71] resulted in durable complete remission.

Antigen-Specific T Cells

Using ex vivo expanded tumor-infiltrating lymphocytes after chemotherapy-induced lymphocyte depletion in patients with metastatic melanoma is probably the most successful example of adoptive cell transfer of activated but otherwise unmanipulated T cells.[72,73] However, it has not been replicated in any other types of cancer. Reasons

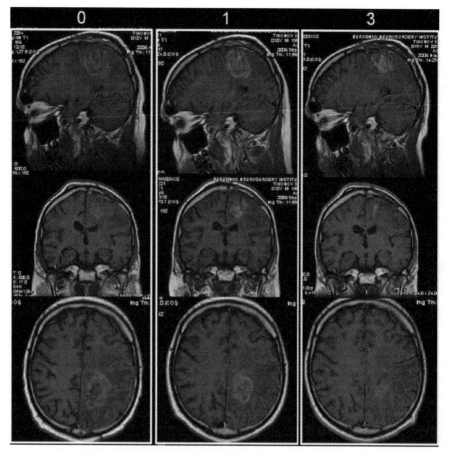

Fig. 1. Partial response after dendritic cell vaccination in a teenager with gliobastoma multiforme recurring after radiation treatment, temozolomide, and Gamma Knife radiosurgery. The patient is currently alive 6 years after recurrence (personal observation, M. Yankelevich).

for low anticancer activity of ex vivo expanded polyclonal T cells could be the absence of tumor-specific high-affinity T-cell receptors and the presence of Tregs or myeloid-derived suppressor cells, and other secreted factors from stroma surrounding the tumor.

Chimeric Antigen Receptor T Cells

Chimeric antigen receptor (CAR) T cells are genetically modified to express a T-cell receptor via fusion of single-chain variable fragment of monoclonal antibody that targets a TAA and transmembrane signaling domain derived from the CD3-ζ chain. Clinical success has been achieved with second-generation anti-CD19 CARs, with induction of ALL responses and depletion of normal CD19-positive B cells.[73–76] Grupp and colleagues[73] reported complete remission after second-generation CD19-specific CAR T cells against heavily pretreated relapsed B-precursor ALL; however, CD19-negative ALL relapse can occur. Several clinical trials of CD19-specific CAR T cells in children with leukemia are currently open, including fourth-generation CD19 CAR T cells at Seattle Children's Hospital (NCT02028455) and allogeneic UCB-derived CD19 CAR T cells at MD Anderson Cancer Center (NCT01362452).

Recently EBV-specific T cells engineered to coexpress ganglioside GD2-specific CAR in children with high-risk neuroblastoma demonstrated significant antitumor activity, with prolonged persistence of transfected cells and a durable clinical response.[77–79]

T Cells Armed with Bispecific Antibodies

Cross-linking T-cell receptors (TCRs) with anti-CD3 monoclonal antibody leads to T-cell activation and proliferation, cytokine secretion, and immune responses.[80] Blinatumomab, a CD3-CD19 bispecific antibody, was evaluated in the AALL1121 phase II pilot study, and is now integrated in COG trials for relapsed ALL after showing significant activity in both adult and pediatric ALL as a single agent. Other studies have evaluated bispecific antibodies linking CD3 to TAAs.[81] Bispecific antibodies are being developed against several pediatric targets including anti-Her2, anti-EGFR, anti-CD20, and anti-GD2.[79,82–84] GD2 bispecific antibodies show activity against GD2-positive neuroblastoma and osteosarcoma in vitro and in vivo.[79] The clinical studies for neuroblastoma and osteosarcoma are currently open for enrollment at the Children's Hospital of Michigan, Detroit (NCT021173093).

Natural Killer Cell Therapies

The antitumor activity of NK cells was best described in the settings of allogeneic HCT in leukemia patients,[85] as ADCC effector cells during monoclonal antibody therapy, for example, GD2 monoclonal antibody therapy for children with neuroblastoma and as post-HCT infusions of purified donor NK cells.[85–88] KIR genotype and donor-recipient mismatch in alloreactive NK cells can mediate the GVL/T effect, with significant clinical responses after repeated infusions. At present the studies of allogeneic NK cell infusions after hematopoietic stem cell transplantation in children with hematologic malignancies are open at St. Jude Children's Research Hospital (NCT00145626, NCT01807611, and NCT01621477) and Fred Hutchinson Cancer Research Center (NCT00789776), and at the Medical College of Wisconsin (NCT02100891) for children with solid tumors.

NK cells are major mediators of ADCC via activation of their CD16 receptor by monoclonal antibodies, so the combination of monoclonal antibodies and purified NK cell infusions is potentially synergistic. The studies of allogeneic NK cell infusions in combination with anti-GD2 antibodies 3F8 and hu14.18k322A for children with neuroblastoma are open at Memorial Sloan-Kettering Cancer Center (NCT0087710) and St. Jude Children's Research Hospital (NCT01576692). Another approach is to engineer autologous NK cells to express built-in ADCC-like activity using anticancer CAR, which was demonstrated by Esser and colleagues[89] in their preclinical study of efficacy of GD2-specific CAR NK cells in neuroblastoma cells. A recent report also demonstrated that human NK T cells engineered to express a CAR specific to the GD2, which is overexpressed by malignant neuroblasts, became highly cytotoxic against neuroblastoma cells and had potent antitumor activity in NSG mice with metastatic xenografts of human neuroblastoma.[90]

Adverse Effects of T-Cell Therapies

Ex vivo expanded and activated T cells are complex biological therapeutics prepared using genetic manipulations, complex media, and activating cytokines, all of which not only increase the risk for infusion reactions but also convert these cells into highly potent sources of proinflammatory cytokines for days after the initial infusion, as some of these cellular products can proliferate in vivo more than 1000 times after infusions.[91] A spectrum of clinical conditions varying from febrile reactions, nausea, and muscle aches in milder cases, to multiple organ failure has been observed in patients receiving T-cell infusions, thought to be related to the cytokines released by the cells. In the second-generation CD19 CAR T cells trials from the University of Pennsylvania and Memorial Sloan Kettering Cancer Center for adult and pediatric patients with leukemia, all responding patients experienced a cytokine release syndrome corresponding to engineered T-cell proliferation and killing of leukemia cells.[92] The pediatric patients reported by Grupp and colleagues[73] and Maus and colleagues[91] both developed grade III to IV reactions with fevers, respiratory/cardiovascular failure, and confusion on days 4 to 6 after cell infusions. One of them required ventilator and vasopressor support, but responded quickly to anticytokine therapy with IL6-R monoclonal antibody tocilizumab.

SUMMARY

Although great progress has been made to improve the curative outcomes treating childhood malignancies with allogeneic HCT, further progress with the development of novel therapeutic approaches is important. Immunotherapy with alternative mechanisms may offer curative results with targeted control. These therapies, with or without subsequent HCT, may provide a cure, limiting the transplant-related mortality and long-term effects. As with HCT, cellular immunotherapy has its own limited nonspecific toxicity, and current trials are under way to determine the feasibility of this therapy. Systematic study of multiple immune-based therapies is necessary to determine the optimal treatment approach.

REFERENCES

1. Thomas ED, Buckner CD, Banaji M, et al. One hundred patients with acute leukemia treated by chemotherapy, total body irradiation, and allogeneic marrow transplantation. Blood 1977;49(4):511–33.
2. Weiden PL, Flournoy N, Thomas ED, et al. Antileukemic effect of graft-versus-host disease in human recipients of allogeneic-marrow grafts. N Engl J Med 1979; 300(19):1068–73.
3. Handgretinger R, Kurtzberg J, Egeler RM. Indications and donor selections for allogeneic stem cell transplantation in children with hematologic malignancies. Pediatr Clin North Am 2008;55(1):71–96, x.
4. Shaw PJ, Kan F, Woo Ahn K, et al. Outcomes of pediatric bone marrow transplantation for leukemia and myelodysplasia using matched sibling, mismatched related, or matched unrelated donors. Blood 2010;116(19):4007–15.
5. Cutler C, Giri S, Jeyapalan S, et al. Acute and chronic graft-versus-host disease after allogeneic peripheral-blood stem-cell and bone marrow transplantation: a meta-analysis. J Clin Oncol 2001;19(16):3685–91.
6. Eapen M, Horowitz MM, Klein JP, et al. Higher mortality after allogeneic peripheral-blood transplantation compared with bone marrow in children and adolescents: the Histocompatibility and Alternate Stem Cell Source Working Committee of the International Bone Marrow Transplant Registry. J Clin Oncol 2004; 22(24):4872–80.
7. Meisel R, Klingebiel T, Dilloo D. Peripheral blood stem cells versus bone marrow in pediatric unrelated donor stem cell transplantation. Blood 2013;121(5):863–5.
8. Wagner JE, Barker JN, DeFor TE, et al. Transplantation of unrelated donor umbilical cord blood in 102 patients with malignant and nonmalignant diseases: influence of CD34 cell dose and HLA disparity on treatment-related mortality and survival. Blood 2002;100(5):1611–8.

9. Eapen M, Rubinstein P, Zhang MJ, et al. Outcomes of transplantation of unrelated donor umbilical cord blood and bone marrow in children with acute leukaemia: a comparison study. Lancet 2007;369(9577):1947–54.

10. Sawczyn KK, Quinones R, Malcolm J, et al. Cord blood transplant in childhood ALL. Pediatr Blood Cancer 2005;45(7):964–70.

11. Delaney C, Heimfeld S, Brashem-Stein C, et al. Notch-mediated expansion of human cord blood progenitor cells capable of rapid myeloid reconstitution. Nat Med 2010;16(2):232–6.

12. Mo XD, Zhao XY, Liu DH, et al. Umbilical cord blood transplantation and unmanipulated haploidentical hematopoietic SCT for pediatric hematologic malignances. Bone Marrow Transplant 2014;49(8):1070–5.

13. Davies SM, Ramsay NK, Klein JP, et al. Comparison of preparative regimens in transplants for children with acute lymphoblastic leukemia. J Clin Oncol 2000; 18(2):340–7.

14. Bunin N, Aplenc R, Kamani N, et al. Randomized trial of busulfan vs total body irradiation containing conditioning regimens for children with acute lymphoblastic leukemia: a Pediatric Blood and Marrow Transplant Consortium study. Bone Marrow Transplant 2003;32(6):543–8.

15. Ferry C, Gemayel G, Rocha V, et al. Long-term outcomes after allogeneic stem cell transplantation for children with hematological malignancies. Bone Marrow Transplant 2007;40(3):219–24.

16. Pulsipher MA, Boucher KM, Wall D, et al. Reduced-intensity allogeneic transplantation in pediatric patients ineligible for myeloablative therapy: results of the Pediatric Blood and Marrow Transplant Consortium Study ONC0313. Blood 2009; 114(7):1429–36.

17. Verneris MR, Eapen M, Duerst R, et al. Reduced-intensity conditioning regimens for allogeneic transplantation in children with acute lymphoblastic leukemia. Biol Blood Marrow Transplant 2010;16(9):1237–44.

18. Bitan M, He W, Zhang MJ, et al. Transplantation for children with acute myeloid leukemia: a comparison of outcomes with reduced intensity and myeloablative regimens. Blood 2014;123(10):1615–20.

19. Kumar A, Mhaskar AR, Reljic T, et al. Antithymocyte globulin for acute-graft-versus-host-disease prophylaxis in patients undergoing allogeneic hematopoietic cell transplantation: a systematic review. Leukemia 2012;26(4):582–8.

20. Shah AJ, Kapoor N, Crooks GM, et al. The effects of Campath 1H upon graft-versus-host disease, infection, relapse, and immune reconstitution in recipients of pediatric unrelated transplants. Biol Blood Marrow Transplant 2007;13(5): 584–93.

21. Satwani P, Morris E, Bradley B, et al. Reduced intensity and non-myeloablative allogeneic stem cell transplantation in children and adolescents with malignant and non-malignant diseases. Pediatr Blood Cancer 2008;50(1):1–8.

22. Satwani P, Jin Z, Duffy D, et al. Transplantation-related mortality, graft failure, and survival after reduced-toxicity conditioning and allogeneic hematopoietic stem cell transplantation in 100 consecutive pediatric recipients. Biol Blood Marrow Transplant 2013;19(4):552–61.

23. Barredo JC, Devidas M, Lauer SJ, et al. Isolated CNS relapse of acute lymphoblastic leukemia treated with intensive systemic chemotherapy and delayed CNS radiation: a pediatric oncology group study. J Clin Oncol 2006;24(19): 3142–9.

24. Balduzzi A, Valsecchi MG, Uderzo C, et al. Chemotherapy versus allogeneic transplantation for very-high-risk childhood acute lymphoblastic leukaemia in first

complete remission: comparison by genetic randomisation in an international prospective study. Lancet 2005;366(9486):635–42.

25. Satwani P, Sather H, Ozkaynak F, et al. Allogeneic bone marrow transplantation in first remission for children with ultra-high-risk features of acute lymphoblastic leukemia: a children's oncology group study report. Biol Blood Marrow Transplant 2007;13(2):218–27.

26. Alonzo TA, Wells RJ, Woods WG, et al. Postremission therapy for children with acute myeloid leukemia: the children's cancer group experience in the transplant era. Leukemia 2005;19(6):965–70.

27. Neudorf S, Sanders J, Kobrinsky N, et al. Allogeneic bone marrow transplantation for children with acute myelocytic leukemia in first remission demonstrates a role for graft versus leukemia in the maintenance of disease-free survival. Blood 2004; 103(10):3655–61.

28. Ravindranath Y, Yeager AM, Chang MN, et al. Autologous bone marrow transplantation versus intensive consolidation chemotherapy for acute myeloid leukemia in childhood. Pediatric Oncology Group. N Engl J Med 1996;334(22): 1428–34.

29. Horan JT, Alonzo TA, Lyman GH, et al. Impact of disease risk on efficacy of matched related bone marrow transplantation for pediatric acute myeloid leukemia: the Children's Oncology Group. J Clin Oncol 2008;26(35):5797–801.

30. Oliansky DM, Rizzo JD, Aplan PD, et al. The role of cytotoxic therapy with hematopoietic stem cell transplantation in the therapy of acute myeloid leukemia in children: an evidence-based review. Biol Blood Marrow Transplant 2007; 13(1):1–25.

31. Cwynarski K, Roberts IA, Iacobelli S, et al. Stem cell transplantation for chronic myeloid leukemia in children. Blood 2003;102:1224–31.

32. Suttorp M, Yaniv I, Schultz KR. Controversies in the Treatment of CML in Children and Adolescents: TKIs versus BMT? Biol Blood Marrow Transplant 2011;17: S115–22.

33. Muramatsu H, Kojima S, Yoshimi A, et al. Outcome of 125 children with chronic myelogenous leukemia who received transplants from unrelated donors: the Japan Marrow Donor Program. Biol Blood Marrow Transplant 2010;16:231–8.

34. Smith AR, Christiansen EC, Wagner JE, et al. Early hematopoietic stem cell transplant is associated with favorable outcomes in children with MDS. Pediatr Blood Cancer 2013;60(4):705–10.

35. Locatelli F, Nollke P, Zecca M, et al. Hematopoietic stem cell transplantation (HSCT) in children with juvenile myelomonocytic leukemia (JMML): results of the EWOG-MDS/EBMT trial. Blood 2005;105(1):410–9.

36. Filipovich AH, Weisdorf D, Pavletic S, et al. National Institutes of Health consensus development project on criteria for clinical trials in chronic graft-versus-host disease: I. Diagnosis and staging working group report. Biol Blood Marrow Transplant 2005;11(12):945–56.

37. Claviez A, Canals C, Dierickx D, et al. Allogeneic hematopoietic stem cell transplantation in children and adolescents with recurrent and refractory Hodgkin lymphoma: an analysis of the European Group for Blood and Marrow Transplantation. Blood 2009;114(10):2060–7.

38. Gross TG, Hale GA, He W, et al. Hematopoietic stem cell transplantation for refractory or recurrent non-Hodgkin lymphoma in children and adolescents. Biol Blood Marrow Transplant 2010;16(2):223–30.

39. Sano H, et al. Risk factor analysis of idiopathic pneumonia syndrome after allogeneic hematopoietic SCT in children. Bone Marrow Transplant 2014;49(1):38–41.

40. Cooke KR, Yanik G. Acute lung injury after allogeneic stem cell transplantation: is the lung a target of acute graft-versus-host disease? Bone Marrow Transplant 2004;34(9):753–65.

41. Yanik G, Hellerstedt B, Custer J, et al. Etanercept (Enbrel) administration for idiopathic pneumonia syndrome after allogeneic hematopoietic stem cell transplantation. Biol Blood Marrow Transplant 2002;8(7):395–400.

42. Spitzer TR. Engraftment syndrome following hematopoietic stem cell transplantation. Bone Marrow Transplant 2001;27(9):893–8.

43. DeLeve LD, Shulman HM, McDonald GB. Toxic injury to hepatic sinusoids: sinusoidal obstruction syndrome (veno-occlusive disease). Semin Liver Dis 2002; 22(1):27–42.

44. Kallianpur AR, Hall LD, Yadav M, et al. The hemochromatosis C282Y allele: a risk factor for hepatic veno-occlusive disease after hematopoietic stem cell transplantation. Bone Marrow Transplant 2005;35(12):1155–64.

45. Srivastava A, Poonkuzhali B, Shaji RV, et al. Glutathione S-transferase M1 polymorphism: a risk factor for hepatic venoocclusive disease in bone marrow transplantation. Blood 2004;104(5):1574–7.

46. Hill GR, Ferrara JL. The primacy of the gastrointestinal tract as a target organ of acute graft-versus-host disease: rationale for the use of cytokine shields in allogeneic bone marrow transplantation. Blood 2000;95(9):2754–9.

47. Lin MT, Storer B, Martin PJ, et al. Relation of an interleukin-10 promoter polymorphism to graft-versus-host disease and survival after hematopoietic-cell transplantation. N Engl J Med 2003;349(23):2201–10.

48. Rocha V, Franco RF, Porcher R, et al. Host defense and inflammatory gene polymorphisms are associated with outcomes after HLA-identical sibling bone marrow transplantation. Blood 2002;100(12):3908–18.

49. Jacobsohn DA. Acute graft-versus-host disease in children. Bone Marrow Transplant 2008;41(2):215–21.

50. Dhir S, Slatter M, Skinner R. Recent advances in the management of graft-versus-host disease. Arch Dis Child 2014. [Epub ahead of print].

51. Dall'Amico R, Messina C. Extracorporeal photochemotherapy for the treatment of graft-versus-host disease. Ther Apher 2002;6(4):296–304.

52. Calore E, Calò A, Tridello G, et al. Extracorporeal photochemotherapy may improve outcome in children with acute GVHD. Bone Marrow Transplant 2008; 42(6):421–5.

53. Baird K, Cooke K, Schultz KR. Chronic graft-versus-host disease (GVHD) in children. Pediatr Clin North Am 2010;57(1):297–322.

54. Baker KS, Bresters D, Sande JE. The burden of cure: long-term side effects following hematopoietic stem cell transplantation (HSCT) in children. Pediatr Clin North Am 2010;57(1):323–42.

55. Pulsipher MA, Skinner R, McDonald GB, et al. National Cancer Institute, National Heart, Lung and Blood Institute/Pediatric Blood and Marrow Transplantation Consortium First International Consensus Conference on late effects after pediatric hematopoietic cell transplantation: the need for pediatric-specific long-term follow-up guidelines. Biol Blood Marrow Transplant 2012;18(3):334–47.

56. Warren EH, Deeg HJ. Dissecting graft-versus-leukemia from graft-versus-host disease using novel strategies. Tissue Antigens 2013;81(4):183–93.

57. Horowitz MM, Gale RP, Sondel PM, et al. Graft-versus-leukemia reactions after bone marrow transplantation. Blood 1990;75(3):555–62.

58. Curtis RE, Rowlings PA, Deeg HJ, et al. Solid cancers after bone marrow transplantation. N Engl J Med 1997;336(13):897–904.

59. Bader P, Kreyenberg H, Henze GH, et al. Prognostic value of minimal residual disease quantification before allogeneic stem-cell transplantation in relapsed childhood acute lymphoblastic leukemia: the ALL-REZ BFM Study Group. J Clin Oncol 2009;27(3):377–84.

60. Leung W, Pui CH, Coustan-Smith E, et al. Detectable minimal residual disease before hematopoietic cell transplantation is prognostic but does not preclude cure for children with very-high-risk leukemia. Blood 2012;120(2):468–72.

61. Locatelli F, Pende D, Mingari MC, et al. Cellular and molecular basis of haploidentical hematopoietic stem cell transplantation in the successful treatment of high-risk leukemias: role of alloreactive NK cells. Front Immunol 2013;4:15.

62. Pende D, Marcenaro S, Falco M, et al. Anti-leukemia activity of alloreactive NK cells in KIR ligand-mismatched haploidentical HSCT for pediatric patients: evaluation of the functional role of activating KIR and redefinition of inhibitory KIR specificity. Blood 2009;113(13):3119–29.

63. Olson JA, Leveson-Gower DB, Gill S, et al. NK cells mediate reduction of GVHD by inhibiting activated, alloreactive T cells while retaining GVT effects. Blood 2010;115(21):4293–301.

64. Lankester AC, Locatelli F, Bader P, et al. Will post-transplantation cell therapies for pediatric patients become standard of care? Biol Blood Marrow Transplant 2014. [Epub ahead of print].

65. Yu AL, Gilman AL, Ozkaynak MF, et al. Anti-GD2 antibody with GM-CSF, interleukin-2, and isotretinoin for neuroblastoma. N Engl J Med 2010;363(14):1324–34.

66. Flamand V, Sornasse T, Thielemans K, et al. Murine dendritic cells pulsed in vitro with tumor antigen induce tumor resistance in vivo. Eur J Immunol 1994;24(3):605–10.

67. Honsik CJ, Jung G, Reisfeld RA. Lymphokine-activated killer cells targeted by monoclonal antibodies to the disialogangliosides GD2 and GD3 specifically lyse human tumor cells of neuroectodermal origin. Proc Natl Acad Sci U S A 1986;83(20):7893–7.

68. Mukherji B, Chakraborty NG, Yamasaki S, et al. Induction of antigen-specific cytolytic T cells in situ in human melanoma by immunization with synthetic peptide-pulsed autologous antigen presenting cells. Proc Natl Acad Sci U S A 1995;92(17):8078–82.

69. Geiger JD, Hutchinson RJ, Hohenkirk LF, et al. Vaccination of pediatric solid tumor patients with tumor lysate-pulsed dendritic cells can expand specific T cells and mediate tumor regression. Cancer Res 2001;61(23):8513–9.

70. Ardon H, De VS, Van CF, et al. Adjuvant dendritic cell-based tumour vaccination for children with malignant brain tumours. Pediatr Blood Cancer 2010;54(4):519–25.

71. Krishnadas DK, Shapiro T, Lucas K. Complete remission following decitabine/dendritic cell vaccine for relapsed neuroblastoma. Pediatrics 2013;131(1):e336–41.

72. Rosenberg SA, Dudley ME. Adoptive cell therapy for the treatment of patients with metastatic melanoma. Curr Opin Immunol 2009;21(2):233–40.

73. Grupp SA, Kalos M, Barrett D, et al. Chimeric antigen receptor-modified T cells for acute lymphoid leukemia. N Engl J Med 2013;368(16):1509–18.

74. Brentjens RJ, Davila ML, Riviere I, et al. CD19-targeted T cells rapidly induce molecular remissions in adults with chemotherapy-refractory acute lymphoblastic leukemia. Sci Transl Med 2013;5(177):177ra38.

75. Brentjens RJ, Riviere I, Park JH, et al. Safety and persistence of adoptively transferred autologous CD19-targeted T cells in patients with relapsed or chemotherapy refractory B-cell leukemias. Blood 2011;118(18):4817–28.

76. Kalos M, Levine BL, Porter DL, et al. T cells with chimeric antigen receptors have potent antitumor effects and can establish memory in patients with advanced leukemia. Sci Transl Med 2011;3(95):95ra73.
77. Modak S, Cheung NK. Disialoganglioside directed immunotherapy of neuroblastoma. Cancer Invest 2007;25(1):67–77.
78. Pule MA, Savoldo B, Myers GD, et al. Virus-specific T cells engineered to coexpress tumor-specific receptors: persistence and antitumor activity in individuals with neuroblastoma. Nat Med 2008;14(11):1264–70.
79. Yankelevich M, Kondadasula SV, Thakur A, et al. Anti-CD3 x anti-GD2 bispecific antibody redirects T-cell cytolytic activity to neuroblastoma targets. Pediatr Blood Cancer 2012;59(7):1198–205.
80. Portell CA, Advani AS. Novel targeted therapies in acute lymphoblastic leukemia. Leuk Lymphoma 2014;55(4):737–48.
81. Lum LG, Thakur A. Targeting T cells with bispecific antibodies for cancer therapy. BioDrugs 2011;25(6):365–79.
82. Grabert RC, Cousens LP, Smith JA, et al. Human T cells armed with Her2/neu bispecific antibodies divide, are cytotoxic, and secrete cytokines with repeated stimulation. Clin Cancer Res 2006;12(2):569–76.
83. Lum LG, Thakur A, Liu Q, et al. CD20-targeted T cells after stem cell transplantation for high risk and refractory non-Hodgkin's lymphoma. Biol Blood Marrow Transplant 2013;19(6):925–33.
84. Reusch U, Sundaram M, Davol PA, et al. Anti-CD3 x anti-epidermal growth factor receptor (EGFR) bispecific antibody redirects T-cell cytolytic activity to EGFR-positive cancers in vitro and in an animal model. Clin Cancer Res 2006;12(1):183–90.
85. Ruggeri L, Capanni M, Casucci M, et al. Role of natural killer cell alloreactivity in HLA-mismatched hematopoietic stem cell transplantation. Blood 1999;94(1):333–9.
86. Koehl U, Sorensen J, Esser R, et al. IL-2 activated NK cell immunotherapy of three children after haploidentical stem cell transplantation. Blood Cells Mol Dis 2004;33(3):261–6.
87. Leung W, Sorensen J, Esser R, et al. Inhibitory KIR-HLA receptor-ligand mismatch in autologous haematopoietic stem cell transplantation for solid tumour and lymphoma. Br J Cancer 2007;97(4):539–42.
88. Stern M, Passweg JR, Meyer-Monard S, et al. Pre-emptive immunotherapy with purified natural killer cells after haploidentical SCT: a prospective phase II study in two centers. Bone Marrow Transplant 2013;48(3):433–8.
89. Esser R, Muller T, Stefes D, et al. NK cells engineered to express a GD2 -specific antigen receptor display built-in ADCC-like activity against tumour cells of neuroectodermal origin. J Cell Mol Med 2012;16(3):569–81.
90. Heczey A, Liu D, Tian G, et al. Invariant NKT cells with chimeric antigen receptor provide a novel platform for safe and effective cancer immunotherapy. Blood 2014. [Epub ahead of print].
91. Maus MV, Grupp SA, Porter DL, et al. Antibody-modified T cells: CARs take the front seat for hematologic malignancies. Blood 2014;123(17):2625–35.
92. Teachey DT, Rheingold SR, Maude SL, et al. Cytokine release syndrome after blinatumomab treatment related to abnormal macrophage activation and ameliorated with cytokine-directed therapy. Blood 2013;121(26):5154–7.

Late Effects of Childhood Cancer and Its Treatment

Wendy Landier, PhD, RN, Saro Armenian, DO, MPH, Smita Bhatia, MD, MPH*

KEYWORDS

• Childhood • Cancer • Late effects • Treatment

KEY POINTS

• As survival rates for pediatric cancers continue to improve, the number of childhood cancer survivors continues to increase.
• The burden of long-term therapy-related morbidity experienced by childhood cancer survivors is substantial.
• Childhood cancer survivors require lifelong follow-up care to monitor for late treatment-related sequelae.

INTRODUCTION

With advances in therapeutic strategies for common childhood malignancies such as leukemia, lymphoma, and central nervous system (CNS) tumors, the number of childhood cancer survivors in the United States continues to increase, and is estimated to exceed 500,000 by 2020.[1] About 1 of every 530 young adults between 20 and 39 years of age in the United States is a childhood cancer survivor.[2] Treatment of childhood cancer with chemotherapy, radiation, or hematopoietic cell transplant (HCT) can result in adverse sequelae, which may not become evident for many years. In this article, commonly occurring late effects associated with childhood cancer treatment are reviewed.

BURDEN OF MORBIDITY

The burden of morbidity experienced by childhood cancer survivors is substantial, as shown by the fact that approximately 40% of childhood cancer survivors experience a late effect that is severe, life threatening, disabling, or fatal at 30 years from diagnosis.[3] A primary diagnosis of Hodgkin lymphoma (HL) or brain tumors and exposure to chest radiation or anthracyclines increases the risk of these chronic health conditions. Furthermore, the burden of morbidity increases as the cohort ages.[4] HCT recipients experience a higher burden of morbidity when compared with childhood cancer

Department of Population Sciences, City of Hope, 1500 E. Duarte Rd., DPS-173, Duarte, CA 91010, USA
* Corresponding author.
E-mail address: sbhatia@coh.org

survivors treated with conventional therapy.[5] The potential for serious therapy-related sequelae provide the rationale for ongoing follow-up of childhood cancer survivors into adult life.

STANDARDIZED RECOMMENDATIONS FOR FOLLOW-UP OF CHILDHOOD CANCER

In response to a call from the Institute of Medicine for a systematic plan for lifelong surveillance of cancer survivors,[6] the Children's Oncology Group (COG) developed exposure-related, risk-based guidelines (Long-Term Follow-Up Guidelines for Survivors of Childhood, Adolescent, and Young Adult Cancers)[7] for follow-up of patients treated for pediatric malignancies. Specially tailored patient education materials, known as Health Links, accompany the Guidelines to enhance health promotion in this population. The Guidelines and the Health Links can be downloaded from http://www.survivorshipguidelines.org.[8] Recommendations for screening of specific treatment-related late effects are summarized in **Table 1**. The COG Guideline group, along with several other guideline groups addressing survivorship care,[9–11] have initiated the international harmonization of long-term follow-up guidelines for childhood cancer survivors.[12] To use these guidelines, the first step entails the development of a treatment summary (**Box 1**). This treatment summary allows the survivor and their health care provider to determine recommended follow-up care according to the guidelines. In this article, the more commonly occurring late effects in survivors of childhood cancer, and the relationship between these late effects and specific therapeutic exposures, are reviewed, to suggest reasonable starting points for evaluation of specific long-term problems using the screening recommendations from the COG Long-Term Follow-Up Guidelines.

AUDITORY IMPAIRMENT

Children with cancer often require therapy with potentially ototoxic agents, including platinum-based chemotherapy, aminoglycoside antibiotics, loop diuretics, and radiation therapy. These agents are all capable of causing sensorineural hearing loss.[13,14] Risk for hearing loss is increased with higher doses of platinum-based chemotherapy, particularly cisplatin in cumulative doses exceeding 360 mg/m^2 and myeloablative doses of carboplatin,[15–18] combining platinum chemotherapy with cranial irradiation,[13] treatment with multiple ototoxic agents,[19] age younger than 5 years at treatment,[20] and surgery that involves cranial nerve VIII.[21] Radiation-related hearing loss may be multifactorial. Although sensorineural loss increases in association with high doses of radiation involving the ear, treatment with higher doses of radiation has also been associated with conductive hearing loss.[22,23]

COGNITIVE SEQUELAE

Childhood cancer survivors are at risk for impaired cognition. Cranial radiation is a well-established risk factor for cognitive impairment,[24–26] although corticosteroids and antimetabolite chemotherapy have been implicated as contributors.[27] Cognitive impairment usually become evident within 1 to 2 years after cranial radiation and is progressive, likely because of the child's failure to acquire new abilities at a rate similar to peers. Affected children experience academic difficulties, resulting in problems with receptive and expressive language and attention span. Fatigue and sleep disruption also serve as contributors to the cognitive impairment observed in childhood cancer survivors.[28]

Table 1
Exposure-based screening recommendations for commonly occurring late effects in childhood cancer survivors

Adverse Outcome	Therapeutic Exposures Associated with Increased Risk	Factors Associated with Highest Risk	Recommended Screening
Adverse psychosocial effects	Any cancer experience	CNS tumors Cranial irradiation Hearing loss Older age at diagnosis	Psychosocial assessment Yearly
Neurocognitive deficits	Cranial irradiation Methotrexate (intrathecal, high-dose IV) Cytarabine (high-dose IV)	Female sex Younger age at treatment Cranial irradiation Intrathecal methotrexate	Review of educational or vocational progress Yearly Neuropsychological evaluation Baseline and as clinically indicated
Hearing loss	Cranial irradiation Cisplatin Carboplatin (at myeloablative doses or if given during infancy)	Younger age at treatment Higher doses of chemotherapy and radiation	Complete audiologic evaluation for patients who received: Platinum: baseline and as clinically indicated Cranial radiation ≥30 Gy: Every 5 y
Cataracts	Cranial irradiation Total body irradiation Corticosteroids	Higher radiation dose Single daily radiation fraction Combination of corticosteroids and radiation	Visual acuity and fundoscopic examination Yearly Patients who received radiation only: Evaluation by ophthalmologist Yearly if dose ≥30 Gy or TBI; every 3 y if dose <30 Gy
Dental abnormalities	Cranial irradiation Receipt of any chemotherapy before development of permanent dentition	Younger age at treatment	Dental examination and cleaning Every 6 mo

(continued on next page)

Table 1
(continued)

Adverse Outcome	Therapeutic Exposures Associated with Increased Risk	Factors Associated with Highest Risk	Recommended Screening
Cardiomyopathy Congestive heart failure	Anthracycline chemotherapy Chest and spinal irradiation	Anthracycline cumulative dose >500 mg/m^2 Female sex Younger age at treatment Mediastinal irradiation	Echocardiogram Every 1 to 5 y (frequency based on age at treatment, anthracycline dose, and history of radiation) Electrocardiogram Baseline and as clinically indicated
Atherosclerotic heart disease Myocardial infarction Valvular disease	Chest and spinal irradiation		Patients who received radiation only: Fasting blood glucose or HgA$_{1C}$ and lipid profile Every 2 y; if abnormal, refer for ongoing management
Pulmonary fibrosis Interstitial pneumonitis	Bleomycin, carmustine, lomustine, busulfan Chest or whole lung irradiation	Younger age at treatment Bleomycin dose >400 U/m^2	Pulmonary function tests Baseline and as clinically indicated
Hepatic dysfunction	Methotrexate Mercaptopurine Thioguanine Liver irradiation	Previous veno-occlusive disease of the liver Chronic viral hepatitis	ALT, AST, total bilirubin Baseline and as clinically indicated
Renal dysfunction (glomerular or tubular)	Cisplatin Carboplatin Ifosfamide High-dose methotrexate Abdominal irradiation Nephrectomy	High-dose chemotherapy Younger age at treatment Abdominal radiation	Blood pressure, urinalysis Yearly Serum BUN, creatinine, and electrolytes Baseline and as clinically indicated
Bladder complications	Alkylating agents Abdominal/pelvic irradiation Surgery involving the bladder	Higher-dose alkylating agents administered without bladder uroprophylaxis Abdominal/pelvic irradiation	Urinalysis and targeted history Yearly

Late effect	Treatment	Risk factors	Screening/evaluation
Obesity	Cranial irradiation; Neurosurgery involving the hypothalamic-pituitary axis	Younger age at treatment; Female sex; Cranial irradiation >20 Gy	Height, weight, BMI; Yearly
Hypothyroidism	Radiation impacting the thyroid gland (eg, neck, mantle)	Increasing radiation dose; Female sex; Older age at treatment	Free T4, TSH; Yearly
Precocious puberty	Cranial irradiation	Female sex; Younger age at treatment; Cranial irradiation >18 Gy	Height, weight, Tanner staging; Yearly until sexually mature
Hypogonadism (Leydig cell dysfunction in males; acute or premature ovarian failure in females)	Alkylating agents; Craniospinal irradiation; Abdominopelvic irradiation; Gonadal irradiation	Higher cumulative doses of alkylating agents; Gonadal irradiation; Females: treatment during the peripubertal or postpubertal period	Pubertal onset, tempo, Tanner staging; Yearly until sexually mature; Females: Serum FSH, LH, estradiol; Baseline at age 13 y, and as clinically indicated; Males: Serum testosterone; Baseline at age 14 y, and as clinically indicated
Infertility	Alkylating agents; Craniospinal irradiation; Adominopelvic irradiation; Gonadal irradiation	Male sex; Higher doses of alkylating agents; Gonadal irradiation; Total body irradiation	Females: targeted history and physical examination; Yearly; Males: semen analysis; At request of sexually mature patient; Males: FSH; If unable to obtain semen analysis
Growth hormone deficiency	Cranial irradiation	Cranial irradiation ≥18 Gy	Height, weight, BMI, Tanner staging; Every 6 mo until growth is completed, then yearly
Short stature; Musculoskeletal growth problems	Cranial irradiation; Corticosteroids; Total body irradiation	Younger age at treatment; Cranial radiation dose >18 Gy; Unfractionated (10 Gy) total body irradiation	Standing and sitting height; Yearly until growth completed
Scoliosis/kyphosis	Radiation involving the chest, abdomen, or spine; Thoracic surgery; Neurosurgery involving the spine	Younger age at irradiation; Higher radiation doses; Hemithoracic, abdominal, or spinal surgery	Spine examination for scoliosis and kyphosis; Yearly until growth completed; more frequent assessment during puberty

(continued on next page)

Table 1
(continued)

Adverse Outcome	Therapeutic Exposures Associated with Increased Risk	Factors Associated with Highest Risk	Recommended Screening
Reduced bone mineral density	Corticosteroids Craniospinal irradiation Gonadal irradiation Total body irradiation	Hypothyroidism Hypogonadism Growth hormone deficiency	Bone density evaluation (DEXA or quantitative CT) Baseline and repeat as clinically indicated
Osteonecrosis	Corticosteroids High-dose radiation to any bone	Dexamethasone Adolescent age at treatment Female sex	Targeted history and physical examination Yearly
Life-threatening infection	Splenectomy Radiation impacting the spleen (≥40 Gy) Chronic active graft-versus-host disease	Anatomic asplenia Higher radiation doses to the spleen Ongoing immunsuppression Hypogammaglobulinemia	Blood culture When febrile, temperature ≥38.3°C (≥101°F)
Chronic HCV infection and HCV-related sequelae	Transfusions before 1993	Living in hyperendemic area	Hepatitis C antibody Once if treated before 1993 (date may vary for international patients) Hepatitis C PCR Once in patients with positive hepatitis C antibody
Therapy-related myelodysplasia Therapy-related acute myeloid leukemia	Alkylating agents Epipodophyllotoxins Anthracyclines	Increasing dose of chemotherapeutic agents Older age at treatment Autologous hematopoietic cell transplant	Targeted history/physical examination Yearly

Late effect	Radiation exposure	Risk factors	Surveillance
Skin cancer (basal cell, squamous cell, melanoma)	Radiation (any field)	Orthovoltage radiation (before 1970): delivery of greater dose to skin; Additional excessive exposure to sun or tanning booths	Physical examination Yearly
Secondary brain tumor	Cranial irradiation	Increasing radiation dose; Younger age at treatment	Targeted history and neurologic examination Yearly
Thyroid cancer	Radiation impacting the thyroid gland (eg, neck, mantle)	Increasing radiation dose up to 29 Gy; Female sex; Younger age at radiation	Physical examination Yearly
Breast cancer	Chest irradiation	Increasing radiation dose; Female sex; Longer time because radiation	Females: clinical breast examination Yearly beginning at puberty until age 25 y, then every 6 mo; Mammogram and breast MRI Yearly for patients who received $\geq$20 Gy beginning 8 y after radiation or at age 25 y, whichever occurs last. For patients who received 10–19 Gy, clinician should discuss benefits and risks/harms of screening with patient; if decision made to screen, then follow recommendations for $\geq$20 Gy
Colorectal cancer	Abdominal/pelvic irradiation; Spinal irradiation	Higher radiation dose to bowel; Higher daily dose fraction; Combined with chemotherapy (especially alkylating agents)	Colonoscopy Every 5 y (minimum) for patients who received $\geq$30 Gy, beginning 10 y after radiation or at age 35 y, whichever occurs last; more frequently if indicated based on colonoscopy results. Monitoring of patients who received total body irradiation without additional radiation potentially affecting the colon/rectum should be determined on an individual basis

Abbreviations: ALT, alanine aminotransferase; AST, aspartate aminotransferase; BMI, body mass index; BUN, blood urea nitrogen; CT, computed tomography; DEXA, dual x-ray absorptiometry; FSH, follicle-stimulating hormone; HCV, hepatitis C virus; HgA$_{1C}$, hemoglobin A1C; IV, intravenous; LH, luteinizing hormone; PCR, polymerase chain reaction; T$_4$, thyroxine; TSH, thyroid-stimulating hormone.

Data from Children's Oncology Group long-term follow-up guidelines, version 4.0. 2013. Available at: www.survivorshipguidelines.org. Accessed September 15, 2014.

Box 1
Basic elements of a childhood cancer survivor treatment summary

Key Elements	Details
Demographics	Name, sex, date of birth, treating institution and key team members
Diagnosis	Diagnosis, date, site, stage
	Relapse(s), if applicable, with date(s) and site(s)
	Subsequent malignant neoplasm(s), if applicable, with type(s) and site(s)
	Completion of therapy date(s)
Therapeutic Exposures	
Chemotherapy	Names of chemotherapy agents received
	Routes of administration
	Cumulative doses (per m²) for alkylators, anthracyclines, and bleomycin (at minimum)
	Intermediate/high ($\geq$1000 mg/m²) vs standard dosing for intravenous methotrexate and cytarabine
	Standard vs myeloablative dosing for carboplatin
Radiation	Dates, type, field(s), total dose, number of fractions, dose per fraction
Surgical procedures	Type(s), date(s)
Hematopoietic cell transplant	Type(s), date(s), graft-versus-host disease prophylaxis/treatment

---

Brain tumor survivors are especially vulnerable to impairment in neurocognitive functioning; young age at exposure to cranial radiation, cerebrovascular events, and hearing or motor disabilities contribute to the vulnerability.[29–32] Cranial radiation dose has a direct association with cognitive impairment.[33,34] Cognitive impairment manifests as slow processing and psychomotor speed, inattention, memory impairment, and deficits in verbal and visual-spatial skills.[31,35–40] These impairments have a negative impact on societal reintegration, such as education, employment, income, and marital status.[36]

Survivors of childhood acute lymphoblastic leukemia (ALL) are also at risk for cognitive impairment, presenting as inattention, and impaired processing speed, executive function, and global intellectual function.[41,42] Exposure to 24-Gy cranial radiation,[43] younger age at radiation exposure, and female sex[44,45] are associated with increased risk. This impairment is associated with reduced educational attainment, unemployment,[41,46] and independent living.[47] Cognitive deficits have been observed after treatment with chemotherapy alone[48,49] and include deficits in attention, executive function, and complex fine-motor functioning; global intellectual function is relatively preserved.[41,48,50–52]

CARDIOVASCULAR FUNCTION

Cardiovascular complications such as coronary artery disease, stroke, and especially heart failure have emerged as a leading cause of morbidity and mortality in aging survivors of childhood cancer.[53] These survivors are at a 9-fold risk of having a stroke, 10-fold risk of developing coronary artery disease, and 15-fold risk of developing heart failure when compared with the general population.[3] This increased risk is caused by the combined effects of cardiotoxic cancer treatments (anthracycline chemotherapy, radiation) and traditional cardiovascular risk factors (hypertension, diabetes, dyslipidemia, obesity) that emerge later in life.[53]

Anthracycline chemotherapy increases the risk of developing heart failure in a dose-dependent manner; the incidence of heart failure is less than 5%, with cumulative anthracycline dose of less than 250 mg/m^2; approaches 10% at doses between 250 and 600 mg/m^2; and exceeds 30% for doses greater than 600 mg/m^2.[53,54] Chest radiation, when the heart is in the treatment field, and cardiovascular risk factors, such as hypertension and diabetes, can substantially increase the risk of anthracycline-related heart failure. In cancer survivors, heart failure is associated with a poor prognosis; 5-year overall survival rates are reported to be less than 50%.[55]

Different anthracycline analogues with potential for decreased cardiotoxicity have been studied, but long-term data regarding their efficacy in heart failure risk reduction are lacking.[56–58] Cardioprotectants such as dexrazoxane have been shown to minimize cardiac injury shortly after anthracycline administration without compromising its antitumor efficacy.[56,59] As in anthracycline analogues, long-term data on efficacy of dexrazoxane are lacking, and certain subgroups, particularly children, who have the greatest potential number of life years after cancer therapy, remain understudied.[56] On the other hand, advances in cardiac imaging have helped set the stage for the development of novel prevention strategies in asymptomatic survivors at high risk for therapy-related heart failure. These advances include closer monitoring, better management of cardiovascular risk factors such as hypertension and diabetes, and consideration of pharmacologic therapy (angiotensin-converting enzyme inhibitors or β-blockers) in high-risk individuals with early changes in cardiac function.[60]

Chest radiation therapy has been implicated in the development of constrictive pericarditis, valvular heart disease, coronary artery disease, conduction abnormalities, and heart failure.[53] Clinically evident heart failure, although rare after chest radiation alone, is primarily manifested as left ventricular diastolic dysfunction, in contrast to the systolic dysfunction typically seen after anthracycline exposure.[53,61] On the other hand, premature coronary artery disease is a well-recognized complication of radiation therapy, with a reported cumulative incidence of 21% at 20 years in individuals treated with chest radiation.[53] However, clinically significant coronary artery disease rarely occurs in the absence of other cardiovascular risk factors such as obesity, hypertension, and dyslipidemia, emphasizing the importance of management of these risk factors to reduce subsequent coronary artery disease risk.

PULMONARY FUNCTION

The lungs are exceptionally susceptible to radiation-related damage. The prevalence and extent of radiation-related lung injury are dependent on several factors, including age at exposure, total radiation dose, number of fractions, radiation type, and total lung volume in the radiation field.[62] In very young children, the basis for respiratory damage seems to differ from that seen in adolescents or adults and is likely the result of hypoplasia of the chest wall and compromised growth of the lung parenchyma, as shown by deficits in total lung capacity, forced vital capacity, and diffusion capacity of the lung.[63,64] Although refined radiation therapy techniques have resulted in a dramatically decreased incidence of pulmonary toxicity over the past 2 decades, patients who have received pulmonary radiation during childhood continue to remain at risk for declining pulmonary function over time.[62,63,65]

Several chemotherapeutic agents are also associated with pulmonary damage, including bleomycin, busulfan, lomustine, and carmustine. The pulmonary toxicity of these agents may be increased when combined with radiation.[65] Contemporary pediatric cancer therapy rarely includes high doses of bleomycin, decreasing the likelihood that the growing population of childhood cancer survivors will be at risk for clinically significant bleomycin-induced pulmonary disease later in life.

On the other hand, pulmonary complications remain a leading cause of morbidity and mortality in long-term survivors of HCT.[66,67] This situation is largely because of the additive effects of therapy delivered before transplant and the intensity of therapy required during HCT, which magnify the risk. Obliterative bronchiolitis (BO) is an irreversible chronic obstructive lung disorder, which may occur months to years after allogeneic HCT.[67] Radiographic imaging of patients with BO is characteristic for lung hyperinflation, and parenchymal hypoattenuation and air trapping are apparent on chest computed tomography scans. The treatment of BO remains challenging, and many patients with BO develop end-stage pulmonary disease and do not survive.[67]

THYROID ABNORMALITIES

Thyroid-related complications in childhood cancer survivors include primary or central hypothyroidism, benign or malignant thyroid tumors, and (rarely) hyperthyroidism.[68] Complications related to the thyroid gland are primarily seen in survivors who were treated with radiation to the head, nasopharynx, oropharynx, or total body or those who received radiation involving the cervical, supraclavicular, or mantle fields.[68]

The risk for hypothyroidism or thyroid nodules is especially high for those treated with radiation doses in excess of 20 Gy.[68] Strategies to decrease risk include shielding of the thyroid gland during radiation, use of lower-dose radiation (or elimination of radiation when possible), and avoidance of concurrent use of radiation and iodide-containing contrast materials. Central hypothyroidism related to cranial radiation is typically seen only in survivors who received radiation to the hypothalamic-pituitary axis at doses of 30 Gy or higher.[68,69] The risk of central hypothyroidism in patients who receive lower doses of cranial radiation (such as is typically given in patients with ALL), is very low.[70]

GONADAL FUNCTION
Males

Abnormalities of both germ (Sertoli) cell and gonadal endocrine (Leydig cell) function can result from exposure to chemotherapy, radiation, or surgery in male cancer survivors. Germ cell-producing Sertoli cells are more sensitive to the cytotoxic effects of radiation and chemotherapy than the testosterone-producing Leydig cells. Thus, males may experience impaired germ cell function (oligospermia or azoospermia) without having evidence of gonadal endocrine dysfunction (testosterone insufficiency or deficiency).

Testicular radiation is known to result in decreased testicular volume, reduced or absent production of semen, and increased follicle-stimulating hormone. The effects are dose dependent, with potentially reversible azoospermia at doses of 1 to 3 Gy; azoospermia that is less likely to be reversible at doses of 3 to 6 Gy, and azoospermia that is typically irreversible at doses greater than 6 to 8 Gy.[71–73] Data regarding semen production in males treated with testicular radiation alone before puberty are limited, although there is some evidence that germ cells in the prepubertal testes may be more radiosensitive than those in males who receive testicular radiation after puberty.[74]

Chemotherapy agents with the potential to cause germ cell injury in males include alkylating agents (particularly busulfan, procarbazine, and mechlorethamine), heavy metals (such as platinum compounds), and nonclassic alkylators (such as procarbazine and dacarbazine).[75] Many of these agents affect spermatogenesis in a dose-dependent manner. Effects on spermatogenesis may be reversible in up to 70% of males who receive cumulative cyclophosphamide doses lower than 7.5 gm/m^2[76]; however, doses greater than 7.5 gm/m^2 may result in permanent azoospermia.[73,75,76]

In male survivors of childhood cancer exposed to gonadotoxic chemotherapy, preservation of Leydig cell function in the setting of oligospermia or azoospermia is not uncommon. Similarly, Leydig cell injury is dose dependent, inversely related to age at treatment, and typically associated with radiation doses higher than those causing germ cell injury.[77] Thus, males treated with higher doses of testicular radiation (>20 Gy) when prepubertal or peripubertal are at high risk of both infertility and testosterone deficiency or insufficiency, with resultant delayed or absent sexual maturation.[77] Prepubertal males who receive fractionated doses of testicular radiation lower than 12 Gy are typically able to attain sexual maturity without intervention, although these males often experience compensated Leydig cell failure (normal testosterone with increased luteinizing hormone levels).[77,78] Males in the adolescent and young adult age range at the time of testicular radiation are typically able to tolerate higher doses with lower risk for Leydig cell failure, when compared with younger males.[77]

Surgical effects on male gonadal function include secondary hypogonadism in patients undergoing resection of brain tumors involving the hypothalamus or pituitary,[79] impotence or retrograde ejaculation in patients undergoing partial or complete pelvic exenteration or bilateral retroperitoneal lymph node dissection,[80] and hydrocele associated with nephrectomy.[81]

Females

Two types of ovarian failure have been described in female childhood cancer survivors. Acute ovarian failure occurs when a female loses ovarian function during or shortly after completion of cancer treatment. Premature ovarian failure (POF) occurs when a female survivor retains ovarian function after childhood cancer treatment, but experiences menopause before reaching age 40 years.[82,83] Increased risk for ovarian failure is associated with alkylating chemotherapy, older age at treatment, and pelvic or abdominal radiation.[77,82,83] Conventional fractionated total body irradiation (TBI) is associated with ovarian failure in 50% of prepubertal females and nearly all females older than 10 years at exposure.[84,85]

Ovarian failure associated with alkylating chemotherapy results in dose-dependent and age-dependent toxicity, with gonadal toxicity increasing with chronologic age. However, myeloablative doses of alkylating agents are strongly associated with permanent ovarian failure in females, regardless of age at exposure.[86] There is increasing evidence supporting the risk for the development of POF in female survivors who do not develop amenorrhea after exposure to ovarian radiation or alkylating chemotherapy.[82] In addition to infertility, POF is also associated with increased risks for cardiovascular disease, osteoporosis, and psychosexual dysfunction.

Surgical effects on female gonadal function include secondary hypogonadism in patients undergoing resection of brain tumors involving the hypothalamus or pituitary,[79] hypogonadism requiring replacement therapy and associated infertility in females undergoing bilateral oophorectomy, and increased risk for POF associated with unilateral oophorectomy, as a result of reduced ovarian reserve.[87]

Growth

Decreased linear growth is a common occurrence during therapy in children with cancer, but most children are able to experience catch-up growth after completion of therapy. In some instances, such as after cranial or spinal radiation exposure, short stature is permanent or even progressive.

Cranial irradiation can cause alterations in growth hormone function and secretion, resulting in short stature.[88] The effects of cranial irradiation are age related, and children younger than 5 years at therapy are particularly susceptible.[89,90] Severe growth retardation (standing height <5%) is seen in more than 50% of patients with brain tumors, when radiation doses exceed 30 Gy to the hypothalamus or pituitary gland.[91] In ALL survivors, 24 Gy of cranial irradiation has been shown to result in a decrease in median height of about 5 to 10 cm.[92]

Direct inhibition of vertebral growth by spinal irradiation also contributes to short stature. This change is seen most commonly in patients with brain tumors whose entire spinal columns have received doses in excess of 35 Gy.[93,94] Children who are very young (<5 years) or are undergoing their adolescent growth spurt at the time of radiation therapy are at especially high risk.

The long-term effects of TBI on height in survivors of HCT are well described.[95] After 10 Gy given as a single fraction, long-term, severe decreases in growth rates appear in most children. Fractionation of TBI seems to decrease growth retardation. The pathogenesis of short stature in children who receive conventional fractionated TBI is likely multifactorial and may be exacerbated by HCT-related complications such as graft-versus-host disease and its management.[95]

Current approaches to cancer therapy in children include attempts to spare adverse effects on growth.[96] Leukemia protocols are attempting to use high-dose methotrexate, cytosine arabinoside, or both, or intrathecal chemotherapy alone in lieu of radiation for CNS prophylaxis.[96] Hyperfractionation schedules for radiation therapy and chemotherapy-only regimens are being implemented for treatment of brain tumors and as conditioning regimens for HCT. Whether these changes will permit long-term survivors to have normal growth remains to be seen.

Obesity

Obesity, defined as high body mass index (BMI, calculated as weight in kilograms divided by the square of height in meters, >30 kg/m^2), is well recognized among survivors of childhood ALL and brain tumors.[91,97] Among patients with ALL, cranial radiation at 20 Gy or higher before the age of 5 years, African American race, Hispanic ethnicity, and use of antidepressant drugs (paroxetine) are associated with an increased risk of obesity.[97–99] Among female survivors of brain tumors, young age at radiation to the hypothalamic-pituitary axis at doses exceeding 20 Gy is associated with obesity.[91] Onset of obesity during adolescence or young adulthood is strongly associated with the subsequent development of adult-onset diabetes mellitus, hypertension, dyslipidemia, cardiovascular disease, osteoarthritis, and breast and colon cancer.[100,101] High total fat percentage/lean body mass ratio is a reliable predictor of long-term morbidity. Percentage fat is significantly higher among recipients of cranial radiation, and even among individuals with normal BMI,[102] and could explain the high prevalence of insulin resistance in this population.[103–106] Leptin and adiponectin are secreted by the adipocytes and serve as part of a feedback loop between the hypothalamus, the adipocyte, and the gut with respect to hunger, satiety, and energy usage and storage.[107–109] Adiponectin mirrors insulin resistance, whereas leptin reflects insulin resistance as well as anthropomorphic characteristics and body fat. Growth hormone deficiency seems to be a contributor to central obesity, insulin resistance, and dyslipidemia.[110,111] Unrelated to BMI or physical activity, exposure to TBI or abdominal radiation is associated with an increased risk of diabetes.[112]

OSTEOPOROSIS AND OSTEONECROSIS

Osteoporosis is defined as bone mineral density (BMD) greater than 2.5 standard deviations (SD) less than mean and osteopenia is defined as BMD 1 to 2.5 SD less than mean. Exposure to corticosteroids, methotrexate, and alkylating agents is known to cause BMD deficits[113,114]; whites are at greater risk than African Americans.[113,115] Cranial radiation and TBI increase the risk of osteoporosis, likely because of gonadal dysfunction, growth hormone failure, or hypothyroidism.[113,116]

Osteonecrosis (ON) is well recognized in children with ALL. Estimates for the incidence of symptomatic ON range from 1%[117] to 17.6%.[118] ON can develop during therapy or as late as a decade after treatment.[119] The increasing incidence of ON in patients with ALL is attributed to the incorporation of dexamethasone in treatment regimens.[120–122] Dexamethasone is more toxic to the bone than equivalent doses of prednisone, and continuous cumulative exposure conveys higher risk.[117,119,123] Coagulation alterations may be involved in ON. Antithrombin and protein S levels are significantly lower in patients with ON. A dexamethasone-induced hypercoagulable state may contribute to development of symptomatic ON.[124] Other risk factors for ON include older age at exposure, female gender, radiation, white race, and high BMI.[119,125] Weight-bearing joints are affected in 95% of patients (femoral head is the most frequently affected site) and surgical interventions are needed in more than 25% of cases.[123] Lesions occupying more than 30% of the femoral head have high likelihood of joint deterioration, necessitating arthroplasty at a young age.[126]

SUBSEQUENT MALIGNANT NEOPLASMS

Subsequent malignant neoplasms (SMNs) are histologically distinct malignancies developing among patients treated for a primary malignancy. The cumulative incidence of SMNs in childhood cancer survivors exceeds 20% at 30 years after diagnosis of the primary cancer.[127] This finding represents a 6-fold increased risk of SMNs among cancer survivors, when compared with an age-matched and sex-matched general population. SMNs are the leading cause of nonrelapse late mortality.[128] The risk of SMNs remains increased for more than 20 years from diagnosis of the primary cancer. The excess risk of SMN is highest for HL and Ewing sarcoma (8.7-fold and 8.5-fold compared with the general population, respectively). Exposure to radiation and specific chemotherapeutic agents is associated with increased risk. Breast and thyroid cancers are the most common SMNs.[127] Multiple SMNs have been observed among childhood cancer survivors. Cumulative incidence of a second SMN was 47% at 20 years after the first SMN.[129] The unique role played by specific therapeutic exposures in the development of SMNs have resulted in their classification into 2 distinct categories: (1) chemotherapy-related myelodysplasia (t-MDS) and acute myeloid leukemia (t-AML); and (2) radiation-related solid SMNs. Characteristics of t-MDS/AML include a short latency (<3 years from primary cancer diagnosis) and association with alkylating agents or topoisomerase II inhibitors.[130] Solid SMNs have a strong association with radiation and are characterized by a latency that exceeds 10 years.[130]

THERAPY-RELATED LEUKEMIA

t-MDS/AML has been observed in survivors of HL, non-HL, ALL, and bone sarcoma. The cumulative incidence approaches 2% at 15 years after therapy.[130,131] Two types of t-MDS/AML exist according to the World Health Organization classification: alkylating agent–related type and topoisomerase II inhibitor–related type.[132]

Alkylating agent–related t-MDS/AML develops 3 to 5 years after exposure; the risk increases with increasing dose of alkylating agents.[133] Alkylating agent–related t-MDS is typically associated with abnormalities involving chromosomes 5 (−5/del[5q]) and 7 (−7/del[7q]).[133]

Topoisomerase II inhibitor–related t-MDS/AML presents as overt leukemia after a latency of 6 months to 3 years and is associated with balanced translocations involving chromosome bands 11q23 or 21q22.[134]

THERAPY-RELATED SOLID SUBSEQUENT MALIGNANT NEOPLASMS

Therapy-related solid SMNs show a strong relation with ionizing radiation. The risk of solid SMNs is highest when the exposure occurs at a younger age and increases with the total dose of radiation and with increasing follow-up after radiation.[127,135] Some of the well-established radiation-related solid SMNs include breast cancer, thyroid cancer, brain tumors, sarcomas, and nonmelanoma skin cancer (NMSC).[130]

Breast Cancer

Breast cancer is the most common solid SMN, observed most commonly after chest radiation for HL. Female survivors of HL are at a 25-fold to 55-fold increased risk of radiation-related breast cancer when compared with the general population.[127,131,135–144] The cumulative incidence of breast cancer approaches 20% by age 45 years among female HL survivors treated with chest radiation during the perpubertal period.[131] The median latency after chest radiation ranges from 8 to 10 years, and the risk increases linearly with radiation dose, with an estimated relative risk of 6.4 at a dose of 20 Gy and 11.8 at a dose of 40 Gy.[145] Radiation-induced breast cancer is influenced by hormonal stimulation, as shown by the attenuation of risk among women who also received radiation doses of 5 Gy or greater to the ovaries.[145]

Thyroid Cancer

Thyroid cancer is observed after radiation to the neck for treatment of HL, ALL, and brain tumors, and after TBI for HCT.[127,130,135] Survivors exposed to neck radiation are at an 18-fold increased risk of developing thyroid cancer when compared with the general population.[146] A linear dose-response relation between thyroid cancer and radiation is observed up to 20 Gy, with a decline in the odds ratio at higher doses, showing evidence for a cell kill effect.[147,148] Female sex and younger age at exposure modify the risk of radiation-related thyroid cancer.[149]

Sarcoma

Childhood cancer survivors are at a 9-fold increased risk of bone and soft tissue sarcoma when compared with the general population.[150] Radiation therapy increases the risk in a dose-response manner, with increased risks at doses exceeding 10 Gy.[151–158] A primary diagnosis of retinoblastoma or HL and exposure to higher doses of anthracyclines or alkylating agents increase the risk of sarcoma.[150–152,154,159]

Lung Cancer

Lung cancer develops after chest irradiation for HL. The increase in risk of lung cancer with increasing radiation dose is greater among the patients who smoke after exposure to radiation than among nonsmokers.[160]

Brain Tumors

Meningiomas and gliomas develop after cranial radiation.[127,135,161–166] The relation between risk for second brain tumors and radiation dose is linear; the dose response seems weaker for gliomas than for meningiomas.[161,163,167] Increased exposure to intrathecal methotrexate significantly increases risk of meningioma.[167]

Bladder Cancer

The risk of bladder cancer in childhood cancer survivors is increased 3-fold to 5-fold that of the general population.[168–171] Heritable retinoblastoma and exposure to cyclophosphamide and pelvic radiation are associated with an increased risk.[168,172,173]

Renal Cell Carcinoma

Childhood cancer survivors are at an 8-fold increased risk of developing renal cell carcinoma when compared with the general population.[174] The highest risk is observed among neuroblastoma survivors.[174–176] Radiation to the renal bed at doses greater than 5 Gy and platinum-based therapy increase the risk.[174,175]

Salivary Gland Tumors

Childhood cancer survivors are at a 39-fold increased risk of developing a salivary gland tumor, when compared with the general population.[177] Risk of salivary gland tumors increases linearly with radiation dose and remained increased after 20 years.[177] Young age at exposure to radiation increases the risk of related salivary gland tumors.[178,179]

Melanoma

Childhood cancer survivors have a 2.5-fold increased risk of developing melanoma when compared with the general population.[180,181] Hereditary retinoblastoma survivors also have a higher risk of melanoma.[182]

Nonmelanoma Skin Cancer

Childhood cancer survivors are at a 5-fold increased risk of NMSC compared with the general population.[169] Radiation is associated with a 6-fold increase in risk.[183] Most tumors develop within the radiation field.

SUBSEQUENT MALIGNANT NEOPLASMS AND GENETIC SUSCEPTIBILITY

The risk of SMNs could be modified by mutations in high-penetrance genes that lead to genetic diseases, such as Li-Fraumeni syndrome. However, the attributable risk is small because of their low prevalence. The interindividual variability in risk of SMNs is more likely related to common polymorphisms in low-penetrance genes that regulate the availability of active drug metabolite, or those responsible for DNA repair. Gene-environment interactions may magnify subtle functional differences resulting from genetic variations.

LATE MORTALITY AMONG CHILDHOOD CANCER SURVIVORS

Childhood cancer survivors are at an 8-fold increased risk for premature death when compared with the general population.[128,184] Recurrent disease is the most common cause. SMNs, cardiac, and pulmonary causes account for most nonrelapse mortality.

SUMMARY: CANCER SURVIVORSHIP–FUTURE RESEARCH OPPORTUNITIES

A clear understanding of the association between therapeutic exposures and specific long-term complications has guided the design of less toxic therapies. Furthermore, an understanding of the magnitude of the burden of morbidity borne by cancer survivors has led to the development of treatment summaries, survivorship care plans, and efforts to harmonize survivorship guidelines worldwide.[12] However, there is a need for ongoing efforts to reduce this burden of morbidity. Thus, it is important that more recent cohorts of childhood and adolescent patients with cancer continue to be followed to determine how therapy modifications affect the prevalence and spectrum of late effects. It is important to develop, implement, and test interventions that can reduce the impact of treatment-related late effects on morbidity and mortality. There is also a need for research relating to the etiopathogenesis of therapy-related cancers and other late effects. Opportunities also exist to explore gene-environment interactions, which may modify susceptibility to develop adverse outcomes, thus providing insights into the identification of high-risk populations.

REFERENCES

1. Robison LL, Hudson MM. Survivors of childhood and adolescent cancer: life-long risks and responsibilities. Nat Rev Cancer 2014;14:61–70.
2. Ward E, Desantis C, Robbins A, et al. Childhood and adolescent cancer statistics, 2014. CA Cancer J Clin 2014;64:83–103.
3. Oeffinger KC, Mertens AC, Sklar CA, et al. Chronic health conditions in adult survivors of childhood cancer. N Engl J Med 2006;355:1572–82.
4. Hudson MM, Ness KK, Gurney JG, et al. Clinical ascertainment of health outcomes among adults treated for childhood cancer. JAMA 2013;309:2371–81.
5. Armenian SH, Sun CL, Kawashima T, et al. Long-term health-related outcomes in survivors of childhood cancer treated with HSCT versus conventional therapy: a report from the Bone Marrow Transplant Survivor Study (BMTSS) and Childhood Cancer Survivor Study (CCSS). Blood 2011;118: 1413–20.
6. Hewitt M, Weiner SL, Simone JV, editors. Childhood cancer survivorship: improving care and quality of life. Washington, DC: National Academies Press; 2003.
7. Landier W, Bhatia S, Eshelman DA, et al. Development of risk-based guidelines for pediatric cancer survivors: the Children's Oncology Group long-term follow-up guidelines from the Children's Oncology Group Late Effects Committee and Nursing Discipline. J Clin Oncol 2004;22:4979–90.
8. Children's Oncology Group. Long-term follow-up guidelines for survivors of childhood, adolescent, and young adult cancers, version 4.0. Monrovia (CA): Children's Oncology Group; 2013. Available at: http://www. survivorshipguidelines.org. Accessed September 15, 2014.
9. UK Children's Cancer Study Group Late Effects Group. Therapy based long term follow up practice statement, UKCCSG. 2011. Available at: www.cclg. org.uk/dynamic_files/LTFU-full.pdf. Accessed August 5, 2014.
10. Dutch Childhood Oncology Group. Richtlijn follow-up na kinderkanker meer dan 5 jaar na diagnose. Den Haag/Amsterdam, SKION, 2010. [in Dutch]. Available at: http://www.skion.nl/. Accessed August 5, 2014.
11. Scottish Intercollegiate Guidelines Network: long term follow up of survivors of childhood cancer. A national clinical guideline, SIGN. 2013. Available at: www.sign.ac.uk/guidelines/fulltext/132/index.html. Accessed August 5, 2014.
12. Kremer LC, Mulder RL, Oeffinger KC, et al. A worldwide collaboration to harmonize guidelines for the long-term follow-up of childhood and young adult cancer survivors: a report from the International Late Effects of Childhood Cancer Guideline Harmonization Group. Pediatr Blood Cancer 2013;60:543–9.
13. Schell MJ, McHaney VA, Green AA, et al. Hearing loss in children and young adults receiving cisplatin with or without prior cranial irradiation. J Clin Oncol 1989;7:754–60.

14. Bates DE, Beaumont SJ, Baylis BW. Ototoxicity induced by gentamicin and furosemide. Ann Pharmacother 2002;36:446–51.
15. Knight KR, Kraemer DF, Neuwelt EA. Ototoxicity in children receiving platinum chemotherapy: underestimating a commonly occurring toxicity that may influence academic and social development. J Clin Oncol 2005;23:8588–96.
16. Landier W, Knight K, Wong FL, et al. Ototoxicity in children with high-risk neuroblastoma: prevalence, risk factors, and concordance of grading scales–a report from the Children's Oncology Group. J Clin Oncol 2014;32:527–34.
17. Brock PR, Bellman SC, Yeomans EC, et al. Cisplatin ototoxicity in children: a practical grading system. Med Pediatr Oncol 1991;19:295–300.
18. Parsons SK, Neault MW, Lehmann LE, et al. Severe ototoxicity following carboplatin-containing conditioning regimen for autologous marrow transplantation for neuroblastoma. Bone Marrow Transplant 1998;22:669–74.
19. Ilveskoski I, Saarinen UM, Wiklund T, et al. Ototoxicity in children with malignant brain tumors treated with the "8 in 1" chemotherapy protocol. Med Pediatr Oncol 1996;27:26–31.
20. Weatherly RA, Owens JJ, Catlin FI, et al. cis-platinum ototoxicity in children. Laryngoscope 1991;101:917–24.
21. Simon MV. Neurophysiologic intraoperative monitoring of the vestibulocochlear nerve. J Clin Neurophysiol 2011;28:566–81.
22. Paulino AC, Simon JH, Zhen W, et al. Long-term effects in children treated with radiotherapy for head and neck rhabdomyosarcoma. Int J Radiat Oncol Biol Phys 2000;48:1489–95.
23. Young YH, Lu YC. Mechanism of hearing loss in irradiated ears: a long-term longitudinal study. Ann Otol Rhinol Laryngol 2001;110:904–6.
24. Moleski M. Neuropsychological, neuroanatomical, and neurophysiological consequences of CNS chemotherapy for acute lymphoblastic leukemia. Arch Clin Neuropsychol 2000;15:603–30.
25. Mulhern RK, Fairclough D, Ochs J. A prospective comparison of neuropsychological performance of children surviving leukemia who received 18-Gy, 24-Gy, or no cranial irradiation. J Clin Oncol 1991;9:1348–56.
26. Butler RW, Haser JK. Neurocognitive effects of treatment for childhood cancer. Ment Retard Dev Disabil Res Rev 2006;12:184–91.
27. Peterson CC, Johnson CE, Ramirez LY, et al. A meta-analysis of the neuropsychological sequelae of chemotherapy-only treatment for pediatric acute lymphoblastic leukemia. Pediatr Blood Cancer 2008;51:99–104.
28. Clanton NR, Klosky JL, Li C, et al. Fatigue, vitality, sleep, and neurocognitive functioning in adult survivors of childhood cancer: a report from the Childhood Cancer Survivor Study. Cancer 2011;117:2559–68.
29. Reimers TS, Ehrenfels S, Mortensen EL, et al. Cognitive deficits in long-term survivors of childhood brain tumors: identification of predictive factors. Med Pediatr Oncol 2003;40:26–34.
30. Walter AW, Mulhern RK, Gajjar A, et al. Survival and neurodevelopmental outcome of young children with medulloblastoma at St Jude Children's Research Hospital. J Clin Oncol 1999;17:3720–8.
31. Palmer SL, Gajjar A, Reddick WE, et al. Predicting intellectual outcome among children treated with 35-40 Gy craniospinal irradiation for medulloblastoma. Neuropsychology 2003;17:548–55.
32. Silber JH, Radcliffe J, Peckham V, et al. Whole-brain irradiation and decline in intelligence: the influence of dose and age on IQ score. J Clin Oncol 1992;10:1390–6.

33. Ris MD, Packer R, Goldwein J, et al. Intellectual outcome after reduced-dose radiation therapy plus adjuvant chemotherapy for medulloblastoma: a Children's Cancer Group study. J Clin Oncol 2001;19:3470–6.

34. Mulhern RK, Kepner JL, Thomas PR, et al. Neuropsychologic functioning of survivors of childhood medulloblastoma randomized to receive conventional or reduced-dose craniospinal irradiation: a Pediatric Oncology Group study. J Clin Oncol 1998;16:1723–8.

35. Ellenberg L, McComb JG, Siegel SE, et al. Factors affecting intellectual outcome in pediatric brain tumor patients. Neurosurgery 1987;21:638–44.

36. Ellenberg L, Liu Q, Gioia G, et al. Neurocognitive status in long-term survivors of childhood CNS malignancies: a report from the Childhood Cancer Survivor Study. Neuropsychology 2009;23:705–17.

37. Kiehna EN, Mulhern RK, Li C, et al. Changes in attentional performance of children and young adults with localized primary brain tumors after conformal radiation therapy. J Clin Oncol 2006;24:5283–90.

38. Mabbott DJ, Penkman L, Witol A, et al. Core neurocognitive functions in children treated for posterior fossa tumors. Neuropsychology 2008;22:159–68.

39. Mulhern RK, Merchant TE, Gajjar A, et al. Late neurocognitive sequelae in survivors of brain tumours in childhood. Lancet Oncol 2004;5:399–408.

40. Nagel BJ, Delis DC, Palmer SL, et al. Early patterns of verbal memory impairment in children treated for medulloblastoma. Neuropsychology 2006;20:105–12.

41. Krull KR, Brinkman TM, Li C, et al. Neurocognitive outcomes decades after treatment for childhood acute lymphoblastic leukemia: a report from the St Jude lifetime cohort study. J Clin Oncol 2013;31:4407–15.

42. Krull KR, Okcu MF, Potter B, et al. Screening for neurocognitive impairment in pediatric cancer long-term survivors. J Clin Oncol 2008;26:4138–43.

43. Campbell LK, Scaduto M, Sharp W, et al. A meta-analysis of the neurocognitive sequelae of treatment for childhood acute lymphocytic leukemia. Pediatr Blood Cancer 2007;49:65–73.

44. Jain N, Brouwers P, Okcu MF, et al. Sex-specific attention problems in long-term survivors of pediatric acute lymphoblastic leukemia. Cancer 2009;115:4238–45.

45. Kadan-Lottick NS, Zeltzer LK, Liu Q, et al. Neurocognitive functioning in adult survivors of childhood non-central nervous system cancers. J Natl Cancer Inst 2010;102:881–93.

46. Kirchhoff AC, Krull KR, Ness KK, et al. Physical, mental, and neurocognitive status and employment outcomes in the childhood cancer survivor study cohort. Cancer Epidemiol Biomarkers Prev 2011;20:1838–49.

47. Krull KR, Annett RD, Pan Z, et al. Neurocognitive functioning and health-related behaviours in adult survivors of childhood cancer: a report from the Childhood Cancer Survivor Study. Eur J Cancer 2011;47:1380–8.

48. Kadan-Lottick NS, Brouwers P, Breiger D, et al. Comparison of neurocognitive functioning in children previously randomly assigned to intrathecal methotrexate compared with triple intrathecal therapy for the treatment of childhood acute lymphoblastic leukemia. J Clin Oncol 2009;27:5986–92.

49. Conklin HM, Krull KR, Reddick WE, et al. Cognitive outcomes following contemporary treatment without cranial irradiation for childhood acute lymphoblastic leukemia. J Natl Cancer Inst 2012;104:1386–95.

50. Buizer AI, de Sonneville LM, Veerman AJ. Effects of chemotherapy on neurocognitive function in children with acute lymphoblastic leukemia: a critical review of the literature. Pediatr Blood Cancer 2009;52:447–54.

51. Spiegler BJ, Kennedy K, Maze R, et al. Comparison of long-term neurocognitive outcomes in young children with acute lymphoblastic leukemia treated with cranial radiation or high-dose or very high-dose intravenous methotrexate. J Clin Oncol 2006;24:3858–64.
52. Waber DP, Turek J, Catania L, et al. Neuropsychological outcomes from a randomized trial of triple intrathecal chemotherapy compared with 18 Gy cranial radiation as CNS treatment in acute lymphoblastic leukemia: findings from Dana-Farber Cancer Institute ALL consortium protocol 95-01. J Clin Oncol 2007;25:4914–21.
53. Lipshultz SE, Adams MJ, Colan SD, et al. Long-term cardiovascular toxicity in children, adolescents, and young adults who receive cancer therapy: pathophysiology, course, monitoring, management, prevention, and research directions: a scientific statement from the American Heart Association. Circulation 2013;128:1927–95.
54. Mulrooney DA, Yeazel MW, Kawashima T, et al. Cardiac outcomes in a cohort of adult survivors of childhood and adolescent cancer: retrospective analysis of the Childhood Cancer Survivor Study cohort. BMJ 2009;339:b4606.
55. Felker GM, Thompson RE, Hare JM, et al. Underlying causes and long-term survival in patients with initially unexplained cardiomyopathy. N Engl J Med 2000;342:1077–84.
56. van Dalen EC, Caron HN, Dickinson HO, et al. Cardioprotective interventions for cancer patients receiving anthracyclines. Cochrane Database Syst Rev 2008;(2):CD003917.
57. van Dalen EC, van der Pal HJ, Caron HN, et al. Different dosage schedules for reducing cardiotoxicity in cancer patients receiving anthracycline chemotherapy. Cochrane Database Syst Rev 2009;(4):CD005008.
58. van Dalen EC, Michiels EM, Caron HN, et al. Different anthracycline derivates for reducing cardiotoxicity in cancer patients. Cochrane Database Syst Rev 2010;(3):CD005006.
59. Lipshultz SE, Scully RE, Lipsitz SR, et al. Assessment of dexrazoxane as a cardioprotectant in doxorubicin-treated children with high-risk acute lymphoblastic leukaemia: long-term follow-up of a prospective, randomised, multicentre trial. Lancet Oncol 2010;11:950–61.
60. Magnano LC, Martinez Cibrian N, Andrade Gonzalez X, et al. Cardiac complications of chemotherapy: role of prevention. Curr Treat Options Cardiovasc Med 2014;16:312.
61. Adams MJ, Lipsitz SR, Colan SD, et al. Cardiovascular status in long-term survivors of Hodgkin's disease treated with chest radiotherapy. J Clin Oncol 2004;22:3139–48.
62. Liles A, Blatt J, Morris D, et al. Monitoring pulmonary complications in long-term childhood cancer survivors: guidelines for the primary care physician. Cleve Clin J Med 2008;75:531–9.
63. Motosue MS, Zhu L, Srivastava K, et al. Pulmonary function after whole lung irradiation in pediatric patients with solid malignancies. Cancer 2012;118:1450–6.
64. Weiner DJ, Maity A, Carlson CA, et al. Pulmonary function abnormalities in children treated with whole lung irradiation. Pediatr Blood Cancer 2006;46:222–7.
65. Mulder RL, Thonissen NM, van der Pal HJ, et al. Pulmonary function impairment measured by pulmonary function tests in long-term survivors of childhood cancer. Thorax 2011;66:1065–71.

66. Collaco JM, Gower WA, Mogayzel PJ Jr. Pulmonary dysfunction in pediatric hematopoietic stem cell transplant patients: overview, diagnostic considerations, and infectious complications. Pediatr Blood Cancer 2007;49:117–26.

67. Gower WA, Collaco JM, Mogayzel PJ Jr. Pulmonary dysfunction in pediatric hematopoietic stem cell transplant patients: non-infectious and long-term complications. Pediatr Blood Cancer 2007;49:225–33.

68. Chemaitilly W, Hudson MM. Update on endocrine and metabolic therapy-related late effects observed in survivors of childhood neoplasia. Curr Opin Endocrinol Diabetes Obes 2014;21:71–6.

69. Gurney JG, Kadan-Lottick NS, Packer RJ, et al. Endocrine and cardiovascular late effects among adult survivors of childhood brain tumors–Childhood Cancer Survivor Study. Cancer 2003;97:663–73.

70. Chow EJ, Friedman DL, Stovall M, et al. Risk of thyroid dysfunction and subsequent thyroid cancer among survivors of acute lymphoblastic leukemia: a report from the childhood cancer survivor study. Pediatr Blood Cancer 2009; 53:432–7.

71. Clifton DK, Bremner WJ. The effect of testicular x-irradiation on spermatogenesis in man. A comparison with the mouse. J Androl 1983;4:387–92.

72. Nandagopal R, Laverdiere C, Mulrooney D, et al. Endocrine late effects of childhood cancer therapy: a report from the Children's Oncology Group. Horm Res 2008;69:65–74.

73. Green DM, Kawashima T, Stovall M, et al. Fertility of male survivors of childhood cancer: a report from the Childhood Cancer Survivor Study. J Clin Oncol 2010; 28:332–9.

74. Shalet SM, Beardwell CG, Jacobs HS, et al. Testicular function following irradiation of the human prepubertal testis. Clin Endocrinol (Oxf) 1978;9:483–90.

75. Meistrich ML. Male gonadal toxicity. Pediatr Blood Cancer 2009;53:261–6.

76. Rivkees SA, Crawford JD. The relationship of gonadal activity and chemotherapy-induced gonadal damage. JAMA 1988;259:2123–5.

77. Sklar C. Reproductive physiology and treatment-related loss of sex hormone production. Med Pediatr Oncol 1999;33:2–8.

78. Couto-Silva AC, Trivin C, Thibaud E, et al. Factors affecting gonadal function after bone marrow transplantation during childhood. Bone Marrow Transplant 2001;28:67–75.

79. Thomsett MJ, Conte FA, Kaplan SL, et al. Endocrine and neurologic outcome in childhood craniopharyngioma: review of effect of treatment in 42 patients. J Pediatr 1980;97:728–35.

80. Jacobsen KD, Ous S, Waehre H, et al. Ejaculation in testicular cancer patients after post-chemotherapy retroperitoneal lymph node dissection. Br J Cancer 1999;80:249–55.

81. Ginsberg JP, Hobbie WL, Ogle SK, et al. Prevalence of and risk factors for hydrocele in survivors of Wilms tumor. Pediatr Blood Cancer 2004;42:361–3.

82. Green DM, Sklar CA, Boice JD Jr, et al. Ovarian failure and reproductive outcomes after childhood cancer treatment: results from the Childhood Cancer Survivor Study. J Clin Oncol 2009;27:2374–81.

83. Chemaitilly W, Mertens AC, Mitby P, et al. Acute ovarian failure in the childhood cancer survivor study. J Clin Endocrinol Metab 2006;91:1723–8.

84. Chemaitilly W, Sklar CA. Endocrine complications of hematopoietic stem cell transplantation. Endocrinol Metab Clin North Am 2007;36:983–98, ix.

85. Sarafoglou K, Boulad F, Gillio A, et al. Gonadal function after bone marrow transplantation for acute leukemia during childhood. J Pediatr 1997;130:210–6.

86. Afify Z, Shaw PJ, Clavano-Harding A, et al. Growth and endocrine function in children with acute myeloid leukaemia after bone marrow transplantation using busulfan/cyclophosphamide. Bone Marrow Transplant 2000;25:1087–92.
87. Read MD, Edey KA, Hapeshi J, et al. The age of ovarian failure following premenopausal hysterectomy with ovarian conservation. Menopause Int 2010; 16:56–9.
88. Sklar C, Wolden S. Therapy for pediatric brain tumors and the risk of growth hormone deficiency. J Clin Oncol 2011;29:4743–4.
89. Chow EJ, Friedman DL, Yasui Y, et al. Decreased adult height in survivors of childhood acute lymphoblastic leukemia: a report from the Childhood Cancer Survivor Study. J Pediatr 2007;150:370–5, 375.e1.
90. Viana MB, Vilela MI. Height deficit during and many years after treatment for acute lymphoblastic leukemia in children: a review. Pediatr Blood Cancer 2008;50:509–16 [discussion: 517].
91. Gurney JG, Ness KK, Stovall M, et al. Final height and body mass index among adult survivors of childhood brain cancer: childhood cancer survivor study. J Clin Endocrinol Metab 2003;88:4731–9.
92. Schriock EA, Schell MJ, Carter M, et al. Abnormal growth patterns and adult short stature in 115 long-term survivors of childhood leukemia. J Clin Oncol 1991;9:400–5.
93. Laughton SJ, Merchant TE, Sklar CA, et al. Endocrine outcomes for children with embryonal brain tumors after risk-adapted craniospinal and conformal primary-site irradiation and high-dose chemotherapy with stem-cell rescue on the SJMB-96 trial. J Clin Oncol 2008;26:1112–8.
94. Kiltie AE, Lashford LS, Gattamaneni HR. Survival and late effects in medullo-blastoma patients treated with craniospinal irradiation under three years old. Med Pediatr Oncol 1997;28:348–54.
95. Sanders JE. Growth and development after hematopoietic cell transplant in children. Bone Marrow Transplant 2008;41:223–7.
96. Hudson MM, Neglia JP, Woods WG, et al. Lessons from the past: opportunities to improve childhood cancer survivor care through outcomes investigations of historical therapeutic approaches for pediatric hematological malignancies. Pediatr Blood Cancer 2012;58:334–43.
97. Oeffinger KC, Mertens AC, Sklar CA, et al. Obesity in adult survivors of childhood acute lymphoblastic leukemia: a report from the Childhood Cancer Survivor Study. J Clin Oncol 2003;21:1359–65.
98. Garmey EG, Liu Q, Sklar CA, et al. Longitudinal changes in obesity and body mass index among adult survivors of childhood acute lymphoblastic leukemia: a report from the Childhood Cancer Survivor Study. J Clin Oncol 2008;26: 4639–45.
99. Green DM, Cox CL, Zhu L, et al. Risk factors for obesity in adult survivors of childhood cancer: a report from the Childhood Cancer Survivor Study. J Clin Oncol 2012;30:246–55.
100. Rogers PC, Meacham LR, Oeffinger KC, et al. Obesity in pediatric oncology. Pediatr Blood Cancer 2005;45:881–91.
101. Armstrong GT, Oeffinger KC, Chen Y, et al. Modifiable risk factors and major cardiac events among adult survivors of childhood cancer. J Clin Oncol 2013; 31:3673–80.
102. Blijdorp K, van den Heuvel-Eibrink MM, Pieters R, et al. Obesity is underestimated using body mass index and waist-hip ratio in long-term adult survivors of childhood cancer. PLoS One 2012;7:e43269.

103. Gurney JG, Ness KK, Sibley SD, et al. Metabolic syndrome and growth hormone deficiency in adult survivors of childhood acute lymphoblastic leukemia. Cancer 2006;107:1303–12.

104. Oeffinger KC, Adams-Huet B, Victor RG, et al. Insulin resistance and risk factors for cardiovascular disease in young adult survivors of childhood acute lymphoblastic leukemia. J Clin Oncol 2009;27:3698–704.

105. Kourti M, Tragiannidis A, Makedou A, et al. Metabolic syndrome in children and adolescents with acute lymphoblastic leukemia after the completion of chemotherapy. J Pediatr Hematol Oncol 2005;27:499–501.

106. Florin TA, Fryer GE, Miyoshi T, et al. Physical inactivity in adult survivors of childhood acute lymphoblastic leukemia: a report from the childhood cancer survivor study. Cancer Epidemiol Biomarkers Prev 2007;16:1356–63.

107. Moller DE, Flier JS. Insulin resistance–mechanisms, syndromes, and implications. N Engl J Med 1991;325:938–48.

108. Lustig RH. Autonomic dysfunction of the beta-cell and the pathogenesis of obesity. Rev Endocr Metab Disord 2003;4:23–32.

109. Askari H, Tykodi G, Liu JM, et al. Fasting plasma leptin level is a surrogate measure of insulin sensitivity. J Clin Endocrinol Metab 2010;95:3836–43.

110. Link K, Moell C, Garwicz S, et al. Growth hormone deficiency predicts cardiovascular risk in young adults treated for acute lymphoblastic leukemia in childhood. J Clin Endocrinol Metab 2004;89:5003–12.

111. Ness KK, Oakes JM, Punyko JA, et al. Prevalence of the metabolic syndrome in relation to self-reported cancer history. Ann Epidemiol 2005;15:202–6.

112. Meacham LR, Sklar CA, Li S, et al. Diabetes mellitus in long-term survivors of childhood cancer. Increased risk associated with radiation therapy: a report for the childhood cancer survivor study. Arch Intern Med 2009;169:1381–8.

113. Wasilewski-Masker K, Kaste SC, Hudson MM, et al. Bone mineral density deficits in survivors of childhood cancer: long-term follow-up guidelines and review of the literature. Pediatrics 2008;121:e705–13.

114. Haddy TB, Mosher RB, Reaman GH. Osteoporosis in survivors of acute lymphoblastic leukemia. Oncologist 2001;6:278–85.

115. Kaste SC, Jones-Wallace D, Rose SR, et al. Bone mineral decrements in survivors of childhood acute lymphoblastic leukemia: frequency of occurrence and risk factors for their development. Leukemia 2001;15:728–34.

116. Krishnamoorthy P, Freeman C, Bernstein ML, et al. Osteopenia in children who have undergone posterior fossa or craniospinal irradiation for brain tumors. Arch Pediatr Adolesc Med 2004;158:491–6.

117. Kadan-Lottick NS, Dinu I, Wasilewski-Masker K, et al. Osteonecrosis in adult survivors of childhood cancer: a report from the childhood cancer survivor study. J Clin Oncol 2008;26:3038–45.

118. Kawedia JD, Kaste SC, Pei D, et al. Pharmacokinetic, pharmacodynamic, and pharmacogenetic determinants of osteonecrosis in children with acute lymphoblastic leukemia. Blood 2011;117:2340–7 [quiz: 2556].

119. Sala A, Mattano LA Jr, Barr RD. Osteonecrosis in children and adolescents with cancer–an adverse effect of systemic therapy. Eur J Cancer 2007;43: 683–9.

120. Fan C, Cool JC, Scherer MA, et al. Damaging effects of chronic low-dose methotrexate usage on primary bone formation in young rats and potential protective effects of folinic acid supplementary treatment. Bone 2009;44:61–70.

121. Yang L, Boyd K, Kaste SC, et al. A mouse model for glucocorticoid-induced osteonecrosis: effect of a steroid holiday. J Orthop Res 2009;27:169–75.

122. Yang L, Panetta JC, Cai XJ, et al. Asparaginase may influence dexamethasone pharmacokinetics in acute lymphoblastic leukemia. J Clin Oncol 2008;26:1932–9.
123. Mattano LA, Sather HN, Trigg ME, et al. Osteonecrosis as a complication of treating acute lymphoblastic leukemia in children: a report from the children's cancer group. J Clin Oncol 2000;18:3262–72.
124. te Winkel ML, Appel IM, Pieters R, et al. Impaired dexamethasone-related increase of anticoagulants is associated with the development of osteonecrosis in childhood acute lymphoblastic leukemia. Haematologica 2008;93:1570–4.
125. Niinimaki RA, Harila-Saari AH, Jartti AE, et al. High body mass index increases the risk for osteonecrosis in children with acute lymphoblastic leukemia. J Clin Oncol 2007;25:1498–504.
126. Karimova EJ, Rai SN, Howard SC, et al. Femoral head osteonecrosis in pediatric and young adult patients with leukemia or lymphoma. J Clin Oncol 2007;25: 1525–31.
127. Friedman DL, Whitton J, Leisenring W, et al. Subsequent neoplasms in 5-year survivors of childhood cancer: the Childhood Cancer Survivor Study. J Natl Cancer Inst 2010;102:1083–95.
128. Mertens AC, Liu Q, Neglia JP, et al. Cause-specific late mortality among 5-year survivors of childhood cancer: the childhood cancer survivor study. J Natl Cancer Inst 2008;100:1368–79.
129. Armstrong GT, Liu W, Leisenring W, et al. Occurrence of multiple subsequent neoplasms in long-term survivors of childhood cancer: a report from the childhood cancer survivor study. J Clin Oncol 2011;29:3056–64.
130. Bhatia S, Sklar C. Second cancers in survivors of childhood cancer. Nat Rev Cancer 2002;2:124–32.
131. Bhatia S, Yasui Y, Robison LL, et al. High risk of subsequent neoplasms continues with extended follow-up of childhood Hodgkin's disease: report from the Late Effects Study Group. J Clin Oncol 2003;21:4386–94.
132. Vardiman JW, Harris NL, Brunning RD. The World Health Organization (WHO) classification of the myeloid neoplasms. Blood 2002;100:2292–302.
133. Thirman MJ, Larson RA. Therapy-related myeloid leukemia. Hematol Oncol Clin North Am 1996;10:293–320.
134. Pedersen-Bjergaard J, Philip P. Balanced translocations involving chromosome bands 11q23 and 21q22 are highly characteristic of myelodysplasia and leukemia following therapy with cytostatic agents targeting at DNA-topoisomerase II. Blood 1991;78:1147–8.
135. Neglia JP, Friedman DL, Yasui Y, et al. Second malignant neoplasms in five-year survivors of childhood cancer: childhood cancer survivor study. J Natl Cancer Inst 2001;93:618–29.
136. Henderson TO, Amsterdam A, Bhatia S, et al. Systematic review: surveillance for breast cancer in women treated with chest radiation for childhood, adolescent, or young adult cancer. Ann Intern Med 2010;152:444–55 W144–54.
137. Bhatia S, Robison LL, Oberlin O, et al. Breast cancer and other second neoplasms after childhood Hodgkin's disease. N Engl J Med 1996;334:745–51.
138. Guibout C, Adjadj E, Rubino C, et al. Malignant breast tumors after radiotherapy for a first cancer during childhood. J Clin Oncol 2005;23:197–204.
139. Kenney LB, Yasui Y, Inskip PD, et al. Breast cancer after childhood cancer: a report from the Childhood Cancer Survivor Study. Ann Intern Med 2004;141:590–7.
140. Jenkinson HC, Hawkins MM, Stiller CA, et al. Long-term population-based risks of second malignant neoplasms after childhood cancer in Britain. Br J Cancer 2004;91:1905–10.

141. Inskip PD, Curtis RE. New malignancies following childhood cancer in the United States, 1973-2002. Int J Cancer 2007;121:2233–40.

142. Taylor AJ, Winter DL, Stiller CA, et al. Risk of breast cancer in female survivors of childhood Hodgkin's disease in Britain: a population-based study. Int J Cancer 2007;120:384–91.

143. Ng AK, Bernardo MV, Weller E, et al. Second malignancy after Hodgkin disease treated with radiation therapy with or without chemotherapy: long-term risks and risk factors. Blood 2002;100:1989–96.

144. Travis LB, Hill DA, Dores GM, et al. Breast cancer following radiotherapy and chemotherapy among young women with Hodgkin disease. JAMA 2003;290:465–75.

145. Inskip PD, Robison LL, Stovall M, et al. Radiation dose and breast cancer risk in the childhood cancer survivor study. J Clin Oncol 2009;27:3901–7.

146. Sklar C, Whitton J, Mertens A, et al. Abnormalities of the thyroid in survivors of Hodgkin's disease: data from the Childhood Cancer Survivor Study. J Clin Endocrinol Metab 2000;85:3227–32.

147. Sigurdson AJ, Ronckers CM, Mertens AC, et al. Primary thyroid cancer after a first tumour in childhood (the Childhood Cancer Survivor Study): a nested case-control study. Lancet 2005;365:2014–23.

148. Ronckers CM, Sigurdson AJ, Stovall M, et al. Thyroid cancer in childhood cancer survivors: a detailed evaluation of radiation dose response and its modifiers. Radiat Res 2006;166:618–28.

149. Bhatti P, Veiga LH, Ronckers CM, et al. Risk of second primary thyroid cancer after radiotherapy for a childhood cancer in a large cohort study: an update from the childhood cancer survivor study. Radiat Res 2010;174:741–52.

150. Henderson TO, Whitton J, Stovall M, et al. Secondary sarcomas in childhood cancer survivors: a report from the Childhood Cancer Survivor Study. J Natl Cancer Inst 2007;99:300–8.

151. Henderson TO, Rajaraman P, Stovall M, et al. Risk factors associated with secondary sarcomas in childhood cancer survivors: a report from the childhood cancer survivor study. Int J Radiat Oncol Biol Phys 2012;84:224–30.

152. Hawkins MM, Wilson LM, Burton HS, et al. Radiotherapy, alkylating agents, and risk of bone cancer after childhood cancer. J Natl Cancer Inst 1996;88:270–8.

153. Le Vu B, de Vathaire F, Shamsaldin A, et al. Radiation dose, chemotherapy and risk of osteosarcoma after solid tumours during childhood. Int J Cancer 1998;77:370–7.

154. Newton WA Jr, Meadows AT, Shimada H, et al. Bone sarcomas as second malignant neoplasms following childhood cancer. Cancer 1991;67:193–201.

155. Bielack SS, Rerin JS, Dickerhoff R, et al. Osteosarcoma after allogeneic bone marrow transplantation. A report of four cases from the Cooperative Osteosarcoma Study Group (COSS). Bone Marrow Transplant 2003;31:353–9.

156. Garwicz S, Anderson H, Olsen JH, et al. Second malignant neoplasms after cancer in childhood and adolescence: a population-based case-control study in the 5 Nordic countries. The Nordic Society for Pediatric Hematology and Oncology. The Association of the Nordic Cancer Registries. Int J Cancer 2000;88:672–8.

157. Kony SJ, de Vathaire F, Chompret A, et al. Radiation and genetic factors in the risk of second malignant neoplasms after a first cancer in childhood. Lancet 1997;350:91–5.

158. Tabone MD, Terrier P, Pacquement H, et al. Outcome of radiation-related osteosarcoma after treatment of childhood and adolescent cancer: a study of 23 cases. J Clin Oncol 1999;17:2789–95.

159. Ferrari C, Bohling T, Benassi MS, et al. Secondary tumors in bone sarcomas after treatment with chemotherapy. Cancer Detect Prev 1999;23:368–74.
160. van Leeuwen FE, Klokman WJ, Stovall M, et al. Roles of radiotherapy and smoking in lung cancer following Hodgkin's disease. J Natl Cancer Inst 1995;87: 1530–7.
161. Neglia JP, Robison LL, Stovall M, et al. New primary neoplasms of the central nervous system in survivors of childhood cancer: a report from the Childhood Cancer Survivor Study. J Natl Cancer Inst 2006;98:1528–37.
162. Bhatia S, Sather HN, Pabustan OB, et al. Low incidence of second neoplasms among children diagnosed with acute lymphoblastic leukemia after 1983. Blood 2002;99:4257–64.
163. Little MP, de Vathaire F, Shamsaldin A, et al. Risks of brain tumour following treatment for cancer in childhood: modification by genetic factors, radiotherapy and chemotherapy. Int J Cancer 1998;78:269–75.
164. Goshen Y, Stark B, Kornreich L, et al. High incidence of meningioma in cranial irradiated survivors of childhood acute lymphoblastic leukemia. Pediatr Blood Cancer 2007;49:294–7.
165. Ron E, Modan B, Boice JD Jr, et al. Tumors of the brain and nervous system after radiotherapy in childhood. N Engl J Med 1988;319:1033–9.
166. Bowers DC, Nathan PC, Constine L, et al. Subsequent neoplasms of the CNS among survivors of childhood cancer: a systematic review. Lancet Oncol 2013;14:E321–8.
167. Taylor AJ, Little MP, Winter DL, et al. Population-based risks of CNS tumors in survivors of childhood cancer: the British Childhood Cancer Survivor Study. J Clin Oncol 2010;28:5287–93.
168. Frobisher C, Gurung PM, Leiper A, et al. Risk of bladder tumours after childhood cancer: the British Childhood Cancer Survivor Study. BJU Int 2010;106:1060–9.
169. Olsen JH, Garwicz S, Hertz H, et al. Second malignant neoplasms after cancer in childhood or adolescence. Nordic Society of Paediatric Haematology and Oncology Association of the Nordic Cancer Registries. BMJ 1993;307:1030–6.
170. Bassal M, Mertens AC, Taylor L, et al. Risk of selected subsequent carcinomas in survivors of childhood cancer: a report from the Childhood Cancer Survivor Study. J Clin Oncol 2006;24:476–83.
171. Metayer C, Lynch CF, Clarke EA, et al. Second cancers among long-term survivors of Hodgkin's disease diagnosed in childhood and adolescence. J Clin Oncol 2000;18:2435–43.
172. Travis LB, Curtis RE, Glimelius B, et al. Bladder and kidney cancer following cyclophosphamide therapy for non-Hodgkin's lymphoma. J Natl Cancer Inst 1995;87:524–30.
173. Kaldor JM, Day NE, Kittelmann B, et al. Bladder tumours following chemotherapy and radiotherapy for ovarian cancer: a case-control study. Int J Cancer 1995;63:1–6.
174. Wilson CL, Ness KK, Neglia JP, et al. Renal carcinoma after childhood cancer: a report from the childhood cancer survivor study. J Natl Cancer Inst 2013;105: 504–8.
175. Fleitz JM, Wootton-Gorges SL, Wyatt-Ashmead J, et al. Renal cell carcinoma in long-term survivors of advanced stage neuroblastoma in early childhood. Pediatr Radiol 2003;33:540–5.
176. Hedgepeth RC, Zhou M, Ross J. Rapid development of metastatic Xp11 translocation renal cell carcinoma in a girl treated for neuroblastoma. J Pediatr Hematol Oncol 2009;31:602–4.

177. Boukheris H, Stovall M, Gilbert ES, et al. Risk of salivary gland cancer after childhood cancer: a report from the Childhood Cancer Survivor Study. Int J Radiat Oncol Biol Phys 2013;85:776–83.

178. Schneider AB, Lubin J, Ron E, et al. Salivary gland tumors after childhood radiation treatment for benign conditions of the head and neck: dose-response relationships. Radiat Res 1998;149:625–30.

179. Curtis RE, Rowlings PA, Deeg HJ, et al. Solid cancers after bone marrow transplantation. N Engl J Med 1997;336:897–904.

180. Pappo AS, Armstrong GT, Liu W, et al. Melanoma as a subsequent neoplasm in adult survivors of childhood cancer: a report from the childhood cancer survivor study. Pediatr Blood Cancer 2013;60:461–6.

181. Braam KI, Overbeek A, Kaspers GJ, et al. Malignant melanoma as second malignant neoplasm in long-term childhood cancer survivors: a systematic review. Pediatr Blood Cancer 2012;58:665–74.

182. Eng C, Li FP, Abramson DH, et al. Mortality from second tumors among long-term survivors of retinoblastoma. J Natl Cancer Inst 1993;85:1121–8.

183. Perkins JL, Liu Y, Mitby PA, et al. Nonmelanoma skin cancer in survivors of childhood and adolescent cancer: a report from the childhood cancer survivor study. J Clin Oncol 2005;23:3733–41.

184. Armstrong GT, Liu Q, Yasui Y, et al. late mortality among 5-year survivors of childhood cancer: a summary from the childhood cancer survivor study. J Clin Oncol 2009;27:2328–38.

Remaining Challenges in Childhood Cancer and Newer Targeted Therapeutics

Malcolm A. Smith, MD, PhD[a],*, Gregory H. Reaman, MD[b]

KEYWORDS

- Targeted therapy • Personalized medicine • Pediatric cancer drug development
- Innovative clinical trials • Preclinical testing

KEY POINTS

- There are only a limited number of druggable molecular targets identified to date in childhood cancers. Nonetheless, evaluation of inhibitors of those that have been identified is warranted in relevant tumor types and subsets of patients.
- The principle of integration of active targeted therapy with best-available therapy has been established and will likely be the basis for future investigations and hopefully advances.
- Strong biologic rationale and preclinical data, particularly from in vivo testing, are central to effective prioritization of agents for clinical evaluation.
- Prioritization of "same-in-class" products will be a persistent challenge, but is essential for effective pediatric cancer drug-development strategies.
- Increased, effective communication and collaboration among clinical investigators, industry, and international regulatory agencies are essential for the development of successful clinical research plans and improved drug-development opportunities.

INTRODUCTION

The remaining challenges for childhood cancer research are best understood in the context of past advances. Treatment of childhood cancer was one of the important success stories of twentieth century medicine as exemplified by the conversion of pediatric acute lymphoblastic leukemia (ALL) from an incurable disease in the 1950s to one in which more than 90% of children survived 5 years from diagnosis, with most of these children cured of their leukemia.[1] Other cancers also have 5-year survival

[a] Cancer Therapy Evaluation Program, National Cancer Institute, 9609 Medical Center Drive, RM 5-W414, MSC 9737, Bethesda, MD 20892, USA; [b] Office of Hematology and Oncology Products, OND, Center for Drug Evaluation and Research, U.S. Food and Drug Administration, White Oak Building 22, Room 2202, 10903 New Hampshire Avenue, Silver Spring, MD 20993, USA
* Corresponding author.
E-mail address: Malcolm.Smith@nih.gov

Pediatr Clin N Am 62 (2015) 301–312
http://dx.doi.org/10.1016/j.pcl.2014.09.018
0031-3955/15/$ – see front matter Published by Elsevier Inc.
pediatric.theclinics.com

rates approaching or exceeding 90%, including Wilms tumor, non-Hodgkin lymphoma (NHL), Hodgkin lymphoma, and germ cell tumors. Importantly, the decline in childhood cancer mortality that began in the 1960s continued through the first decade of the twenty-first century.[1] Research advances averted more than 45,000 childhood cancer deaths from 1975 to 2010.[1]

Despite the successes in identifying effective treatments for many children with cancer, approximately 2000 children and adolescents die of their disease each year in the United States.[1] **Fig. 1** shows the distribution of childhood cancer mortality for children and adolescents, highlighting the contribution of leukemias, brain cancers, and neuroblastoma in younger children and the contribution of leukemias and brain cancers, along with sarcomas and lymphomas, in adolescents. Additionally, for some cancers, progress has been very limited (eg, diffuse intrinsic brainstem gliomas, high-grade gliomas, and metastatic sarcomas). Beyond the number of children who die each year, there is also the burden of long-term morbidity that diminishes quality of life for some childhood cancer survivors.

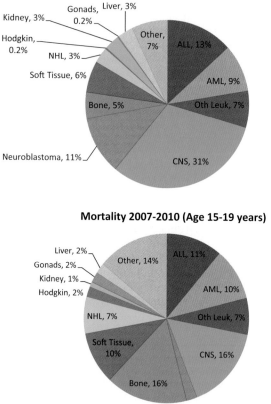

Fig. 1. Patterns of mortality for children and adolescents younger than 15 years and 15 to 19 years for 2007 to 2010. CNS, central nervous system; Oth Leuk, other leukemia. (*Adapted from* Smith MA, Altekruse SF, Adamson PC, et al. Declining childhood and adolescent cancer mortality. Cancer 2014;120(16):2500; with permission.)

The challenge for the future is to discover and implement new strategies that will allow successful treatment of those for whom current therapeutic approaches are suboptimal, either because of insufficient efficacy or because of the damage that the treatments cause to critical normal tissues, resulting in acute morbidity and long-term disability. In addressing this challenge, it is important to acknowledge that most of the anticancer drug and biologic products that will be studied in the context of clinical trials in children will be ones initially developed for adult cancers. Even so, it is critical that pediatric oncologists prioritize these agents independently of their utility for adult cancers, as both the biology and the goals of treatment generally differ between childhood and adult cancers. For example, the primary goal in treating childhood cancers is cure, not palliation, whereas for many adult cancers sustained stable disease aimed at palliation is an important objective. Agents and treatment regimens that only slow tumor growth and prevent disease progression for a finite period may be valuable as adult cancer treatments, assuming that they prolong survival while allowing acceptable quality of life[2]; however, for children, temporarily delaying disease progression is at best a modest success. This critical distinction between the relative benefit of cure versus palliation for children and adults with cancer, coupled with the differences in etiology and biology of pediatric and adult cancers, has implications both in terms of the cellular pathways targeted for intervention and in terms of clinical trial design. Moreover, it highlights the need for pediatric cancer prioritization decisions to focus on the biology of the cancers and on the specific needs of the children afflicted with these cancers.[2] We discuss factors that will play key roles in guiding pediatric oncologists as they select lines of research to pursue in their quest for more effective treatments for children with cancer.

GENOMIC ALTERATIONS AS THERAPEUTIC GUIDEPOSTS

One essential line of research for identifying more effective treatment strategies is understanding in detail the genomic alterations that provide the blueprint for the growth and survival signaling pathways of childhood cancers. These genomic alterations highlight the genes that the cancers are most dependent on, whether for their oncogenic driver effect or for their tumor suppressor role. Oncogenes with genomic alterations have proven among the most useful guideposts for identifying therapeutic targets, as illustrated by the success of imatinib for BCR-ABL leukemias (chronic myeloid leukemia and Philadelphia-positive [Ph+] ALL) and the success of crizotinib for *ALK*-rearranged non–small cell lung cancer. The success of imatinib when added to standard chemotherapy for children with Ph+ ALL is particularly informative. Single-agent imatinib induces remissions of relatively short duration in Ph+ ALL, whereas standard chemotherapy is effective for a minority of children (approximately 30%). However, the combination of imatinib and standard chemotherapy was able to induce and maintain long-term remission in approximately 70% of children with Ph+ ALL.[3]

A decade ago it was possible to hope that targetable oncogenes might be identified in a high percentage of childhood cancers and that the imatinib paradigm described previously could be broadly applied to other childhood cancers. At this point, thousands of childhood cancer specimens have been sequenced so that the vast majority of recurring mutations have now been identified. Targetable activated oncogenes have been identified, including the *NPM-ALK* fusion gene for anaplastic large cell lymphoma, ALK point mutations for a subset of neuroblastoma, BRAF genomic alterations for pediatric gliomas, Hedgehog pathway mutations for a subset of medulloblastoma, and ABL family genes activated by translocation in a subset of Ph-like ALL. However, these examples represent a small minority of all childhood cancers, making it clear that most childhood cancers do not have recurring mutations in genes that are, at the present time, considered targetable.

Two approaches to therapeutically targeting the "untargetable" warrant mention. One is the concept of identifying targetable susceptibilities created by untargetable genomic alterations. This concept is illustrated by the activity of EZH2 inhibitors in rhabdoid tumors. SMARCB1 loss of function through deletion or mutation is the sole recurring genomic alteration in rhabdoid tumors.[4] EZH2 is a member of the Polycomb Repressor Complex 2 (PRC2) that mediates gene silencing through catalyzing trimethylation of histone 3 lysine 27 (H3K27) at the promoters of target genes.[5] Mice with conditional loss of SMARCB1 in their T cells rapidly develop T-cell lymphomas, but tumor development is completely suppressed by concomitant loss of EZH2.[6] Small molecule inhibitors of EZH2 have been developed and have entered clinical evaluation.[7] Treatment of rhabdoid tumor xenografts with an EZH2 inhibitor led to dose-dependent tumor regression, providing evidence for the potential clinical utility of EZH2 inhibitors for cancers with SMARCB1 loss of function.[8] Another example of targetable susceptibilities created by untargetable genomic alterations is the requirement of mixed lineage leukemia (MLL)-rearranged leukemias for the DOT1L methyltransferase.[9,10] A small molecule inhibitor of DOT1L induced complete regressions in a xenograft model of MLL leukemia, and this agent has entered clinical evaluation.[11]

A second approach to targeting the untargetable is applying medicinal chemistry and high-throughput screening methods to identify small molecule inhibitors of pediatric oncogenes. This strategy is illustrated by efforts at developing small molecule inhibitors of EWS-FLI1 activity that resulted in development of YK-4-279, a small molecule that blocks EWS-FLI1 from interacting with RNA Helicase A.[12] Other pediatric oncogenes that are candidates for targeting include the PAX-FKHR fusion proteins of alveolar rhabdomyosarcoma and MYCN, which is amplified in high-risk neuroblastoma in children older than 18 months.

Although genomic alterations are reliable therapeutic guideposts for many targeted agents, the role of the tissue of origin should not be overlooked as a potential guidepost for some targeted agents. As an example, proteasome inhibitors are effective for patients with multiple myeloma, even though mutations in proteasome subunits are exceedingly rare. The susceptibility of myeloma to proteasome inhibition likely relates to the high level of synthesis of immunoglobulins in myeloma cells, which leads to a dependence on proteasome function to process the resulting elevated levels of unfolded proteins.[13] Similarly, inhibitors of PI3K delta are highly active in malignancies of mature B cells, not because of *PIK3CD* mutations, but because of the dependence of these mature B cells on signaling through the B-cell receptor.[14] The favorable therapeutic impact of engaging the glucocorticoid receptor in ALL cells is a pediatric example of the importance of tissue-of-origin effects.

MOLECULARLY DEFINED DISEASE SUBTYPES

A consequence of the detailed molecular characterization of childhood cancers is the recognition that single disease entities actually represent multiple clinically and biologically distinctive subtypes. For example, analysis of gene expression profiles of B-ALL cases identified 8 distinctive subtypes, 1 of which had similar characteristics as Ph+ ALL but lacked the BCR-ABL fusion gene,[15,16] Further investigation of this "Ph-like" ALL subset showed that these cases in turn possess a range of genomic alterations, with most having an alteration in genes involved in growth factor signaling.[17] These alterations include potentially therapeutically relevant fusion genes involving tyrosine kinases (eg, *PDGFRB*, *ABL1*, and *CSF1R*), as well as well as genomic alterations involving *CRLF2*, JAK family members, and RAS pathway alterations.

Detailed investigation of medulloblastoma cases has identified 4 molecular subtypes, each with a distinctive constellation of genomic alterations as well as distinctive demographic and prognostic characteristics. One subtype, the sonic hedgehog (SHH) group, is characterized by mutations in the SHH pathway.[18] The SHH pathway can be activated by genomic alterations in a number of genes, including *PTCH1*, *SUFU*, *GLI2*, *MYCN*, and *SMO*. Only cases with "upstream" mutations in the SHH pathway (eg, *PTCH1* and *SMO*) are susceptible to inhibition by currently available SHH pathway inhibitors that block SMO action (eg, vismodegib and sonidegib). Patients within the SHH subtype of medulloblastoma show distinctive genomic profiles by age, with infants having primarily either *PTCH1* or *SUFU* mutations, older children having *PTCH1* mutations or *GLI2* amplification, and adults having primarily *PTCH1* mutations.[18] For the pediatric age range, up to 50% of cases have lesions downstream of SMO that are inherently nonresponsive to these agents.[18] This example highlights the complexities of targeted therapy development in children, even when a targetable oncogenic pathway is activated in a specific patient population.

Some have proposed that the molecular characterization of cancer heralds the end of the era of histology-defined treatment and the move to an era in which specific genomic alterations rather than histology will define treatment. For childhood cancers, there is reason for a more conservative approach to research strategy in which molecular characterization complements, but does not replace, histologic classification of cancers. One reason for this conservative approach is the remarkable relationship between specific genomic alterations and specific cancer types, as illustrated by the finding of *H3F3A* K27M mutations in midline high-grade gliomas of children but in virtually no other cancers.[19] Similarly, *BRAF* mutations do not occur randomly across childhood cancers, but are found primarily among cases of low-grade gliomas.[20] A second reason for skepticism is that the therapeutic implications of genomic alterations can be cell context dependent, as illustrated by the high activity of BRAF inhibitors for patients with melanoma and *BRAF* V600E mutations, but their low activity in patients with colorectal cancer with the same mutation.[21] A final note of caution that is particularly relevant for childhood cancers is that the development pathway for targeted agents that show single-agent activity will likely be (at least initially) through their integration with standard therapy, as illustrated by the imatinib example for Ph+ ALL described previously. To the extent that different histologies have different standard treatments, the development of targeted agents will be accordingly segregated by histology.

IMMUNOTHERAPY STRATEGIES

Immunotherapeutic approaches to cancer treatment are revolutionizing treatment for some adult cancers. Examples include monoclonal antibodies targeting overexpressed cancer cell proteins (eg, the HER2-targeted agent Herceptin for HER2-amplified breast cancer), antibody-drug conjugates (eg, the CD30-targeted agent brentuximab vedotin for Hodgkin lymphoma and trastuzumab emtansine for HER2-amplified breast cancer), and checkpoint inhibitors (eg, the CTLA-4 targeted agent ipilimumab for advanced melanoma and anti-PD1 targeted agents for non–small cell lung cancer and melanoma). Evaluating immunotherapeutic approaches is an important line of pediatric oncology research; ch14.18 (a monoclonal antibody targeting GD2 on neuroblastoma cells) was identified in a phase 3 trial as effective for children with high-risk neuroblastoma.[22] Brentuximab vedotin is highly active as a single agent against relapsed/refractory CD30-expressing malignancies, such as Hodgkin lymphoma and anaplastic large cell lymphoma, and clinical trials in children evaluating its contribution when added to standard chemotherapy for each of these conditions are under way. A number of other pediatric-relevant antibody-drug conjugates have entered clinical trials for adult cancers, including agents targeting CD19, CD22, CD33, and CD56. It is anticipated that these agents will be evaluated in children with cancers expressing these antigens. Checkpoint inhibitors entered pediatric evaluation through a phase 1 evaluation of ipilimumab, and clinical trials to evaluate efficacy in specific pediatric cancers are planned. Early-phase clinical trials for other checkpoint inhibitors in children are under way or being planned. Given the remarkable activity observed for checkpoint inhibitors for several disparate adult cancers, it will be important to determine whether there are comparable pediatric populations that can benefit from checkpoint inhibition. Given the nonoverlapping toxicity profiles of this class of drugs when compared with conventional cytotoxic agents, the potential for combinatorial approaches to therapy is significant.

Other immunotherapy strategies that have entered pediatric evaluation include bispecific T-cell engager (BiTE) antibodies and chimeric antigen receptor (CAR) T cells. Proof of principle for each of these strategies has been achieved through clinical trials for CD19-expressing B-ALL in adults and children. Blinatumomab is a BiTE antibody with 2 binding sites: one for CD3 on T cells and the other for CD19 on the surface of B-ALL cells. The close juxtaposition of the T cell and leukemia cell is sufficient to trigger T-cell–mediated cytotoxicity. Blinatumomab induces remission in a substantial proportion of adults and children with multiply relapsed B-ALL.[23] A phase 3 clinical trial is evaluating its incorporation into salvage therapy for children with ALL in first relapse. CARs are engineered receptors that can target surface molecules and that can engage molecular structures independent of MHC. CAR T cells targeting CD19 have shown high complete remission rates in children and adults with relapsed/refractory B-ALL.[24]

PRIORITIZING AGENTS FOR CLINICAL EVALUATION

Childhood cancer clinical research is limited by the thankfully relatively small numbers of children with any individual type of cancer. As a result, only a small subset of the hundreds of anticancer agents under development for adult cancers will ever be studied in children. For individual cancers, no more than 2 agents can undergo definitive testing through phase 3 evaluations in a decade. Hence, successful prioritization decisions that move truly effective agents to definitive testing are critical to curing more children, as moving ineffective agents forward for definitive testing blocks progress during the period in which they are tested.

One aspect of prioritization is identifying the target/pathway that is of highest priority for clinical evaluation for a specific childhood cancer. As noted earlier, recurring genomic alterations identify targets/pathways that cancer cells are dependent on and have been good guideposts for successful prioritization. A second aspect of prioritization of targets/pathways is the preclinical testing of agents against childhood cancer models, although multiple caveats apply. Although in vitro testing can be informative, it provides limited evidence for therapeutic window. The potential for overprediction for clinical activity is high when claims are made for sensitivity to the test agent based on sustained in vitro exposure to concentrations of the agent that are not achievable in humans (or if achievable, are maintained for only brief periods).

In vivo testing, using either xenografts or genetically engineered models, can make important contributions to the prioritization process, although cautionary notes apply here as well. The preclinical models used for testing need to replicate the key molecular characteristics of the cancers that they are meant to represent. The detailed molecular profiling of preclinical models is essential in the era of molecularly targeted therapies, as particular agents are likely to have activity only against models with corresponding specific genomic alterations. The testing results for a MEK inhibitor evaluated against a large panel of pediatric xenografts illustrates this point, as the only responding xenograft was one with a *BRAF* V600E mutation.[25] A second caveat for in vivo testing using xenografts is that the drug exposures observed in mice at the dose/schedule of the agent used preclinically need to match those achievable in humans. A common cause for overprediction of clinical activity by in vivo testing results is the tolerance of mice to higher drug exposures for the tested agent compared with those tolerated in humans. It is possible to minimize false-positive predictions of clinical activity resulting from greater tolerance of mice for anticancer agents by reducing the dose of the tested agents so that the drug levels in mice more closely approximate those achievable in humans.[26,27] Pharmacokinetic-pharmacodynamic (PK-PD) models also can be developed that characterize the relationship between drug concentration and antitumor activity in dose-ranging xenograft experiments, with the PK-PD models then used to assess whether drug exposure profiles observed in humans match those associated with activity in rodents.[28,29] A final cautionary note regarding the predictive value of in vivo preclinical models to predict for clinical activity relates to the use of clinically relevant criteria for claiming antitumor activity. Publications describing preclinical testing results often include claims of agent activity based on tumor growth delay (sometimes very modest delay), which in the clinical setting would be defined as progressive disease. For childhood cancer in vivo preclinical testing, tumor regressions are felt to be the best predictor of likely clinically relevant activity. As noted earlier, the goal of treatment for childhood cancers is cure, and the pathway to cure must go through complete response, whether achieved by chemotherapy, radiotherapy, or surgery. Pediatric-relevant examples of agents that induce objective responses both in preclinical models and in the clinic include topoisomerase I inhibitors for neuroblastoma,[27] crizotinib for *ALK*-rearranged tumors,[30,31] dasatinib for BCR-ABL ALL,[32] sorafenib for *FLT3*-ITD leukemias,[33–35] and MEK inhibitors for *BRAF* mutated cancers.[25,36]

It is critical for prioritization to not only occur between agents targeting different pathways but also between agents within the same therapeutic class. For example, at one time, more than a dozen IGF-1R targeted agents were in clinical development, and Ewing sarcoma was an obvious disease of interest for these agents. Conducting single-agent phase 1 and even phase 2 trials for Ewing sarcoma was possible for several of these agents, as only 20 to 30 patients were needed per agent for these clinical trials. However, conducting a definitive study to show that one of these agents improved outcome when added to standard therapy for patients with Ewing sarcoma would have required hundreds of patients, such that no more than one agent could have been feasibly studied in North America. The IGF-1R pathway is not unique in having multiple agents targeting it enter clinical development, as the same issue applies to checkpoint inhibitors, MEK inhibitors, ALK inhibitors, BRAF inhibitors, SMO inhibitors, immunoconjugates, and other classes of agents including CAR T cells. The issue of prioritization within class will have to be addressed for each of these classes of agents as they move further into pediatric testing.

CLINICAL TRIALS IN THE ERA OF PRECISION MEDICINE

Pediatric oncologists have been at the forefront of applying the "precision medicine" concept in the clinic. As noted in a National Academy of Sciences report,[37] precision medicine "does not literally mean the creation of drugs or medical devices that are unique to a patient, but rather the ability to classify individuals into subpopulations that differ in their susceptibility to a particular disease, in the biology and/or prognosis of those diseases they may develop, or in their response to a specific treatment." Childhood cancer clinical trials have for years used molecular characteristics of cancers to assign patients to particular clinical trials and to particular treatments (eg, MYCN for neuroblastoma, and hyperdiploidy and *ETV6-RUNX1* for ALL, and *FLT3*-ITD for acute myeloid leukemia [AML]). A consequence of applying precision medicine concepts to childhood cancers is that the patient populations appropriate for evaluation get smaller and smaller, which has important consequences for clinical trial design.

The development of imatinib for Ph+ ALL in children illustrates one approach to addressing the challenge of smaller and smaller patient populations.[38] In this case, results from a single-arm study demonstrated that imatinib added benefit to standard therapy. The extent to which this example can be replicated for other agent/biomarker combinations will depend in part on the extent to which the following factors are similarly represented:

- Imatinib had substantial single-agent activity for the target patient population, increasing confidence that any effects observed with its addition to standard therapy were likely to be true effects.
- There was a reasonably large, recent historical control population that allowed a comparison to be made between outcome for standard therapy with and without the addition of imatinib.
- The treatment effect observed with the addition of imatinib was large (3-year event-free survival (EFS) of 80% ± 11% vs 35% ± 4% for the addition of imatinib compared with historical controls, respectively).[38]

An example of applying the historical control approach to identify the contribution of novel agents added to standard therapy is ANHL12P1 (NCT01979536), a randomized phase 2 clinical trial for children with anaplastic large cell lymphoma. This population is characterized by their genomic lesion (an *ALK* fusion gene) and by their uniform expression of the surface protein CD30, making these patients responsive to both crizotinib and brentuximab vedotin.[39,40] Patients enrolled on ANHL12P1 receive standard therapy plus either crizotinib or brentuximab vedotin, and a total of approximately 140 patients are to be enrolled. The primary outcome measure is a comparison of the EFS for each arm to the estimated EFS for chemotherapy alone, such that with 70 or fewer patients per arm, one or both arms may be identified as superior to chemotherapy alone.

Often sufficiently large historical controls will not be available for molecularly defined patient populations, and so alternative trial designs will need to be considered when targeted agents are evaluated for these patient populations. One alternative design for small patient populations is randomization, with reductions in the number of patients required achieved by either targeting large treatment effects, or by using inflated type I error rates, or both. When large treatment effects are targeted, the number of patients required can be markedly reduced, as illustrated by a clinical trial of a scorpion antivenom in children using a randomized design with a minimum sample size of 14 patients.[41] Likewise, inflating type I error rates beyond the standard 2-sided 0.05 reduces the numbers of patients required for any given targeted effect size.[42]

A requirement for pediatric precision medicine is a childhood cancer clinical trials infrastructure proficient in evaluating new therapies in genomically defined subtypes of childhood cancers. Pediatric oncologists have a history of rapidly adopting new technologies that provide prognostic and/or therapeutic insights for their patients, and so adoption of next-generation sequencing methods to clinical specimens to molecularly define relevant patient populations will likely occur quickly. The greater challenge will be addressing the relatively limited numbers of children with genomically defined subtypes of a given cancer diagnosis. More than ever, cohesion within the pediatric oncology community will be needed, as clinical trials for small populations that would be challenging with widespread participation will become impossible if the population is fragmented by multiple research teams all trying to study the same small group of patients. International collaborations will be increasingly needed so that sufficient patients with specific genomic characteristics can be enrolled onto clinical trials to define the contribution of novel agents for these patient populations.

INCENTIVIZING DEVELOPMENT OF PEDIATRIC-SPECIFIC AGENTS

A corollary of the observation that distinctive genomic alterations not found in adult cancers drive some childhood cancers is that mechanisms need to be developed to identify and develop agents that selectively block the oncogenic activity of these unique childhood cancer therapeutic targets. Development of ch14.18 for neuroblastoma may provide a blueprint for how such agents can be developed.[22] In this case, public funds were used to discover the therapeutic target and develop the agent through phase 1, 2, and 3 clinical trials. The successful phase 3 trial sufficiently "de-risked" ch14.18 to the extent that a biotechnology company could commit to supporting the multiple additional steps required for submitting a Biologics License Application (BLA). As well, recent legislative initiatives, such as the "Creating Hope Act," may stimulate development of childhood cancer–specific agents by providing an incentive to industry by issuing transferrable priority review vouchers when drugs are developed and approved for specific pediatric rare diseases including cancers.[43] The first priority review voucher was recently sold for $67.5 million, supporting the utility of the program as a means for incentivizing pharmaceutical companies to develop "pediatric-specific" agents.

More generally regarding the role of Food and Drug Administration (FDA), provisions of the 2012 FDA Safety and Innovation Act (FDASIA), including the permanent reauthorization of the Best Pharmaceuticals for Children Act and the Pediatric Research Equity Act, have the potential to accelerate the evaluation of new therapies for childhood cancers, because there is now a requirement to consider and discuss pediatric development plans at "end of phase 2 meetings" for new agents under development for adult malignancies. This should lead to the generation and issuance of Written Requests for pediatric evaluations at an earlier point in the drug-development timeline.

SUMMARY

The genomic discoveries of the past decade have provided biological insights that were hardly imaginable even 2 decades ago. Translating these insights into more effective treatments is well advanced for some patient populations, but barely initiated for others. A multitude of challenges will need to be addressed, ranging from prioritizing from among agents under development for adult cancers to developing agents specific for pediatric cancer targets. More than ever, a unified effort is needed for the definitive testing of agents for their ability to cure more children with cancer. Future progress will require the ingenuity, insight, and dedication of a new generation of pediatric oncologists to build on past discoveries and to make critical new discoveries so that the goal of curative therapy for every child with cancer is achieved.

REFERENCES

1. Smith MA, Altekruse SF, Adamson PC, et al. Declining childhood and adolescent cancer mortality. Cancer 2014;120(16):2497–506.
2. Smith MA. Lessons learned from adult clinical experience to inform evaluations of VEGF pathway inhibitors in children with cancer. Pediatr Blood Cancer 2014; 61(8):1497–505.
3. Schultz KR, Carroll A, Heerema NA, et al. Long-term follow-up of imatinib in pediatric Philadelphia chromosome-positive acute lymphoblastic leukemia: Children's Oncology Group Study AALL0031. Leukemia 2014;28(7):1467–71.
4. Lee RS, Stewart C, Carter SL, et al. A remarkably simple genome underlies highly malignant pediatric rhabdoid cancers. J Clin Invest 2012;122(8):2983–8.
5. Maze I, Noh KM, Soshnev AA, et al. Every amino acid matters: essential contributions of histone variants to mammalian development and disease. Nat Rev Genet 2014;15(4):259–71.
6. Wilson BG, Wang X, Shen X, et al. Epigenetic antagonism between polycomb and SWI/SNF complexes during oncogenic transformation. Cancer Cell 2010; 18(4):316–28.
7. Campbell RM, Tummino PJ. Cancer epigenetics drug discovery and development: the challenge of hitting the mark. J Clin Invest 2014;124(1):64–9.
8. Knutson SK, Warholic NM, Wigle TJ, et al. Durable tumor regression in genetically altered malignant rhabdoid tumors by inhibition of methyltransferase EZH2. Proc Natl Acad Sci U S A 2013;110(19):7922–7.
9. Okada Y, Feng Q, Lin Y, et al. hDOT1L links histone methylation to leukemogenesis. Cell 2005;121(2):167–78.
10. Bernt KM, Zhu N, Sinha AU, et al. MLL-rearranged leukemia is dependent on aberrant H3K79 methylation by DOT1L. Cancer Cell 2011;20(1):66–78.
11. Daigle SR, Olhava EJ, Therkelsen CA, et al. Potent inhibition of DOT1L as treatment of MLL-fusion leukemia. Blood 2013;122(6):1017–25.
12. Hong SH, Youbi SE, Hong SP, et al. Pharmacokinetic modeling optimizes inhibition of the 'undruggable' EWS-FLI1 transcription factor in Ewing sarcoma. Oncotarget 2014;5(2):338–50.
13. Meister S, Schubert U, Neubert K, et al. Extensive immunoglobulin production sensitizes myeloma cells for proteasome inhibition. Cancer Res 2007;67(4): 1783–92.
14. Zhong Y, Byrd JC, Dubovsky JA. The B-cell receptor pathway: a critical component of healthy and malignant immune biology. Semin Hematol 2014;51(3):206–18.
15. Roberts KG, Morin RD, Zhang J, et al. Genetic alterations activating kinase and cytokine receptor signaling in high-risk acute lymphoblastic leukemia. Cancer Cell 2012;22(2):153–66.
16. Harvey RC, Mullighan CG, Wang X, et al. Identification of novel cluster groups in pediatric high-risk B-precursor acute lymphoblastic leukemia with gene expression profiling: correlation with genome-wide DNA copy number alterations, clinical characteristics, and outcome. Blood 2010;116(23):4874–84.
17. Roberts KG, Li Y, Payne-Turner D, et al. The genetic landscape of Ph-like acute lymphoblastic leukemia. Proceedings of the 105th Annual Meeting of the American Association for Cancer Research. San Diego (CA); Philadelphia: AACR; 2014:[abstract: #3083].
18. Kool M, Jones DT, Jager N, et al. Genome sequencing of SHH medulloblastoma predicts genotype-related response to smoothened inhibition. Cancer Cell 2014; 25(3):393–405.

19. Fontebasso AM, Liu XY, Sturm D, et al. Chromatin remodeling defects in pediatric and young adult glioblastoma: a tale of a variant histone 3 tail. Brain Pathol 2013; 23(2):210–6.
20. Kieran MW. Targeting BRAF in pediatric brain tumors. Am Soc Clin Oncol Educ Book 2014;e436–40.
21. Bollag G, Tsai J, Zhang J, et al. Vemurafenib: the first drug approved for BRAF-mutant cancer. Nat Rev Drug Discov 2012;11(11):873–86.
22. Yu AL, Gilman AL, Ozkaynak MF, et al. Anti-GD2 antibody with GM-CSF, interleukin-2, and isotretinoin for neuroblastoma. N Engl J Med 2010;363(14): 1324–34.
23. Hoffman LM, Gore L. Blinatumomab, a bi-specific anti-CD19/CD3 BiTE((R)) antibody for the treatment of acute lymphoblastic leukemia: perspectives and current pediatric applications. Front Oncol 2014;4:63.
24. Maus MV, Grupp SA, Porter DL, et al. Antibody-modified T cells: CARs take the front seat for hematologic malignancies. Blood 2014;123(17):2625–35.
25. Kolb EA, Gorlick R, Houghton PJ, et al. Initial testing (stage 1) of AZD6244 (ARRY-142886) by the Pediatric Preclinical Testing Program. Pediatr Blood Cancer 2010; 55(4):668–77.
26. Zamboni WC, Stewart CF, Thompson J, et al. Relationship between topotecan systemic exposure and tumor response in human neuroblastoma xenografts. J Natl Cancer Inst 1998;90(7):505–11.
27. Santana VM, Furman WL, Billups CA, et al. Improved response in high-risk neuroblastoma with protracted topotecan administration using a pharmacokinetically guided dosing approach. J Clin Oncol 2005;23(18):4039–47.
28. Wong H, Choo EF, Alicke B, et al. Antitumor activity of targeted and cytotoxic agents in murine subcutaneous tumor models correlates with clinical response. Clin Cancer Res 2012;18(14):3846–55.
29. Yamazaki S, Vicini P, Shen Z, et al. Pharmacokinetic/pharmacodynamic modeling of crizotinib for anaplastic lymphoma kinase inhibition and antitumor efficacy in human tumor xenograft mouse models. J Pharmacol Exp Ther 2012;340(3): 549–57.
30. Christensen JG, Zou HY, Arango ME, et al. Cytoreductive antitumor activity of PF-2341066, a novel inhibitor of anaplastic lymphoma kinase and c-Met, in experimental models of anaplastic large-cell lymphoma. Mol Cancer Ther 2007; 6(12 Pt 1):3314–22.
31. Kwak EL, Bang YJ, Camidge DR, et al. Anaplastic lymphoma kinase inhibition in non-small-cell lung cancer. N Engl J Med 2010;363(18):1693–703.
32. Kolb EA, Gorlick R, Houghton PJ, et al. Initial testing of dasatinib by the pediatric preclinical testing program. Pediatr Blood Cancer 2008;50(6):1198–206.
33. Auclair D, Miller D, Yatsula V, et al. Antitumor activity of sorafenib in FLT3-driven leukemic cells. Leukemia 2007;21(3):439–45.
34. Sora F, Chiusolo P, Metafuni E, et al. Sorafenib for refractory FMS-like tyrosine kinase receptor-3 (FLT3/ITD+) acute myeloid leukemia after allogenic stem cell transplantation. Leuk Res 2011;35(3):422–3.
35. Winkler J, Rech D, Kallert S, et al. Sorafenib induces sustained molecular remission in FLT3-ITD positive AML with relapse after second allogeneic stem cell transplantation without exacerbation of acute GVHD: a case report. Leuk Res 2010;34(10):e270–2.
36. Banerjee A, Jakacki R, Onar-Thomas A, et al. A phase 1 study of AZD6244 in children with recurrent or refractory low-grade gliomas: a Pediatric Brain Tumor Consortium report. J Clin Oncol 2014;32(Suppl):5s [abstract: 10065].

37. National Research Council (US) Committee on A Framework for Developing a New Taxonomy of Disease. Toward Precision Medicine: Building a Knowledge Network for Biomedical Research and a New Taxonomy of Disease. Washington (DC): National Academies Press (US); 2011.
38. Schultz KR, Bowman WP, Aledo A, et al. Improved early event-free survival with imatinib in Philadelphia chromosome-positive acute lymphoblastic leukemia: a Children's Oncology Group study. J Clin Oncol 2009;27(31):5175–81.
39. Mosse YP, Lim MS, Voss SD, et al. Safety and activity of crizotinib for paediatric patients with refractory solid tumours or anaplastic large-cell lymphoma: a Children's Oncology Group phase 1 consortium study. Lancet Oncol 2013;14(6): 472–80.
40. Pro B, Advani R, Brice P, et al. Brentuximab vedotin (SGN-35) in patients with relapsed or refractory systemic anaplastic large-cell lymphoma: results of a phase II study. J Clin Oncol 2012;30(18):2190–6.
41. Boyer LV, Theodorou AA, Berg RA, et al. Antivenom for critically ill children with neurotoxicity from scorpion stings. N Engl J Med 2009;360(20):2090–8.
42. Rubinstein LV, Korn EL, Freidlin B, et al. Design issues of randomized phase II trials and a proposal for phase II screening trials. J Clin Oncol 2005;23(28): 7199–206.
43. Connor E, Cure P. "Creating hope" and other incentives for drug development for children. Sci Transl Med 2011;3(66):66cm1.

Index

Note: Page numbers of article titles are in **boldface** type.

A

Pediatr Clin N Am 62 (2015) 313–327
http://dx.doi.org/10.1016/S0031-3955(14)00231-4
0031-3955/15/$ – see front matter © 2015 Elsevier Inc. All rights reserved.

Moving?

Make sure your subscription moves with you!

To notify us of your new address, find your **Clinics Account Number** (located on your mailing label above your name), and contact customer service at:

Email: journalscustomerservice-usa@elsevier.com

800-654-2452 (subscribers in the U.S. & Canada)
314-447-8871 (subscribers outside of the U.S. & Canada)

Fax number: 314-447-8029

Elsevier Health Sciences Division
Subscription Customer Service
3251 Riverport Lane
Maryland Heights, MO 63043

*To ensure uninterrupted delivery of your subscription, please notify us at least 4 weeks in advance of move.